D1521813

STEPCHILDREN OF NATURE

STEPCHILDREN

OF NATURE

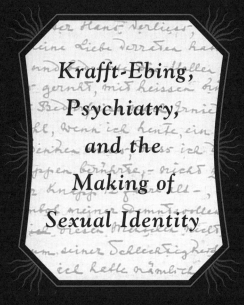

Krafft-Ebing,
Psychiatry,
and the
Making of
Sexual Identity

HARRY OOSTERHUIS

THE UNIVERSITY OF CHICAGO PRESS + CHICAGO AND LONDON

HARRY OOSTERHUIS teaches at the University of Maastricht and is
the author of *Homosexuality and Male Bonding in Pre-Nazi Germany*
(1991) and *Homoseksualiteit in katholiek Nederland* (1992) and
coauthor of *Fascisme en homoseksualiteit* (1985) and *Gay Men and
the Sexual History of the Political Left* (1995).

The University of Chicago Press, Chicago 60637
The University of Chicago Press, Ltd., London
© 2000 by The University of Chicago
All rights reserved. Published 2000
Printed in the United States of America

09 08 07 06 05 04 03 02 01 00   1 2 3 4 5
ISBN: 0-226-63059-5 (cloth)

Library of Congress Cataloging-in-Publication Data
Oosterhuis, Harry.
    Stepchildren of Nature: Krafft-Ebing, psychiatry, and the making
of sexual identity / Harry Oosterhuis.
        p.   cm. — (The Chicago series on sexuality, history, and
society)
    Includes bibliographical references (p.) and index.
    ISBN 0-226-63059-5 (cloth : alk. paper)
    1. Sexual deviation—History—19th century.   2. Sexual
deviation—Treatment—History—19th century.   3. Sexology—
History—19th century.   4. Krafft-Ebing, R. von (Richard),
1840–1902.   5. Psychiatry—History—19th century.   I. Title.
II. Series.

HQ71.O57   2000
616.85'83'009034–dc21

                                                        00-023399

CONTENTS

ACKNOWLEDGMENTS

In 1894 the Viennese psychiatrist Richard von Krafft-Ebing wrote to a friend that after his retirement he planned "to exploit" his "heaped-up treasures," which consisted of "approximately 1,500 case notes" of patients.[1] It is likely that when he finally retired, in 1902, he took these patient files home, planning to use them for publications. However, Krafft-Ebing died at the end of the same year. His "treasures" would be hidden away in an attic for ninety years. Although his family was hardly aware of their historical significance and nobody showed an interest in them, his son, granddaughter, and great-grandson have preserved this archive carefully. In addition to documents such as manuscripts of his publications, summaries and notes, and letters and postcards from friends and colleagues, it contains 1,386 files of Krafft-Ebing's patients, dating from 1871 to 1902. In about two hundred of these case histories, letters and autobiographical accounts of patients or correspondence of third parties (family members, friends, doctors, or lawyers) are included.

The discovery of this unexploited archive has been the major impetus to write this book. Without the support of Dr. Rainer Krafft-Ebing, great-grandson of Richard von Krafft-Ebing, this undertaking would not have been possible. He and his mother, Marion Krafft-Ebing, gave me a warm welcome when, in the summer of 1992, I visited them for the first time in their house in Graz. They were rather surprised that a Dutch historian was interested in the work of their forefather and, along with portraits, photos, and a bust, they showed me three cases full of papers. Not long thereafter they offered me free access to this archive and invited me to stay with them to research it. The kind hospitality of Rainer, his wife Gabrielle, and his mother has been invaluable, and I have very good memories of the time I

1. Autograph 469/16–2, Österreichische Nationalbibliothek, Vienna.

spent in the sunroom of their house, working my way through a mass of papers. Rainer Krafft-Ebing's generosity and concern greatly contributed to the completion of this book. I am also very grateful to him for putting some photos in the Krafft-Ebing family archive at my disposal.

I did not discover the Krafft-Ebing estate on my own. Reading Klaus Müller's dissertation on nineteenth-century homosexual autobiographies and medical case histories (*Aber in meinem Herzen sprach eine Stimme so laut*, 1991) raised my interest in Krafft-Ebing and his patients. I am much obliged to my friend and former colleague Gert Hekma, who, always supportive and encouraging, took the first steps in tracing Krafft-Ebing's descendants and incited me to delve into his work. I am also grateful to Dr. Walter Grünzweig of the University of Graz for his assistance in contacting the Krafft-Ebing family, as well as to Günther Haumann for helping me to find my way in Graz and offering me hospitality when I visited the city for the first time. Dr. Alois Kernbauer, director of the Archives of the University of Graz, was very helpful in finding relevant documents tracing Krafft-Ebing's career as a professor of psychiatry.

Dr. Renate Hauser, who finished a dissertation on Krafft-Ebing when I started my research, has traced many of his little-known writings. Dr. Hauser and the Wellcome Institute for the History of Medicine in London kindly gave me permission to consult her unpublished dissertation. This book builds on her work; her bibliography of Krafft-Ebing's publications was particularly valuable, making it a lot easier for me to trace articles and published case histories by Krafft-Ebing in the library of the Medical Society in Vienna and the Obersteiner library of the Neurological Institute of the University of Vienna. I am obliged to the staff of these libraries for their kind assistance. The staff of the library of the Institute for the History of Medicine in Vienna was also helpful in finding published and unpublished sources. In Vienna Dr. Franz X. Eder was my guide and host; he kindly shared with me his wide knowledge of the history of sexuality in Austria.

I am indebted to Han Israëls for providing me with a privately published article by Peter Swales on the professional relationship between Krafft-Ebing and Freud. He also informed me about some references to Krafft-Ebing in the memoirs of Carl Gustav Jung and Wilhelm Stekel. James Steakley pointed me to the novel *Sind es Frauen?* by Aimée Duc in which the lesbian characters refer to themselves as "Krafft-Ebing people." Manfred Herzer made an effort to trace the Berlin authors of the pamphlet published by a committee "for the liberation of homosexuals from criminal law" that I found in Krafft-Ebing's estate, and Marita Keilson-Lauritz supplied me with bibliographical information on some literary works Krafft-Ebing refers to in one of his articles on homosexuality. Dr. Marlis Kuhlmann of the Ferdinand Enke Publishing House kindly provided me with copies of contracts between the publisher and Krafft-Ebing as well as some letters of Krafft-Ebing to Enke. Mark and Gabi Richartz helped me to decipher some handwritings. The Wellcome Institute gave me permission to illustrate this book with three postcards that I found in Krafft-Ebing's estate. I thank Gert Hekma for allowing me to consult his valuable library.

Over the years many colleagues and friends have contributed to this book by commenting on earlier drafts of its chapters. The discussions with my colleagues in the Department of History of the University of Maastricht and the Huizinga Institute, the Graduate School for Cultural History, were especially fruitful. I also want to thank all who made useful comments on the papers I presented at the universities of Nijmegen, Utrecht, Wisconsin, and Vienna; at the Akademie der Künste in Berlin; at the Second Carleton Conference on the History of the Family in Ottawa; the Triennial Conference of the European Association for the History of Psychiatry in London; the First and Fourth Maastricht-Cambridge Wellcome Workshops on the History of Medicine in Maastricht; the Symposium on Sexual Cultures in Europe at the Institute for Social Sciences in Amsterdam; the Annual Conference of the Dutch Society of Sociology in Amsterdam; the Workshop for the History of Psychiatry at the Trimbos Institute in Utrecht; and the International Conference on Neurosciences and Psychiatry in Zurich. Franz Eder, George Mosse, James Steakley, and Jo Wachelder commented on parts of my work in progress. At the end Ton Brouwers, Marijke Gijswijt-Hofstra, Gert Hekma, Marita Keilson-Lauritz, Lissa Roberts, Jessica Slijkhuis, and Gerlof Verwey read the complete manuscript. I am much obliged to them for their constructive criticism.

Ton Brouwers corrected my English and translated some parts originally written in Dutch. He is not only an excellent translator, but also a conscientious reader and editor whose opinions are always to the point. My text has greatly benefited from his editorial advice. I am also indebted to Erin DeWitt, senior manuscript editor at the University of Chicago Press, for her fine work. John Fout, the editor of the Chicago Series on Sexuality, History, and Society, and Douglas Mitchell, my editor at the University of Chicago Press, must be thanked for their encouragement and help.

The many quotes from Krafft-Ebing's work and his case histories in this book appear in English translation. Apart from some editions of *Psychopathia sexualis* and an article by Krafft-Ebing published in the American psychiatric journal *Alienist and Neurologist* in 1888, no work by Krafft-Ebing on sexuality has been translated into English, as far as I know. I have consulted the most recent American translation of Krafft-Ebing's *Psychopathia sexualis*, edited by Brian King and published by Bloat in 1999. This new edition is based on earlier American editions of *Psychopathia sexualis*: the translation of the seventh German edition by Charles Gilbert Chaddock published in 1893 and that of the twelfth German edition by F. J. Rebman, which appeared in 1906. These two editions contain many flaws. King states in his introduction that he and his associate editor have checked, corrected, and revised the older translations. Yet after checking King's edition against the original German texts, it turns out that, unfortunately, many passages are still inaccurate or incomplete, and sometimes even incorrect. Therefore I have not reproduced them word by word, although for each quotation from *Psychopathia sexualis* I have consulted the Bloat edition before making my own version of the translation. As far as authorized English translations are available for passages I quote, I refer to both the original German source and the Bloat edition or the article in the *Alienist and Neurologist*. Other quotations were translated by Ton Brouwers and by myself. All the references to Krafft-Ebing's works are indicated in the text by the year of their publication; *Psychopathia sexualis* is abbreviated as "*Ps.*"

Two sabbatical terms afforded me with the time and the peace and quiet necessary to finish this book. One was granted by the Faculty of Arts and Culture of the University of Maastricht and the other was made possible by a grant from the Dutch Organisation of Scientific Research (NWO). The Department of History of the University of Maastricht financed various trips to Vienna and Graz.

Over the years, many of my friends frequently had to put up with my worries and moods that the project engendered. I thank all of them for their patience. Vincent van Oss and Gernot Ottink should be mentioned in particular, even more for reminding me that there are more important and enjoyable things in life than writing an academic study.

Unfortunately George Mosse did not live to see the book finished. His encouragement and support in getting it published have been crucial. George was not only an inspiring colleague, but also a dear friend. This book is dedicated to his memory.

INTRODUCTION

Although I fear to annoy you, Sir, with my letter—after all, in the preface of your "Psychopathia sexualis," you mention the "innumerable letters by such stepchildren of nature"—I still trustingly turn to you, hoping
that a layman might report something to the scholar that is not entirely
without interest: even the most inconspicuous thing may gain importance in the right place and may be worthy of scholarly attention.[1]

In 1900 a young Latvian nobleman, Von R, addressed himself in this manner to the renowned German-Austrian psychiatrist Richard von Krafft-
Ebing (1840–1902), author of *Psychopathia sexualis* and one of the founders
of scientific sexology. For the most part, Von R's letter is an elaborate introspection of his problematic sexuality. At the age of ten, he ascertained in
retrospective, his homosexual and masochistic impulses had already revealed themselves in his fantasies, reading habits, and games. The lust he
experienced as a boy, when he made a ceremony out of decapitating flowers
(he was too sensitive for torturing animals) was a clear symptom of his
deep-seated proclivities. In particular, his urge to be humiliated by his male
subordinates—"the idea to be the servant of my servant by my own voli-
tion"—caused inward conflict. Torn between his irresistible sexual desire
and his class prejudice, Von R was weighed down by shame and guilt. At
the same time, in his letter, he meticulously explored and evaluated every
circumstance that might shed light on his anomaly: his particular way of
acting and feeling, his childhood, the fact that before the age of fourteen
he had had no opportunity to mix with females, the way he experienced
puberty and sexual maturity, the fantasies and moral conflicts that accom-

---

1. Letter of Von R to Krafft-Ebing (July 1900), Nachlass Krafft-Ebing.

panied his self-abuse, his failure to copulate with a prostitute, his character
and intellectual faculties, his conscience, his health and mental state, and
his family background. He detected a slight "nervousness" in his behavior
and referred to possible hereditary taints: his brother was suffering from
"dementia paralytica," and he identified some distant relatives afflicted
with mental disorders.

The way Von R framed his autobiographical account is noteworthy as
well. As if to underline its structure and give his very personal confession
a semblance of objectivity, he added notes in the margins of the pages. Von
R's composition of his life story and his marginal comments resemble the
formal and narrative characteristics of many handwritten psychiatric case
histories that I found in Krafft-Ebing's estate. After Krafft-Ebing's assistants
had written down the patient's biography, symptoms, and anamnesis,
Krafft-Ebing added the diagnosis and other remarks in the margins. Thus
the individual case was compared to others, classified, and fitted into his
taxonomy. Although Von R may have never seen a handwritten case history, his letter mirrors the psychiatric model of the individual case description. Analyzing his own self-observation and writing down key words in
the margins of his letter, he made, as it were, a diagnosis of his own condition. He used the format and language of the psychiatric case description,
and his autobiographical account reflected medical explanations of sexuality. Doubtlessly, Von R was inspired by Krafft-Ebing's *Psychopathia sexualis*, which contained many case studies and autobiographies. Offering his
life story as grist for the interpretative mill, he apparently placed his fate
into the hands of the psychiatrist, and his confession seems to be typical
of the process that Michel Foucault and other scholars have designated as
the medical construction of perversion (Foucault 1976; cf. Weeks 1981;
Hekma 1987; Greenberg 1988; Stanton 1992).

Whereas earlier historians have understood the medicalization of sexuality as a change of attitudes and labels only—for them, unchanging deviant sexual behaviors and feelings were no longer regarded as unnatural,
sinful, or criminal but simply became diseases, relabeled or "medicalized"
by physicians—Foucault and other social constructivist historians have
challenged this interpretation. They are not only critical of the view espousing that the medical model was a scientific step forward, but they also
argue that the conception of nonprocreative sexuality as a sign of sickness
was not merely a substitution for earlier denouncements of such activities
as immoral. They emphasize that medical theories entailed a fundamental
metamorphosis of the social and psychological reality of sexual deviants
from a form of behavior to a way of being: irregular sexual acts were not
just viewed as immoral, but as the manifestation of an underlying morbid

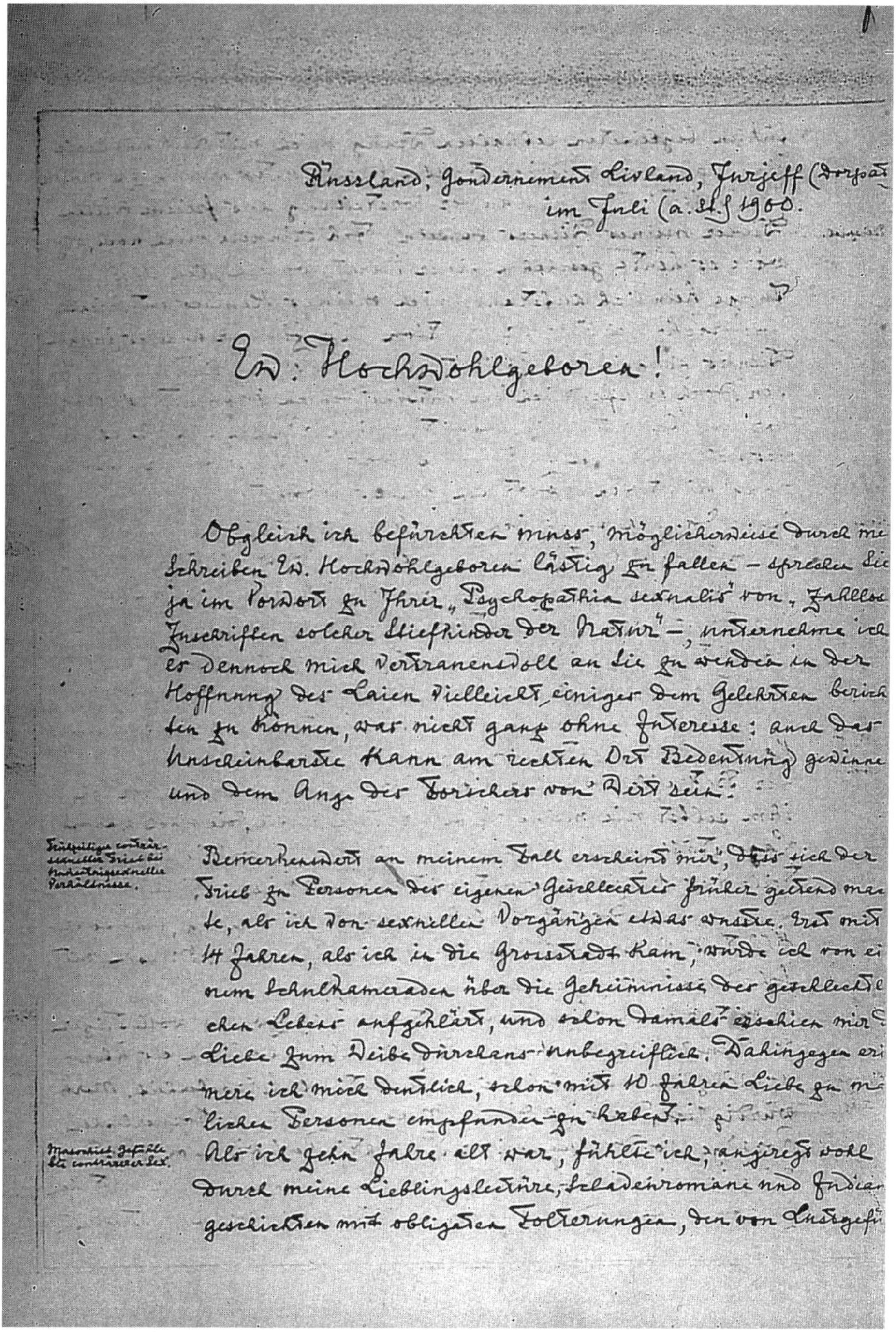

Russland, Gouvernement Livland, Jurjeff (Dorpat)
im Juli (a. St.) 1900.

Ew. Hochwohlgeboren!

Obgleich ich befürchten muss, möglicherweise durch mein Schreiben Ew. Hochwohlgeboren lästig zu fallen – sprechen Sie ja im Vorwort zu Ihrer „Psychopathia sexualis" von „zahllosen Zuschriften solcher Stiefkinder der Natur" –, unternehme ich es dennoch mich vertrauensvoll an Sie zu wenden in der Hoffnung, der Laie vielleicht einiges dem Gelehrten berichten zu können, was nicht ganz ohne Interesse: auch das Unscheinbarste kann am rechten Ort Bedeutung gewinnen und dem Auge des Forschers von Wert sein.

Frühzeitiger conträrsexueller Trieb bei Andersgeschlechtlicher Verhältnisse.

Bemerkenswert an meinem Fall erscheint mir, dass sich der Trieb zu Personen des eigenen Geschlechtes früher geltend machte, als ich von sexuellen Vorgängen etwas wusste. Erst mit 14 Jahren, als ich in die Grossstadt kam, wurde ich von einem Schulkameraden über die Geheimnisse des geschlechtlichen Lebens aufgeklärt, und schon damals erschien mir die Liebe zum Weibe durchaus unbegreiflich. Dahingegen erinnere ich mich deutlich, schon mit 10 Jahren Liebe zu männlichen Personen empfunden zu haben.

Masochist. Gefühle bei conträrer Sex.

Als ich zehn Jahre alt war, fühlte ich, angeregt wohl durch meine Lieblingslectüre, Sclavenromane und Indianergeschichten mit obligaten Folterungen, den von Lustgefü

Figure 1. Fragment of a letter of Von R. (Krafft-Ebing Family Archive, Graz, Austria)

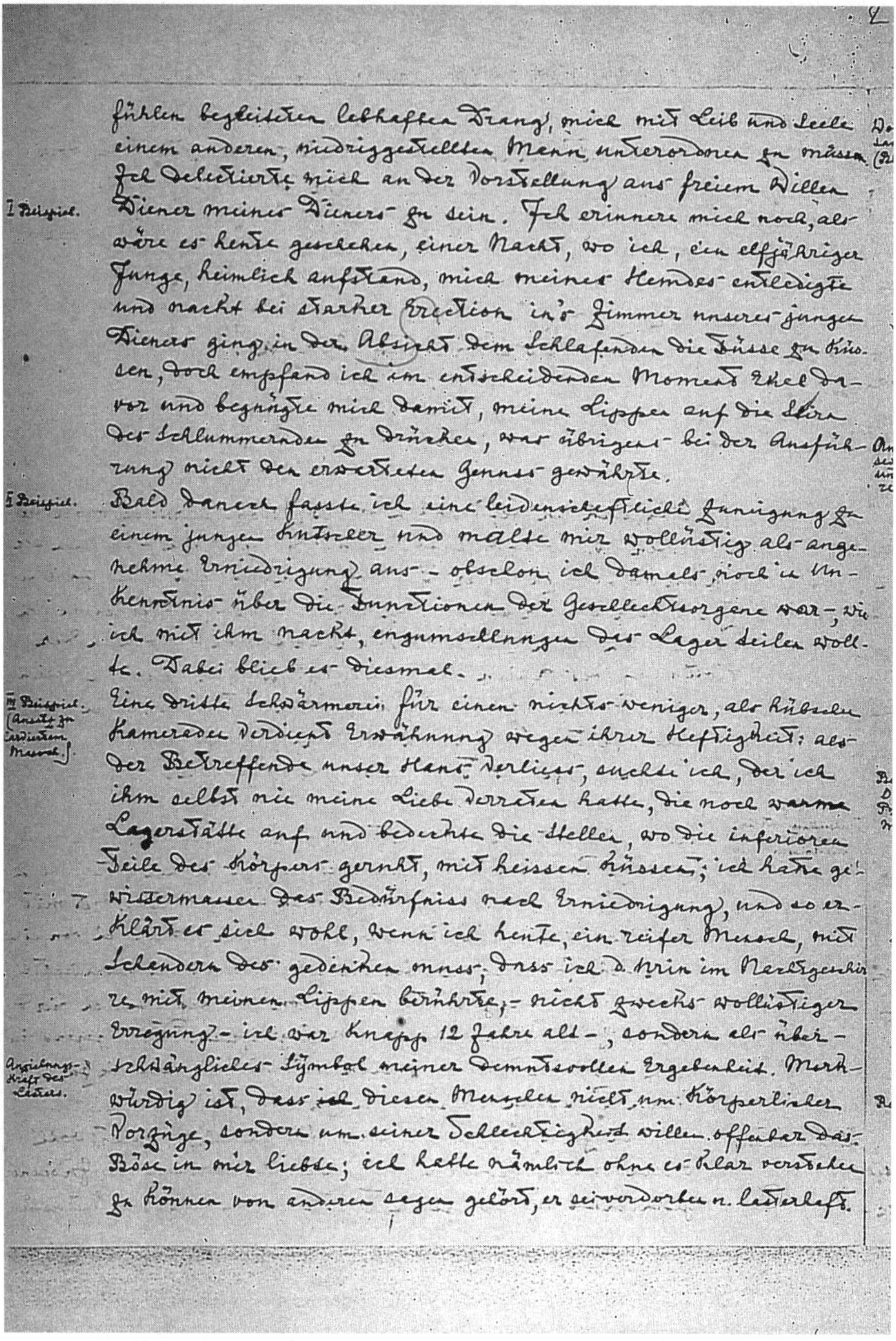

4

fühlen begleiteten lebhaften Drang, mich mit Leib und Seele
einem anderen, niedriggestellten Mann unterordnen zu müssen.
Ich delectierte mich an der Vorstellung aus freiem Willen
I Beispiel. Diener meines Dieners zu sein. Ich erinnere mich noch, als
wäre es heute geschehen, einer Nacht, wo ich, ein elfjähriger
Junge, heimlich aufstand, mich meines Hemdes entledigte
und nackt bei starker Erection in's Zimmer unseres jungen
Dieners ging in der Absicht dem Schlafenden die Füsse zu küssen, doch empfand ich im entscheidenden Moment Ekel da-
vor und begnügte mich damit, meine Lippen auf die Stirn
des Schlummernden zu drücken, was übrigens bei der Ausfüh-
rung nicht den erwarteten Genuss gewährte.
II Beispiel. Bald darauf fasste ich eine leidenschaftliche Zuneigung zu
einem jungen Kutscher und malte mir wollüstig als ange-
nehme Erniedrigung aus – obschon ich damals noch in Un-
kenntnis über die Functionen der Geschlechtsorgane war –, wie
ich mit ihm nackt, engumschlungen das Lager teilen woll-
te. Dabei blieb es diesmal.
III Beispiel. (Ansatz zu [illegible] Masoch.) Eine dritte Schwärmerei für einen nichts weniger als hübschen
Kameraden verdient Erwähnung wegen ihrer Heftigkeit: als
der Betreffende unser Haus verliess, suchte ich, der ich
ihm selbst nie meine Liebe verraten hatte, die noch warme
Lagerstätte auf und bedeckte die Stellen, wo die inferioren
Teile des Körpers geruht, mit heissen Küssen; ich hatte gewissermassen das Bedürfnis nach Erniedrigung, und so er-
klärt es sich wohl, wenn ich heute, ein reifer Mensch, mit
Schaudern des gedenken muss, dass ich d. Urin im Nachtgeschir-
re mit meinen Lippen berührte, – nicht zwecks wollüstiger
Erregung – ich war knapp 12 Jahre alt –, sondern als über-
Anziehungskraft des Lasters. schwängliches Symbol meiner demutsvollen Ergebenheit. Merk-
würdig ist, dass ich diesen Menschen nicht um körperlicher
Vorzüge, sondern um seiner Schlechtigkeit willen, offenbar das
Böse in mir liebte; ich hatte nämlich ohne es klar verstehen
zu können von anderen sagen gehört, er sei verdorben u. lasterhaft.

Figure 2. Fragment of a letter of Von R. (Krafft-Ebing Family Archive, Graz, Austria)

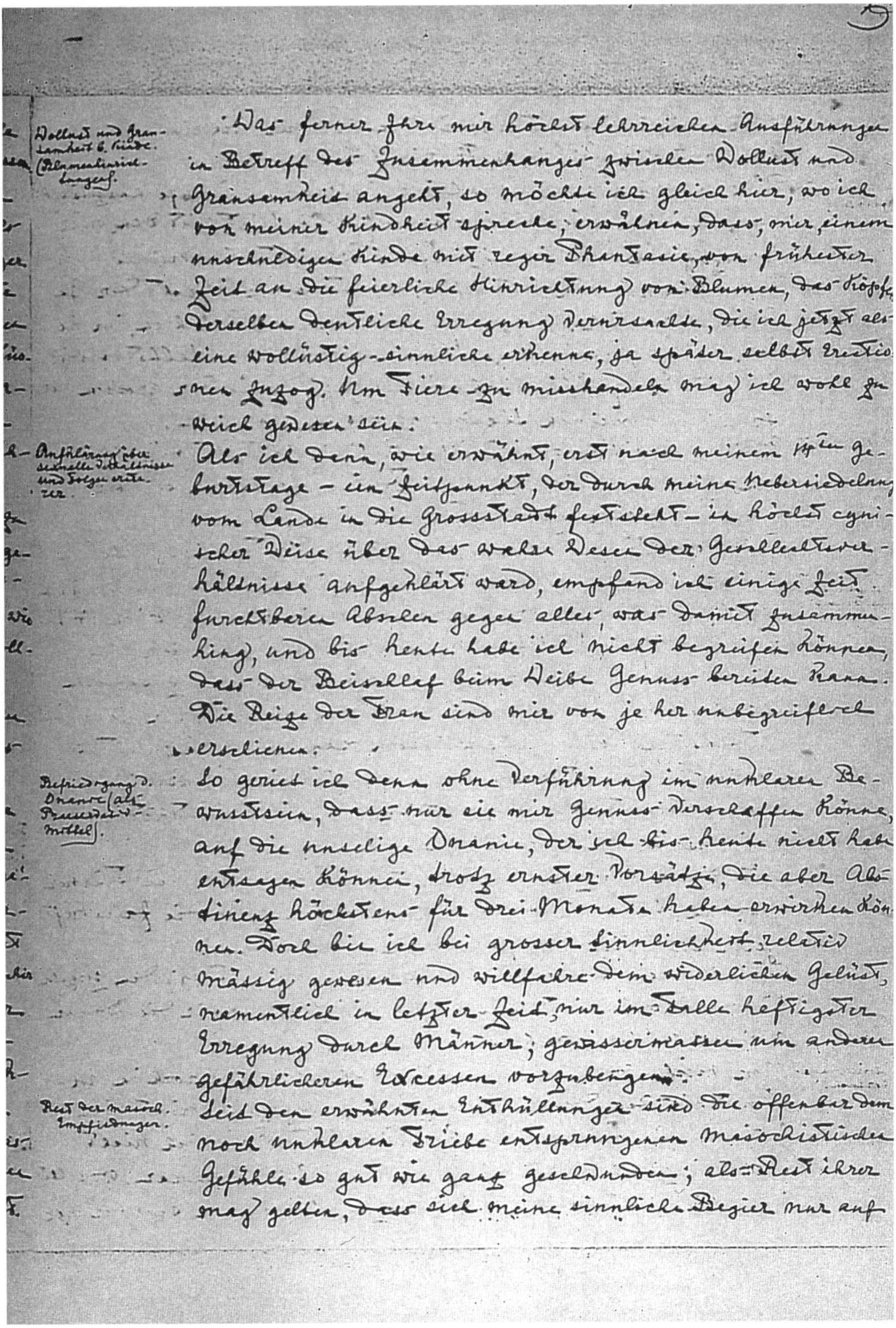

9

Was ferner Ihre mir höchst lehrreichen Ausführungen in Betreff des Zusammenhanges zwischen Wollust und Grausamkeit angeht, so möchte ich gleich hier, wo ich von meiner Kindheit spreche, erwähnen, dass mir, einem unschuldigen Kinde mit reger Phantasie, von frühester Zeit an die feierliche Hinrichtung von Blumen, das Köpfen derselben deutliche Erregung verursachte, die ich jetzt als eine wollüstig-sinnliche erkenne, ja später selbst Erectionen zuzog. Um Tiere zu misshandeln mag ich wohl zu weich gewesen sein.

Als ich denn, wie erwähnt, erst nach meinem 14ten Geburtstage – ein Zeitpunkt, der durch meine Uebersiedelung vom Lande in die Grossstadt feststeht – in höchst cynischer Weise über das wahre Wesen der Geschlechtsverhältnisse aufgeklärt ward, empfand ich einige Zeit furchtbaren Abscheu gegen alles, was damit zusammenhing, und bis heute habe ich nicht begreifen können, dass der Beischlaf beim Weibe Genuss bereiten kann. Die Reize der Frau sind mir von je her unbegreiflich erschienen.

So geriet ich denn ohne Verführung im unklaren Bewusstsein, dass nur sie mir Genuss verschaffen könne, auf die unselige Onanie, der ich bis heute nicht habe entsagen können, trotz ernster Vorsätze, die aber Abstinenz höchstens für drei Monate haben erwirken können. Doch bin ich bei grosser Sinnlichkeit relativ mässig gewesen und willfahre dem widerlichen Gelüst, namentlich in letzter Zeit, nur im Falle heftigster Erregung durch Männer; gewissermassen um anderen gefährlicheren Excessen vorzubeugen.

Seit den erwähnten Enthüllungen sind die offenbar dem noch unklaren Triebe entsprungenen masochistischen Gefühle so gut wie ganz geschwunden; als Rest ihrer mag gelten, dass sich meine sinnliche Begier nur auf

Wollust und Grausamkeit b. Kinde. (Blumenhinrichtungen.)

Aufklärung über sexuelle Verhältnisse und Folgen derselben

Befriedigung d. Onanie (als Präservativmittel).

Rest der masoch. Empfindungen.

Figure 3. Fragment of a letter of Von R. (Krafft-Ebing Family Archive, Graz, Austria)

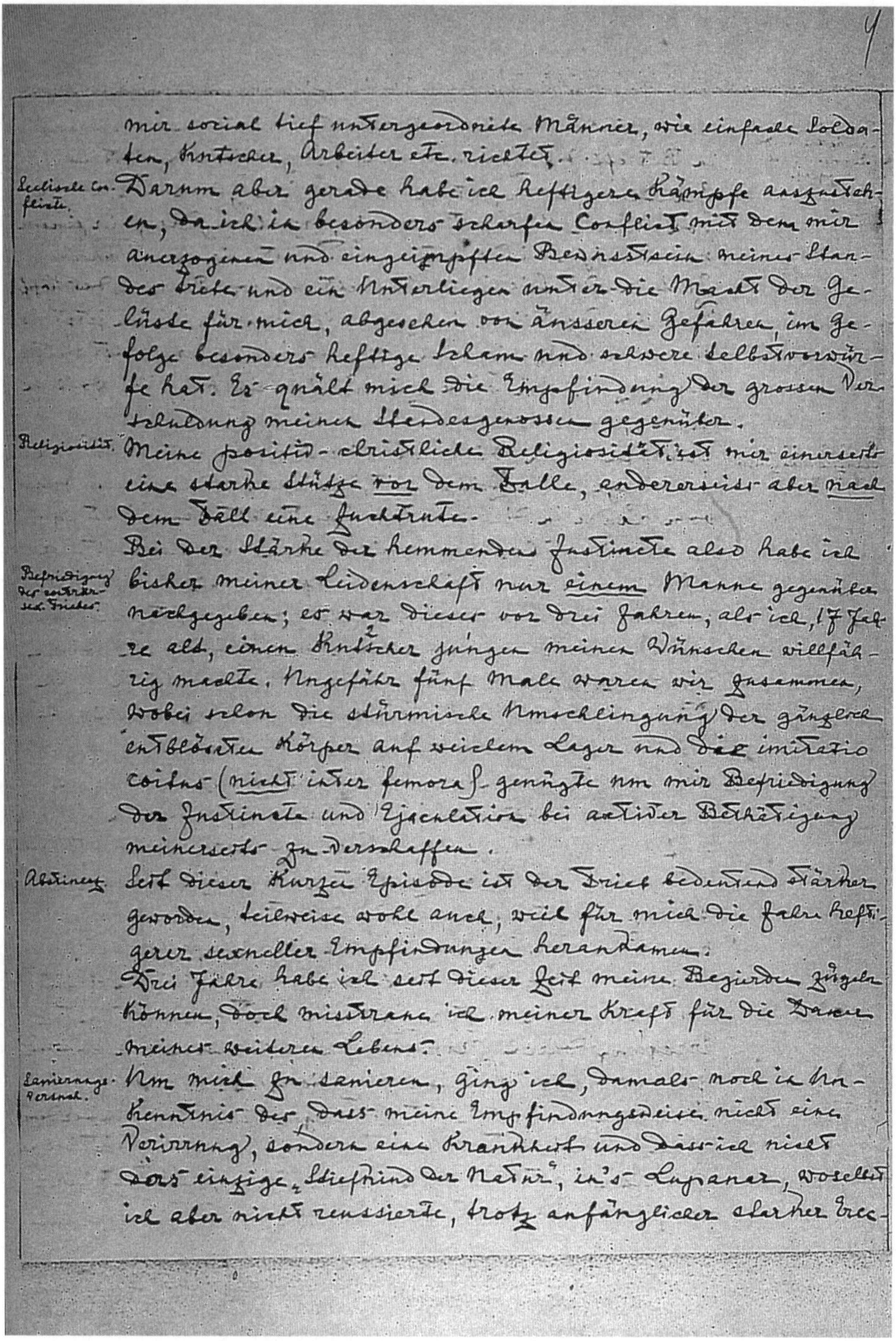

4

mir social tief untergeordnete Männer, wie einfache Solda-
ten, Kutscher, Arbeiter etc. richtet.

Seelische Conflicte.

Darum aber gerade habe ich heftigere Kämpfe auszustehen,
en, da ich in besonders scharfen Conflict mit dem mir
anerzogenen und eingeimpften Bewusstsein meiner Stan-
des Würde und ein Unterliegen unter die Macht der Gelüste für mich, abgesehen von äusseren Gefahren, im Ge-
folge besonders heftige Scham und schwere Selbstvorwür-
fe hat. Es quält mich die Empfindung der grossen Ver-
schuldung meinen Standesgenossen gegenüber.

Religiosität.

Meine positiv-christliche Religiosität ist mir einerseits
eine starke Stütze vor dem Falle, andererseits aber nach
dem Fall eine Fuchtrute.

Bei der Stärke der hemmenden Instincte also habe ich

Befriedigung des contrar-sex. Triebes.

bisher meiner Leidenschaft nur einem Manne gegenüber
nachgegeben; es war dieses vor drei Jahren, als ich, 17 Jahre alt, einen Kutscher jünger meinen Wünschen willfäh-
rig machte. Ungefähr fünf Male waren wir zusammen,
wobei schon die stürmische Umschlingung der gänzlich
entblössten Körper auf weichem Lager und das imitatio
coitus (nicht inter femora!) genügte um mir Befriedigung
des Instincts und Ejaculation bei activer Bethätigung
meinerseits zu verschaffen.

Abstinenz.

Seit dieser kurzen Episode ist der Trieb bedeutend stärker
geworden, teilweise wohl auch, weil für mich die Jahre hefti-
gerer sexueller Empfindungen herankamen.
Drei Jahre habe ich seit dieser Zeit meine Begierden zügeln
können, doch misstraue ich meiner Kraft für die Dauer
meines weiteren Lebens.

Sanierungs-Versuch.

Um mich zu sanieren, ging ich, damals noch in Un-
kenntnis dessen, dass meine Empfindungsweise nicht eine
Verirrung, sondern eine Krankheit und dass ich nicht
das einzige „Stiefkind der Natur", in's Lupanar, woselbst
ich aber nicht reussierte, trotz anfänglicher starker Erec-

Figure 4. Fragment of a letter of Von R. (Krafft-Ebing Family Archive, Graz, Austria)

condition.[2] Inspired by Foucault, a number of sociologists and historians have geared their research toward the "making of the modern homosexual," stressing that in the last decades of the nineteenth century, sexual deviance became a matter of personal identity (Plummer 1981; Hekma 1987; Greenberg 1988; Müller 1991; Rosario 1997).

Foucault argues that the modern idea of sexuality was historically constituted when medical science delimited deviance. Socially created out of disciplining powers and discourses of knowledge, sexuality was a nineteenth-century invention. Before medical theories emerged that lumped together behavior, physical characteristics, and the emotional makeup of individuals, there was no entity, according to Foucault, that could be delineated as sexuality. By differentiating between the normal and the abnormal, and by stigmatizing sexual variance as sickly deviation, physicians, as exponents of an anonymous "biopower," were controlling the free and easy pleasures of the body. Although Foucault stresses that sexuality was shaped rather than repressed by the scientific will to know, the purport of his argument, and even more that of some of his followers, is that perverts were submitted to a medical regime that disseminated a disputable biological determinism. According to Jeffrey Weeks, doctors were "powerful agents in the organisation, and potential control, of the sexual behaviours they sought to describe" (Weeks 1981, 145).

Even before Foucault's *History of Sexuality* had set the tone, historians of sexuality damned Krafft-Ebing's pioneering contribution to medical interference with sexuality as "an unmitigated disaster" and blamed him for "the confusion which continues to surround the subject of sexual variation today" (Brecher 1969, 56). In a similar vein, the prophet of anti-psychiatry, Thomas Szasz, has passed his judgment on Krafft-Ebing. Szasz believes that scientific psychiatry has one overarching social function, and that is control. In his view, psychiatrists are imperialists because, in order to provide an account of mental illness, they transfer the model of physical disease to deviancy, an extrapolation that is unfounded and misguided. For Szasz, it is clear that the self-professed claims made by physicians only disguised their urge for manipulative power.

> Krafft-Ebing was not interested in liberating men and women from the shackles of sexual prejudice or the constraints of anti-sexual legislation. On the contrary, he was interested in supplanting the waning power of the church with the waxing power of medicine. . . . [B]ecause he wrote about sex when polite society was silent about it, and because he wrote about it as if it were a disease or medical problem, Krafft-Ebing has been

2. Throughout this book my use of the terms *deviance* and *deviant*, *perversion* and *pervert*, and *normal* and *abnormal* is merely denotative and does not imply any value judgment.

mistaken as a progressive force in the struggle against sexual prejudice and prudery.

Adding that Krafft-Ebing's *Psychopathia sexualis* is "full of falsehoods pretentiously presented as if they were the fruits of hard-won scientific discoveries," Szasz's opinion is typical of the way several historians have viewed his work from a presentist perspective (Szasz 1980, 19–20). Krafft-Ebing has been criticized for endorsing traditional views of sexuality; for opposing sexual liberation; for espousing the heterosexual standard, homophobia, and Roman Catholic faith in the teleology of sexuality; for representing bourgeois respectability and male chauvinism; for urging the state to control as much as possible all forms of "immorality"; and for overlooking the supposedly political context of his case histories.[3] Edward Shorter, although a fierce critic of the Szaszian and Foucaultian type of history writing, has characterized Krafft-Ebing's *Psychopathia sexualis* as "a classic example of psychiatry run off the rails, of the misuse of scientific authority to demonize cultural preferences" (Shorter 1997, 96). Even historian Vernon Bullough, whose evaluation of Krafft-Ebing is much more balanced, concludes that among the early sexologists, the "key missing ingredient" was

> a willingness to accept sexuality, not just procreation, as a fact of life; a willingness to look on sex as a vital physical force that was capable of doing more good than harm; and a willingness to see it as one of life's pleasures. Krafft-Ebing had struggled to come to terms with a need for change but had not quite succeeded. Though there was a growing middle class willing to accept pleasure as an important element in their lives, the medical community as a whole either saw no need to challenge or were unwilling to challenge traditional ideology. (Bullough 1994, 49)

Clearly, Krafft-Ebing's work has evoked powerful emotions and value judgments, but to this day it has barely been done justice by historians. He hardly appears in the well-known cultural-historical works on fin de siècle Vienna, such as Allan Janik and Stephen Toulmin's *Wittgenstein's Vienna* (1973), Carl Schorske's *Fin-de-Siècle Vienna* (1980), and Jacques Le Rider's *Modernité viennoise et crises de l'identité* (1990). Although his name shows up in many historical studies of sexuality and in some histories of psychiatry and while his *Psychopathia sexualis* is often discussed, Renate Hauser's unpublished dissertation "Sexuality, Neurasthenia and the Law: Richard von Krafft-Ebing (1840–1902)" (1992) is the only intellectual biography available to date. Historians of psychiatry and sexuality have generally given a limited and one-sided view of Krafft-Ebing. I cannot escape the impression

3. Johnston 1972, 233; Gay 1984, 154; Mosse 1985, 10–11, 29; Hacker 1987; Mosse 1988, 18, 23; Fout 1992, 1, 274; Bristow 1997, 26; Noyes 1997, 56.

that many of them base their knowledge of his work on what others have written about it and only a cursory reading of *Psychopathia sexualis* and perhaps two of his other psychiatric textbooks. Krafft-Ebing is usually characterized as a traditional materialist psychiatrist (generally to contrast him in a negative way with Sigmund Freud), a staunch adherent of degeneration theory, a manic classifier, and a harsh Victorian judge of weird sexual perversions. Thus a stereotypical image—often implicitly or explicitly very judgmental—is invoked again and again. The many works that Krafft-Ebing published besides *Psychopathia sexualis*, the institutional settings in which he worked, the role that he played in contemporary psychiatry, and, last but not least, the subjects of his numerous case histories have all been basically neglected.

In this book I will argue that Krafft-Ebing's sexual pathology played a key role in the historical construction of the modern concept of sexuality. As far as the scientific discussion about sexuality is concerned, Sigmund Freud was not the radical pioneer he is often thought to be. Freud built on medical theories of sexuality that had been formulated between 1870 and 1900, Krafft-Ebing's being one of the most influential. Whereas other scholars have defined sexual modernism mainly as a reaction against Victorian prohibitions, in my view it is not only an ideology of sexual liberation, but even more an epistemological transformation, an individualization and psychologization of sexuality (cf. Robinson 1976; Davidson 1987 & 1990; Showalter 1991). The emergence of sexual identity is central to the "modernization" of sexuality. However, to believe that a transformation of such magnitude was caused merely by medical theories and practices would be overrating the power of the medical paradigm.

The rather one-sided and biased picture that historians of sexuality and psychiatry have drawn of Krafft-Ebing can be attributed for a large part to their presentism. Such an approach especially colors interpretations of nineteenth-century medical theories of sexuality, such as Krafft-Ebing's. Not only has he been blamed for the stigmatization of sexual minorities; he has also been criticized because his psychiatric viewpoint on sexual perversion does not stand the test of modern psychology. It seems that the sexual revolution of the 1960s, relegating sexual repression to the dustbin of history, has made it difficult to judge his work in an unbiased way and to consider it in its proper historical context. Another legacy of the 1960s has also contributed to a one-sided picture of Krafft-Ebing. It is no coincidence that Foucault and Szasz stressed the disciplining effects of medical interference with sexuality in which psychiatrists played a leading role. Together with Ronald D. Laing and David Cooper, they set the tone for a "revisionist" history of psychiatry.

The first historians of psychiatry, often psychiatrists themselves, tended to evaluate past psychiatric ideas and practices according to their own contemporary scientific and moral standards; they emphasized the accomplishments of the discipline, suggesting that superstitious beliefs and cruel practices had been replaced by sound medical science and humanitarian treatments. Since the 1960s, however, revisionist historians of psychiatry have rejected these "Whiggish" and internalist histories that highlight scientific enlightenment and humanitarian reform as the driving forces of progress. Stressing that psychiatric theories and practices should not be understood on their own terms but in their institutional and social context, they have taken a critical if not hostile view of medical psychiatry. Inspired directly or indirectly by the anti-psychiatric movement of the 1960s and 1970s, the concepts of social control, repression, and disciplining are central in their interpretative scheme. Revisionist social historians associate psychiatric practice with the development of industrial capitalism and the modern state, and they view professional psychiatrists as agents of the "therapeutic state," intent on marginalizing outsiders and imposing social order and conformity onto bourgeois society. Reducing psychiatric practice to external forces, they come to the conclusion that it was in fact a covert form of social, political, and moral control.[4]

Whereas Foucault, Szasz, and other scholars consider the emergence of the science of sexuality as a deplorable medical colonization, replacing religious and judicial authority with a new form of moral tyranny, contemporaries of Krafft-Ebing like Von R did not experience it as such. He wrote to Krafft-Ebing that reading *Psychopathia sexualis* had made him aware that

> my way of feeling is not an error, but an illness, and that I am not the only "stepchild of nature." . . . If a cure and salvation are possible for me, I will have you to thank for these. I would have never believed that my pride could convince me to make these confessions. Only your work has opened my eyes. It made the world and myself not appear in the gray light of disdain any longer and it gave me confidence in a reassuring and rehabilitating way.

For Von R, Krafft-Ebing's work was an eye-opener. He was not the only pervert writing to Krafft-Ebing who made references to the salutary effects of *Psychopathia sexualis*. Another correspondent wrote to him: "A heavily suffering person turns to the benign and great help of your science. . . . It is incredibly hard for me to expose myself. And I can only do it to you, to you

4. See Foucault 1961; Dörner 1969; Rothman 1971; Szasz 1971 & 1972; Castel 1976; Scull 1979.

alone in the entire world, because I know from your work 'Psychopathia sexualis' that I will not be saying totally strange things."[5] Many others who addressed themselves to Krafft-Ebing and sent him their autobiographies expressed themselves in similar ways. A physician who felt psychologically and physically like a woman explained that Krafft-Ebing's writings had saved him from despair:

> Sir—I must beg your indulgence for troubling you with my communica-
> tion. I lost all control, and thought of myself only as a monster before
> which I myself shuddered. Then your work gave me courage again, and
> I was determined to get to the bottom of the matter, examine my past
> life, and let the results be what they might be. . . . After reading your
> work I hope that . . . I may still count myself among human beings who
> do not merely deserve to be despised. (1890e, 79; Ps 1999, 267–68)

How should these expressions be qualified? Are these individuals, as the Foucaultian interpretation would have it, trapped in a medical discourse through which not only power relations and social control of deviant sexu-alities but also sexual subjects themselves are constituted? The radical im-plication of Foucault's reasoning is that before, say, 1870 deviants like ho-mosexuals, masochists, fetishists, and transsexuals did not exist, nor did their counterparts, "normal" heterosexuals. If this contention can be de-fended at all, it is still problematic that new sexual categories and identities are too easily seen as mere scientific constructions of physicians. In other words, the disciplining effects of medical interference with sexuality are overemphasized. Individuals, labeled as patients and perverts, are mainly presented as passive victims of a medical juggernaut, with no other choice than to conform to medical stereotypes. Yet, the exclusive focus on the disciplinary constructions of medical discourse has resulted in a neglect of individual voices and the sociopsychological formation of sexual subjec-tivity.

It has become a truism that doctors, such as Krafft-Ebing, by describing and categorizing perversion, were instrumental in creating a new discourse on sexuality, but in spite of the extensive debates about the impact of late-nineteenth-century medicine on social attitudes about sexuality, we do not yet have detailed studies of how their theories were popularized within and outside the medical profession, nor do we quite know how they were re-ceived by those concerned. Histories of psychiatry, both traditional and revisionist, and also most works about the medicalization of sexuality tend to focus on institutions, the professional interests of doctors, and their views of mental illness and sexuality, but they say little about the subjective

---

5. Letter of GP to Krafft-Ebing (March 10, 1899), Nachlass Krafft-Ebing.

experiences of their patients. Typically, patients are presented as either the raw and inert "clinical material" on the basis of which medical scientists developed and demonstrated their theories, or as passive victims in an exploitative process, the undifferentiated objects of social control. The emphasis on medical labeling as the major influence in the process of creating deviants presents a social-deterministic model in which individuals essentially appear as pawns of social forces having no will of their own. In theories of medicalization, the relation between doctors and patients is often conceptualized in a one-sided way. The medical profession is generally depicted as a coherent, overpowering social force that imposes its definitions, methods, and techniques on society, making people completely dependent on the whims of physicians. Of course, medically defined categories and symptoms may help individuals to order and make sense of their vague sensations and confusing experiences, but that does not mean that individual meanings automatically and only follow medical thinking.

As I will show in this book, case histories and autobiographical accounts of Krafft-Ebing's patients demonstrate that perverts did not always passively accept external conditions of action; they rather responded to social constraints in different ways, reflected upon them, and reconstituted them in the light of their particular circumstances. The historian should be cautious in accepting medical rhetoric at face value, in privileging medical theory over practice, and placing the scientific enterprise of doctors above the actual treatment and the existential experience of patients (Risse and Warner 1992, 201). Life as concrete experience will inevitably be trapped within the contradictions of constraint and choice, similarity and diversity.

Historians of psychiatry who studied the treatment of psychosomatic illnesses, especially that of hysteria and neuroses, point out that patients often played a highly active role in the interactions with doctors, thus contributing substantially to the development of medical theories (Micale 1990, 72–74; Shorter 1992). In nineteenth-century general medicine, the introduction of methods of physical diagnosis and "objective" physiological signs of disease gradually superseded the patient's own accounts and diminished the need and ability of the sick to give articulate expression to their complaints. By contrast, in late-nineteenth-century psychiatry, stories of individual patients began to influence the production of medical knowledge. The psychiatric theories on sexuality that emerged at the end of the nineteenth century only became established as facts about sexuality because they were directly linked to specific social groups and the larger cultural setting from the beginning. Not only was the relationship between doctors and patients reciprocal; there were also close connections between individual experiences involving sexuality and changes in society. Both patients and doctors were agents of culture at large.

Foucault rightly points out that modern sexual identities were articulated in medical works. Without psychiatrists, the pervert may indeed not have appeared as a specific type of person, but psychiatrists alone were not able to "construct" perversions at will. Unlike what many historians of sexuality and psychiatry have suggested, late-nineteenth-century psychiatrists were anything but powerful agents of social control. Despite the often triumphal rhetoric of the psychiatric profession, the position of psychiatrists within medicine, as well as in society at large, remained precarious. During the first half of the nineteenth century, they had won dominion over the most serious and dangerous forms of mental dysfunction, but their authority was basically confined to the walls of the lunatic asylum, which housed the chronically insane. Moreover, even in the second half of the century, psychiatrists had difficulties in convincing other scholars and the public that as physicians they had an exclusive and scientific insight into the nature of insanity. For psychiatry to be accepted as a distinct branch of modern medical science, it was necessary to emphasize that mental disorder was an organic disease of the brain and the nervous system, and also to prove that they were able to cure insanity. But there was, in fact, hardly any anatomical or physiological evidence of the somatic basis of mental illness, and as a therapeutic institution, the asylum did not meet expectations.

Throughout the nineteenth century, psychiatry's scientific program remained inadequate from a medical point of view and its intellectual and professional weaknesses made it vulnerable to lay criticism. Psychiatrists operated in the margins of medicine as well as of society. When Krafft-Ebing started his career in the 1860s, the professional status of psychiatrists was fragile and it had only slightly improved at the time of his death in 1902. I would suggest therefore that psychiatry's theorizing on and treatment of sexual deviance grew out of its weakness rather than its strength. Consequently, instead of looking for answers to explain how psychiatrists used their power to control and discipline sexual deviants, it seems more appropriate to ask why psychiatrists like Krafft-Ebing directed their attention to sexual issues as a way to promote their specialty and to extend their professional domain, and also how their work on perversion was received in society at that time, especially by those directly concerned. Although psychiatric knowledge is not devoid of social and cultural considerations, it should not be portrayed one-dimensionally as an epiphenomenon of social and cultural trends. One also has to make an effort to understand the content of psychiatry from within and the way contemporaries understood it. In this book I have tried to make a detailed analysis of the contents of Krafft-Ebing's psychiatry, of his motivations and intentions as well as those of his patients, before putting them in their wider social-cultural context.

Foucault and other scholars rightly stress that not only the attitude of people toward sexual behavior but also the concept and meaning of sexuality itself are subject to cultural variation and historical change. They argue that sexuality is a cultural and historical construct that makes no sense except as inscribed in language, discourses, meanings, "representations," and symbols. However, a critical attitude toward the concept of sexuality as a stable, natural psychobiological unity should not lead to losing sight of sexual identity as a sociopsychological phenomenon, as part of real individual experience. The argument that sexual identities are culturally shaped, rather than rooted in a biological or psychological essence, does not mean that they can be constructed and, as many postmodernist scholars seem to believe, deconstructed at will.[6] Sexual identities originated not only as medical inventions; changes in society as well as in the experience of self set the condition for their emergence.

The delineation of sexual perversions and their incorporation in psychiatric classifications required more than the existence of an organized medical profession that interfered with so-called perverts; what was also necessary was a group of people whose experience of sexual deviance had changed in such a way that it was no longer perceived as more or less temporal, fleeting digressions, but as a continuous and essential feature of their lives. In order to explain how sexual identities were shaped, it is necessary to enter the subjective world of individuals who read Krafft-Ebing's work and responded to it, as well as to take their intentions, purposes, and meanings seriously on their own terms. The presentist question of whether Krafft-Ebing's scientific viewpoint on sexuality was right or wrong from the perspective of modern biological or psychological research is not relevant in my historical analysis of the effects of his work, the way it was read and used by contemporaries. Who were the patients and informants of Krafft-Ebing? What were their social and cultural backgrounds? Why did they read Krafft-Ebing's work? How did they interpret medical theories, and how did they come into contact with the psychiatrist? How did they present themselves, and what kind of stories did they tell? In what way did medical theories and individual experiences interact, and how did these interferences between scientific and autobiographical meaning-constructions develop?

Changes in the self-understanding of the individuals who became the object of scientific discourses as well as the development and professionalization of psychiatry have to be taken into account to understand the historical context of medical debates about sexuality. Arguing that new ways of understanding sexuality emerged not only from medical thinking itself,

6. For a discussion of the so-called essentialist-constructionist controversy, see Weeks 1985; Vance 1989; Stein 1990; and Stanton 1992.

I focus on the connections between the cognitive content of Krafft-Ebing's work, his casuistry, the institutional setting of his psychiatry, and the wider social and cultural contexts in which sexual identities evolved. Class and, to a lesser extent, sex are of particular importance to understanding the role perverts themselves played in the modernization of sexuality and how their self-reflections contributed to the formation of sexual identity. This raises the question of which social developments affected the changing experience of sexuality in the nineteenth century. In this book I will put forward some possible explanations. Sexual subjectivity was especially fostered by the growing significance of the middle-class ideal of romantic love, entailing a differentiation of sexuality as a more or less autonomous social sphere. The spread of autobiographical self-analysis among the bourgeoisie was also crucial. Also, economic independence and social and geographical mobility were important social conditions for the emergence of sexual identities.

Part 1 of this book focuses on medical and psychiatric ideas of sexuality in the nineteenth century. First, it offers an overview of the way sexuality became an object of medical interference and research in general and psychiatry in particular in western and central Europe. Secondly, I demonstrate how Krafft-Ebing's work on sexual pathology was part of this broad development. Medical views of sexuality in general and Krafft-Ebing's in particular were far from static and unambiguous. Medical opinion on sexuality was multifaceted: toward the end of the century, doctors vacillated between physiological and psychological approaches as well as between moral disqualification and, albeit prudently, condonation of sexual aberration.

Part 2 deals with Krafft-Ebing's professional strategies—cognitive as well as institutional—to further the cause of psychiatry, and it delineates the changing social settings in which he worked during the last four decades of the nineteenth century. Krafft-Ebing became actively engaged in the process in which the main institutional locus of psychiatry shifted from the asylum to the university and whereby psychiatry was more or less recognized as a scientific discipline in medical faculties. The shaping of psychiatry as a promising medical specialty—an important phase in its professionalization process—as well as the development of private practice entailed a shift in the social background of its patients from the lower to the middle and upper classes. This shift explains why some of Krafft-Ebing's patients and correspondents began to play an active role in the development of his work on sexual pathology—which is the subject of part 3.

To find out how Krafft-Ebing's sexual pathology and the individual experiences of perverts interacted, the case histories and autobiographies of his patients and correspondents are crucial. In part 3 I demonstrate that a specific development can be discerned in the way Krafft-Ebing assembled the hundreds of cases, most of which he published, not only in his main work in this field, *Psychopathia sexualis*, but also in numerous articles. Case histories and autobiographies of Krafft-Ebing's patients make clear that medical knowledge of sexuality could only be successful because it dovetailed with the experiences of specific social groups. Class and sex are the most relevant parameters here. Psychiatrists like Krafft-Ebing and many of his patients—the great majority of which were men—shared the same cultural background and the same bourgeois values. Belief in psychiatric knowledge among Krafft-Ebing's bourgeois clientele was sustained not simply by its possibility to give a satisfactory explanation of abnormal sexual feelings and experiences, but also by its persuasiveness in negotiating social relations between a representative of established science and those who felt and were considered as outsiders, but who, at the same time, wished to be acknowledged.

The immediate institutional setting of psychiatry and the social background of Krafft-Ebing's patients, however, do not provide sufficient explanation of the emergence of sexual identities. Part 4 explores the wider cultural context in which psychiatrists like Krafft-Ebing as well as perverts themselves gave meaning to sexual experiences. The scientific "will to know" moved forward at the same pace as concern for the authentic and voluble self in society. In my view, not only the impact of psychiatry but also the propagation of autobiographical self-reflection and of romantic love should be taken into account to explain why in late-nineteenth-century bourgeois society, sexuality was privileged as the quintessence of privacy and the individual self. More specifically, I will highlight the anxieties and the inconsistencies surrounding sexuality in fin de siècle Vienna to recapture something of the mentality and cultural climate in which Krafft-Ebing worked. In late-nineteenth-century Vienna, intellectuals and artists were obsessed with themes of sexuality. Krafft-Ebing's sexual pathology reflected the preoccupation of the liberal Austrian intelligentsia with sexuality's dangers and pleasures. The intelligentsia's intellectual style was marked by a combination of philosophical irrationalism and scientific materialism, which was especially appropriate to a new way of thinking about sexuality.

Krafft-Ebing's published and unpublished case histories on sexual perversion, including many letters and autobiographies of patients and correspondents, form the core material for this book; I collected around 440 of them. To find out who his patients were and to reconstruct their experiences, I have analyzed these case studies in a systematic, quantitative manner as well as in a qualitative, interpretative way. Most case studies include basic information about the diagnosis, sex, age, profession, and social position of Krafft-Ebing's patients and correspondents. Many of them also contain information about physical and psychological examinations, treatments, the role of degeneration in the diagnosis, and the way in which the subjects of these case studies became patients of Krafft-Ebing by being hospitalized in an asylum, psychiatric clinic, or sanatorium, or by consulting him as a private patient. Especially significant in my qualitative analysis are the voices that can be heard in these case histories, not only that of the psychiatrist but often also those of the clients, directly as well as indirectly. Many case studies put the narratives of the patients themselves center stage, thereby offering valuable information about their lives and inner experiences. The meanings they attached to their condition and the diverging ways in which these meanings relate to the medical discourse about perversions are crucial to understanding how modern sexual identities evolved.

It would be naive, of course, to believe that these case descriptions are direct representations of the "real" lives of their subjects, that they simply mirror their experiences. They are surviving artifacts of doctor-patient interactions, and as such they are conditioned by institutional settings, cultural assumptions, social status, and power relationships (Risse and Warner 1992, 189; cf. Porter 1985). Medical case histories and the autobiographical self-presentations that were modeled on them are also characterized by particular narrative patterns. The case histories and autobiographical accounts are interpretations by Krafft-Ebing and his patients, and therefore can only be comprehended by looking at the wider psychiatric and cultural context in which they originated and functioned. My account can and will only be a form of "thick description," a contextualizing interpretation of the meanings these actors bestowed on their experiences (Geertz 1973).

Since I focus mainly on Krafft-Ebing's patients who were treated for sexual disorders and perversions, I have only used a comparatively small part of the unpublished case histories and correspondence that I found in his estate. Nevertheless it has afforded me with new insights, especially concerning the way Krafft-Ebing dealt with the life stories of perverts. Next to this unique and unexploited archive, I explored all relevant published works by Krafft-Ebing. I also consulted sources in the Austrian State Archives, the archives of the Universities of Graz and Vienna, as well as some unpublished manuscripts in the Institute for the History of Medicine of the University of Vienna and the Austrian National Library. Together with some letters of Krafft-Ebing's colleagues that are part of his estate, these provided me with useful information on Krafft-Ebing's academic career.

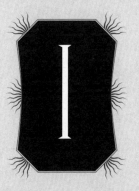

Medical Science
and the
Modernization
of Sexuality

HUMAN REPRODUCTION HAS BEEN AN OBJECT OF INTELLECTUAL reflection in the Western world at least since Aristotle (384–322 B.C.). Traditionally, however, sexuality was viewed more in terms of morality than in terms of knowledge or science. Although Christianity has been far from consistent in its sexual ideology, generally it has stressed the dangers of sexuality, rather than its pleasures. Building on ideas and traditions of Greek and Roman ethics, the church fathers strongly promoted an austere morality. Just like the stoics and the Neoplatonists, Augustine (354–430), the basic theorist of Christian sexual ideology, considered sexual lust as bestial because it could not be controlled by reason or will. In the wake of the Fall, lust became conceptualized as a degenerate emotion, one that proved to be hard to manipulate. To solve this issue, total abstinence was formulated as an ideal, but it never came to function as a norm with which the majority of the believers complied. The evil of lust could only be counterbalanced or partially regulated, Augustine argued, by accepting two principles as fundamental: marriage and procreation. These were the only two contexts in which surrendering to sexual desire became more or less legitimate. Although dominant Christian sexual morality would be slightly modified throughout the centuries, marriage and procreation continued to be the two pillars of its sexual ideology.

Sexual acts not geared toward procreation were commonly referred to as sodomy. In addition to homosexual intercourse, this term might cover anal contact between man and woman, coitus interruptus, bestiality, and even sexual intercourse between Christians and non-Christians (Greenberg 1988, 274–75; Gilbert 1985). By setting up extensive arguments about the essential distinction between natural and unnatural sexual intercourse, theological treatises provided a theoretical foundation for understanding sodomy as a great sin. The most detailed and influential theological justification of Christian sexual morality was formulated by Thomas Aquinas (1228–1274). In his scholastic philosophy, which provided Christian religion with an intellectual basis, reason and free will functioned as central categories. In Thomas's view, plants derived their vitality from metabolism and reproduction, animals had sensory experiences and knew lusts and instincts, but reason and free will were reserved for people only. Everything that conflicted with reason, he argued, was contrary to human nature. Because human beings possessed reason and free will, as prerequisites of moral behavior, they could and should control and channel their drives and lusts.

In the wake of Aristotle and Augustine, Thomas emphasized the goal-orientedness of sexual behavior. God had designed human nature in such a way that new life would be the product of lust, yet the experience of lust for its own sake was sinful. Because, according to Thomas, the raising of the potentially resulting offspring would only be guaranteed in situations where man and woman were united in a fixed relationship, only sexuality within marriage was to be considered moral. Sexual intercourse between man and woman before or outside of marriage, and even rape and incest, could be understood as "natural," since offspring might be the outcome, but it still was not "rational" because in those situations care was not necessarily provided concurrently. In addition to a category of "vice in line with nature," Thomas identified a category of "vice contrary to nature." This included masturbation, same-sex intercourse, bestiality, and sexual intercourse between man and woman whereby conception was actively prevented. Although Thomas differentiated between various forms of "unnatural sex" and although after bestiality he considered sodomy—which he reserved for sexual intercourse between men—as the worst sin against the sixth commandment, he was not so much making a distinction between hetero- and homosexuality as between natural and unnatural, or rational and irrational acts. Thomistic doctrine has strongly determined Roman Catholic sexual ideology, and to secular authorities the views of Thomas—together with the biblical narrative of Sodom—served as legitimization to persecute sodomy for a long time. From the late medieval period to the end of the eighteenth century, in many European countries sodomy was severely punished. Although there was substantial variation in verdicts over time and from place to place, the death penalty was not uncommon.

In the eighteenth century, however, enlightened thinkers began to criticize the Christian morality of sin in general, while also opposing severe punishment of sodomy. They not only favored milder penalties, such as detention or isolation, but they also viewed preventive measures and rehabilitation as more effective means to counter sexual deviations. By 1800, partly as a result of the French Revolution, capital punishment for sodomy was abolished in several European countries. In the nineteenth century, the theological-judicial approach to sexuality was increasingly challenged by new views. Although the ethic of marriage and procreation was left largely intact, the traditional Christian condemnation of sexual aberration in terms of sin and guilt was replaced in part with concerns about depopulization, the weakening of the state, and the undermining of public order; above all, sexual aberration began to be conceived in a medical light. The growth of secular knowledge since the eighteenth century has been accompanied by the faith that science—biomedical science in particular—would have an increasingly significant contribution to make in the understanding of sexual issues. It is this Enlightenment spirit of progress that gave medical scientists of the nineteenth century the idea that they were going to be the ones to reveal the indisputable truth of sexuality.

The Emergence of Sexual Science

The Enlightenment saw the birth of sexual science, which defined women as inherently different from and complementary to men in terms of their anatomy, physiology, temperament, and intellect. In the older one-sex model, man and woman were hierarchically ordered versions of each other, and masculinity and femininity were not viewed as biological opposites but as social and cultural categories. From the eighteenth century on, scientists began to explain the difference between the sexes as one determined by an assumed biological substrate. In the new anthropological model of the emergent biomedical sciences, objective knowledge about individuals could only be derived from their bodies, by observing their anatomy and measuring their physiological functions. The scientific evidence of two fundamentally distinct sexes was located in anatomy and physiology. As political as well as industrial revolutions infringed on traditional status divisions, establishing a more egalitarian social setup, biomedical arguments about "natural" differences began to play an ever greater role in justifying social hierarchies. The belief that the psychological and social differences between men and women were permanently rooted in nature was used to relegate them to distinctive social spheres and to legitimate the exclusion of women from political life as well as from science (Russet 1989; Schiebinger 1989; Laqueur 1990; Honegger 1991).

If modern biomedical thinking on sex differences can be said to have originated in the Enlightenment, the same applies to the scientific interest in sexuality at large. Rationalist criticism of received authority affected sexual mores. Rejecting a transcendental, divine order as the basis of morality, the philosophes replaced the Christian view of sin and virtue with secular, scientific notions of nature. Montesquieu (1689–1755), Voltaire (1694–1778), and especially Julien Offray de Lamettrie (1709–1751) rejected the Christian condemnation of sexual pleasure as an autonomous experience.

Ethical rules had to be accommodated to human nature and actual behavior, not the other way around. They tended to view sexual morals largely as a matter of social convention. Eighteenth-century physiology, especially its vitalist version, stressed that mind and body were not separate spheres, but formed a single integrated system. This naturalization of man entailed a realistic appraisal of human passions.

Thus the Enlightenment had a liberating influence, although mainly men received the benefits (Darnton 1990; Porter 1990). For some, like Giovanni Giacomo Casanova (1725–1798), libertinism seemed to be legitimate because pleasure was pursued under the aegis of a benevolent nature. However, as a natural phenomenon, sexuality was open to different moral meanings. In fact, the philosophes vacillated between two concepts of nature: one referred to a rational and orderly normative principle that replaced divine order, the other to an amoral principle of reality full of irrationality and disorder (Stockinger 1979; Delon 1987). On the one hand, leading Enlightenment thinkers like Denis Diderot (1713–1784) and Jean-Jacques Rousseau (1712–1778) believed that unspoiled nature offered a foundation for both moral behavior and harmonious relations between the individual and society. On the other hand, the Marquis Donatien-Alphonse-Francois de Sade (1740–1814), Baron Paul Dietrich d'Holbach (1723–1789), Pierre Choderlos de Laclos (1741–1803), and others argued that nature was profoundly riven by inner tensions, contradictions, and disruptive forces: natural drives were ethically neutral or even blindly amoral and thus could not provide a foundation on which to build a peaceful society. Given these divergent interpretations of human nature, Enlightenment thinking on sexuality was highly ambivalent. To the extent that sexual activity contributed to procreation and was connected to harmonious heterosexual relations, love, marriage, family, and maternity, it was applauded; but if sexuality was premature, illicit, excessive, or motivated by sheer lust, it was considered socially subversive (Jordanova 1986; Pilkington 1986).

Although the philosophes rejected Christian morality, it was still difficult for most of them to regard sexuality as a positive force in life. Lamettrie and the Marquis de Sade used the idea that nature was amoral to defend idiosyncratic sexual desires, but they belonged to a minority. Most Enlightenment thinkers were ambivalent on sexuality and held on to a narrow view of sexual freedom. Social utilitarianism, the duties individuals were supposed to have toward the common good, set limits on the free expression of natural urges. Even radical materialist thinkers like Dietrich d'Holbach, Diderot, and Claude-Adrien Helvétius (1715–1771), who advocated a naturalist ethics in which sexual variation had its place, gave the interest of society priority over individual desire. The philosophes did not fundamentally overturn existing sexual norms. Most of them took the reproductive pairing of male and female to be the unquestioned norm and goal of sexuality, while nonprocreative activities like masturbation and sodomy were taken to be a manifestation of bad habits, a faulty education, an inflamed fantasy, poor moral conditions, and, above all, a sign of antisocial and unhealthy behavior. The practice of sexuality outside of the private sphere of heterosexual intimacy and marriage challenged normative and reassuring readings of nature as a source of virtue and social order. As a basically irrational, unproductive, and egoistic drive, it undermined the optimistic idea of moral nature and posed a potential risk to social harmony. Therefore, sexuality could only be integrated in society if its practice was brought under rational control.

Already in the eighteenth century, many popular medical and paramedical works on sexuality were circulating in which scientific and practical information was mixed with titillating passages and unconventional behavior received ample attention; especially for the medical fringe, this was a tempting way to make money (P. Wagner 1987). In spite of some tolerance of sexual libertinism, the enlightened eighteenth century also saw the beginnings of the pathological model of sexuality. For the late eighteenth and early nineteenth centuries, the major sexual deviancy was masturbation, which supposedly caused a corruption of sexual behavior, in particular when it started at an early age. Masturbation had been condemned since the first half of the eighteenth century, but Samuel August Tissot (1728–1797), author of the popular *De l'onanisme, ou dissertation physique sur les maladies, produites par la masturbation* (1760), was one of the first physicians to argue that it weakened and eventually damaged both the nervous system and the brain. The causal link between onanism and nervous and mental diseases would be reiterated again and again in the nineteenth century. The preoccupation with the dangers of masturbation was typical of the Enlightenment approach to sexuality: there could be no clearer contrast than that between the fundamentally asocial "solitary vice" and vital, socially constructive heterosexual intercourse. The philosophes put their faith in sanitary solutions and the beneficial effects of education, a healthy lifestyle, moderation, hard work, self-mastery, sublimation, and marriage. A sound education, geared toward implanting mental control mechanisms that suppressed the individual's sexual impulses, was seen as the key to preventing counterproductive and harmful sexual conduct.

However, nineteenth-century medical interest in sexuality was dictated by wider social anxieties. In his influential *Essay on the Principle of Population* (1798), Thomas Robert Malthus (1766–1834) problematized sex in a new way by linking it to economic and social problems. Whereas the dominant eighteenth-century value system expressed a belief in the pleasures of procreation, Malthus felt that it was necessary to bridle sexual drives because of the disastrous social consequences of unlimited propagation: overpopulation, poverty, famine, diseases, and war (Porter and Hall 1995, 127). He shifted the debate away from sexual pleasure in reproduction toward fear of the power of sexual desire as a threat to social well-being. Yet the awareness of the danger of overpopulation also would add a new, albeit semi-legal, dimension to sexual discourse: the case for contraception. In the course of the nineteenth century, contraception became more widely practiced, especially among middle-class couples. From the 1860s, the Neo-Malthusian movement turned birth control into a public issue.

Next to an economic purport, sexuality was also invested with social and political meanings: the middle class used its standard of morality as a means to propagate its respectability and to differentiate itself from the frivolous aristocracy as well as the dissipated lower orders. The fear of sexual license was connected to social questions such as the role of the family, public morality, and social reform, and the concept of utility was invoked to justify self-discipline and social responsibility. Not so much penal law, but medicine, education, and social hygiene were seen as the means to prevent debauchery and create a socially acceptable sexual standard. The state's noninterference in citizens' private lives was a crucial legal principle of both Enlightenment thought and nineteenth-century liberalism. Opposing the union of church and state, Enlightenment and liberal thinkers emphasized the distinction between sin, as the province of the church, and crime, as a concern of the state. They argued that any sexual practice that failed to infringe upon the rights of individuals or society as a whole belonged to the sacrosanct sphere of private life, a world where the state had no dealings. When it came to the actual practice of noninterference in individual sexual life, however, the liberal separation of private and public spheres ran up against its limits in the course of the nineteenth century and obvious inconsistencies came to light. Prostitution, for instance, was a chronic social concern, not only because it was public sexuality, but also because of the transmission of venereal diseases. As a practice, however, it was upheld by a double standard: lower-class women provided a "necessary outlet" for male bourgeois promiscuity (which was tacitly condoned), thus protecting bourgeois women from the sexual urges of the men of their own class. Furthermore, many liberal thinkers still regarded same-sex practices of men as troublesome, particularly when taking place in public places in cities or in institutional settings like barracks, prisons, ships, schools, and dormitories.

Confronted with forms of irregular sexual behavior in the public sphere, liberals debated the proper scope of the state's role. They wavered uneasily between the principles of utilitarianism, seeking the greatest good for the greatest number, and laissez-faire, allowing individuals to pursue their own interests. Advocates of utilitarianism widely agreed that prophylaxis and public hygiene were valid rationales for political and medical intervention in the sexual realm. The more liberalism allied itself with nationalism, the more the right of the state to set standards governing collective survival overrode the claims of private interests (Nye 1984; Mosse 1985; Mort 1987; Fout 1992). Sexual conduct and its possible consequence, procreation, came to be seen as critical social and political issues, since they involved the health and strength of nations. By the late nineteenth century, the concern over depopulation and biological decline became something of an obsession affecting many nations, France in particular, but also Great Britain and Germany. National rivalries—the one between France and Germany, for example—were framed in Darwinian terms of demographic battles for the survival of the fittest. The willingness and ability of the nation to defend its vitality against internal social pathologies became the criterion for its external security. Sexuality played a central role in various "sociobiological" ideologies and disciplines that flourished in the last decades of the nineteenth century; some of them, like social Darwinism and degeneration theory, tended to rationalize social and political inequalities as facts of nature and lent themselves to the arsenals of racism and nationalism. Around the turn of the century especially, the precepts of eugenics seemed to promise a rational mastery of the natural laws of evolution by linking genetics, demographics, and medicine. Racial hygiene and advance were important concerns behind numerous medical works on sexuality.

Next to the economic and political worries over the size and health of the population, the growing concern over public health issues in the nineteenth century fostered interest in sexual problems, that of venereal diseases, prostitution, and public indecency in particular. In the course of the century, systems for registering prostitutes and compulsory medical examination were implemented throughout Europe. While the aim of these regulationist systems was the medical control of sexually transmittable diseases, they were also used for surveillance of the demimonde of prostitution. At the same time, the police apparatus, which became more efficiently organized, increasingly took strong action against other forms of disorderly sexual conduct. The interference with prostitution and deviant sexualities marked a transformation of private activity into conduct that could be legitimately condemned by standards of bourgeois respectability and public health (Weeks 1981; Hekma 1987).

The sexual body occupied a central position in the prevailing discourse about health and sanitation. Sexual immorality and disease were classic targets of public health campaigns, which were rooted in the emergent medical professionalism as well as in moral politics and were aimed at the surveillance and regulation of the urban poor. In the ethical discourse of the public health movement of the mid-nineteenth century, immorality, poverty, and the spread of contagious diseases like cholera became conflated. Sexual immorality was understood as a class issue, specifically linked to the habits and living environment of the urban poor and seen in direct relation to the themes of disease, filth, depravity, overcrowding, bad housing, crime, and disruptive behavior in working-class culture. Immoral conduct was viewed, on the one hand, as a direct result of diseases and unsanitary conditions in working-class milieus, but, on the other hand, it was also cited as one of the main causes of disease. The medical profession—which collaborated with philanthropists campaigning for moral reform and expounding the belief that the health of the population was the key to good government—was an influential pressure group that provided the intellectual rationale for state intervention in working-class culture. Because during the last decades of the nineteenth century physicians embraced a hygienic role in the interventionist state, they were politically sanctioned to expand their domain by claiming expertise in formerly nonmedical issues such as alcoholism, crime, sexual perversion, and other social pathologies.

In addition to class, gender was a crucial variable in nineteenth-century sexual politics. Scientists made radical claims for sexual incommensurability between men and women, and sex became understood as one of the key determinants of personality. Professional medicine reinforced a strict differentiation of gender roles, which was part of the general separation of spheres and duties for men and women within the bourgeoisie. The emerging new medical discourse on sexuality prioritized the fundamental difference between male and female physiology, and hence it saw male and female sexuality as radically different from each other. In the medical paradigm, male sexuality was an independent, powerful force that builds itself up inside the body until it is released in orgasm and ejaculation. Echoing the typical nineteenth-century model of the closed energy system, the (male) sexual drive was conceptualized as energy accumulated and generated through internal physical processes and released in sexual arousal and discharge. This conceptualization of sexuality was part of the "drive model" in nineteenth-century physiological and psychological thinking that was rooted in the Romantic understanding of human self-expression as well as in the materialist-mechanical view of the body as a steam engine or motor (Russelman 1983; Rabinbach 1990). While from a moral viewpoint male continence was seen as desirable, in practice it could hardly be guaranteed because of the assumed strength of the male drive.

In contrast to men, women were defined as essentially asexual beings. Before the 1860s doctors usually had some conception of acceptable pleasure for women, but dominant medical opinion held that motherhood and domesticity made such vital demands on a woman's energy that her sexual desire was basically extinguished. Women were supposedly driven not by lust, but by the desire for love. From this, many doctors concluded that a prostitute's sexual desire was unnatural, and thus they established a sharp distinction between normal respectable women and abnormal depraved prostitutes. When in the middle of the nineteenth century medical attention began to focus on prostitution and venereal diseases, women rather than men were singled out as the human agents of infection, posing a threat to national health. In medical theories the prostitute, who challenged the social order by her active and autonomous sexuality, was imputed with impurity and pathology.

The problems of prostitution and venereal disease opened up the question of sexuality to wider public scrutiny, culminating in a public debate, in the final decades of the nineteenth century, over public morality, the double standard, and private vice. More and more, in fact, the double standard was challenged, and in the same period in which the medical profession grew stronger, its female counterpart gained ground as well: charity and philanthropy became regarded as appropriate activities for middle-class women. Female social reformers, the forerunners of the early women's movement, began to oppose male professional expertise in the field of prostitution. Feminists, supported by socialists and purity movements, contested the regulation of prostitution. These groups claimed that the regulationist systems not only infringed upon the civil liberties of all women, but also sanctioned male vice and the exploitation of working-class women. In contrast to the medical world's approach, this movement viewed male sexuality as the fundamental problem: prostitution was the direct result of men's immorality (Mort 1987, 94–95). They rejected the medical belief that the male sexual urge was uncontrollable and that frequent intercourse was necessary for men's health. Stressing that working-class prostitutes were hapless, passive victims of men and manipulative doctors, these abolitionists isolated male sexuality as the target for reforming intervention, in the interest of creating a higher standard of purity and personal morality. Purity movements, which garnered much support in predominantly Protestant countries like Britain and Germany, stressed the need to promote morality and to outlaw obscenity, indecency, and the victimization of prostitutes.

In the nineteenth century, the scientific discussion about sexuality was dominated by physicians. This was caused in part by the fact that reproduction and the workings of sexual organs were subjects of biomedical research; since the 1830s, for instance, significant new knowledge was discovered about the process of ovulation, menstruation, and fertilization, and in the 1880s the foundations of endocrinology were laid (Farley 1982). But a more important explanation of the strong medical presence in the debate on sexual matters was the enhanced scientific and social status of medicine. Physicians professionalized quite successfully in the second half of the nineteenth century, especially in France and Germany, where they were directly linked to the state and new medical specialties such as public hygiene and psychiatry rapidly expanded. More and more, physicians, acting as mediators between science and the vexing problems of everyday life, succeeded in convincing the public of the indispensability of their expertise, and gradually they began to replace the clergy as authoritative personal consultants in the realm of sexuality. In the public's eyes, it was science that so distinctively separated the modern doctor from the traditional one, and by the end of the nineteenth century, medicine had acquired significant social authority. However, there were still huge disparities in scientific sophistication among individual doctors, and many of them still held quite traditional opinions on sexuality that were relatively akin to lay belief. Many of the more or less sensational medical works on sexuality were intended not so much as scientific studies but to make money, from the book's proceeds as well as from the clientele it might draw to the author's consultation room. Nevertheless, the long-established tradition and the scientific aura of medical writing on sexuality gave the physician the status of expert in a society that was often ambivalent about openly discussing sexual matters.

Biomedical interest in sexuality was stimulated by the theory of Charles Darwin (1809–1882), especially by his idea that sex existed for the good of the species and that sexual selection was a key to evolution. In particular, the publication of Darwin's The Descent of Man (1871) provoked questions on the place of sexuality in the evolution of mankind. Darwinism fostered the idea that sexual activity was natural and biologically inevitable, but at the same time it was looked upon with suspicion: the sexual instinct was beset by dangers that could only be countered or alleviated by social conventions, self-control, sanitary prescriptions, and sex education. For this reason, the British authors Patrick Geddes and J. Arthur Thomson, who in their popular The Evolution of Sex (1889) reassuringly explained that from an evolutionary perspective, cooperation—rather than competition—determined sexuality, at the same time noted a volcanic element in sexuality that would shake the foundation of the social order again and again, possibly leading to catastrophe.

Although hunger and aggression were equally seen as vital instincts in human life, popular medical experts tended to write more about the sexual drives and the need to control them. In the course of the second half of the nineteenth century, sexuality increasingly became a perplexing phenomenon. On the one hand, doctors could not fail to acknowledge that sexual passion was an essential part of human nature. Male sexuality was defined as a powerful, inevitable instinctual urge that was hard to control through personal and social constraints and that could only be gratified by discharge. Many believed that unfulfilled drives, in males in particular, would lead to (nervous) illness. But on the other hand, giving oneself up to uncontrolled impulses was considered dangerous for the health of the individual as well as that of society at large. Sexual morality bore the imprint of economic preoccupations: overexpenditure was presented as leading to exhaustion and physical as well as psychological bankruptcy. In the hydraulic energy-control model, the focus was on limitation rather than on potential. The human sexual economy was believed to function according to a quantitative model of energy flow in which the "spending" of the vital spermatic fluid meant a loss of energy in other areas of life and "moderate" expenditures were most consonant with health and fertility. In this view, energy conservation had to govern sexual life (Barker-Benfield 1973).

Although there was much diversity of opinion in medical literature on what should be considered a healthy sexual order, the keynotes resounding in professional advice to the bourgeoisie were ordered living, moderation, and willpower. Echoing the values that permeated the economic and political rhetoric of liberal individualism, doctors saw the will as the determinant of permanent character. Moderation and willpower counted as the crucial basis of a healthy and moral lifestyle. Just as in other normative areas concerning behavior and personal habits, doctors emphasized the obtainment of a self-controlled and well-ordered expression of the sexual instinct. In their perception of the origin of sexual disease, some of them focused on psychological interpretations, believing, for instance, that seductive fantasies and daydreams could lead the will astray, while others understood the struggle as one between innate nature and exterior civilization. However, "nature" and "civilization" were ambiguous categories. It proved not easy to agree on what was natural as opposed to what was a product of civilization, and one could point to both as the source of sexual health or disease. On the one hand, it was believed that much evil and disorder resided in mankind's natural state: it was hard-won civilization that subdued the human potential for wildness, the primitive animalism so pervasive in nature. Yet, on the other hand, the medical how-to literature, condemning modern civilization as corrupt and decadent, stressed moral and physical adjustment to an unspoiled natural order as the best way to keep sexual derailment and diseases at bay.

Thus, neither nature nor civilization seemed to provide a stable moral basis in the quest for a well-ordered sexuality; biological as well as cultural factors interfered with sexual moderation. Some conceptualized a healthy sexual order as informed by the law of nature; others regarded such order as a potential product of civilization. Medical literature on sexuality tended to underline fears of human inadequacy in both realms. Not only were "natural" instincts often contorted by modern civilization: it was also dreaded that nature itself might be amoral. Apart from the haunting fear that in modern society the will would fail after all (because of improper socialization or subversive elements such as alcohol and other intoxicants) and that an individual's fearsome lower propensities would overwhelm the self, the proper meaning of the will itself was ambivalent and subject to debate. Although experts viewed the will as a product of natural evolution, thus offering the best defense of civilization, the assertion of the will was also interpreted more negatively as an imposed, second-best compensation for the loss of good instincts. Moreover, in a corrupted environment, volitional power could be turned to evil as well as to good. A widespread belief held that the growing complexities of modern civilization and the higher evolutionary development of humanity had made sexual activity much more dangerous than it had ever been before.

As a group, physicians tended to be ambivalent, and sometimes even contradictory, as far as their opinion on what constituted a healthy sexual order was concerned. Regarding the possibilities of male sexual continence, the medical profession had no clear-cut answers, and its advice could be pro- as well as anti-sensual in tendency (Mason 1994, 179, 226–27). Moreover, it is questionable whether the medical profession as a whole did impose a sexual ideology on the lay public. Many anxieties expressed by medical men were probably first shared with or first absorbed from bourgeois patients who consulted them. Often, it was lay opinion, rather than medical science, that by and large determined the dominant sexual ethic. Most doctors were dependent on the approval of their bourgeois clients. As the nineteenth century progressed, in many European countries the medical profession became competitive while many doctors were still seriously underpaid—two conditions that contained powerful inducements for general practitioners to respect lay opinion (Mason 1994, 180–81). In his *Education of the Senses* (1984), Peter Gay has shown that the stereotype of Victorian prudery cannot be sustained: moderate and sensible views of sexuality circulated among bourgeois men and women, while sexual pleasure was experienced by many of them (cf. Johnson 1979). To dole out unfamiliar ideas or unwelcome moralistic advice could be risky, since middle-class men and women all but hesitated to compare and change doctors. The spread of contraceptives, which the majority of doctors opposed, is striking proof of the failure of the medical profession to exert moral hegemony over the lay public (McLaren 1983).

Although physicians were recognized as experts on sexuality, they did not establish a medical hegemony in this field. Many prominent physicians opposed, for instance, the criminalization of deviant sexualities, but in Britain, Germany, and Austria, a criminalizing approach was upheld to safeguard public decency. In 1869 the Prussian medical association, for example, recommended to the government the abolishment of article 143 of the penal code, which made homosexuality and bestiality punishable, but the government did not follow this recommendation; article 143 was upheld and introduced in the unified German Empire as article 175 (Sievert 1984, 15; Sommer 1998, 62–64). In the closing decades of the nineteenth century, other groups in society—moralists and feminists, be they organized in private purity organizations or not—often criticized the medical profession for its "amoral" biological determinism. Developments in Britain illustrate that there was no continuous, uninterrupted growth of medical control over sexuality throughout the nineteenth century (Mason 1994). Much less than in France and Germany, British doctors formed a monolithic professional group that was both willing and able to interfere with the sexuality of its patients. The medical approach to sexuality was successfully challenged by moralists and feminists alike. Singling out the perceived growth in child prostitution and the traffic in girls to the continent, they called for fresh legislation. The result was the 1885 Criminal Law Amendment Act, extending legal control over public indecency, prostitution, and brothel-keeping, and creating new offenses involving male homosexuality and incest (Mort 1987, 101–50).

Notwithstanding the growing secularization in the nineteenth century, the Catholic and Protestant churches continued to be influential on sexual issues. In Great Britain, Germany, and other predominantly Protestant countries, the moral purity campaigns launched during the century's closing decades drew much support from churches and religious groups. Protestant congregations were among the first to raise their voices against the perceived immoralities in modern society, including prostitution, the double standard, pornography, and sexual perversion, homosexuality in particular. In that same period, the Catholic Church also adopted a firmer stance against new developments in the field of sexuality. Reacting to Neo-Malthusianism and the growing practice of contraception, Rome decreed a more active interference of priests in the sexual life of Catholics. Since the French Revolution, the Catholic Church had been losing some of its social authority and political clout, and partly for this reason it increasingly began to focus its attention on the private sphere of family life and sexuality. To underline the assumed objective basis of its moral system, the Catholic leadership regenerated the views of Thomas Aquinas. In the encyclical letter *Aeterni Patris* (1879), Pope Leo XIII proclaimed this medieval doctrine as the official Church philosophy. Because of its emphasis on the intellect and a rationally ordered nature, Thomism offered a system that seemed suited to bringing religion and positivist science into line with one another. However, as far as sexuality was concerned, it was difficult to reconcile new medical views with Christian doctrine. Catholic doctrine was hardly affected by biomedical knowledge. In canon law and in guidelines for spiritual care, for example, the age-old concept of sodomy as referring to sinful homosexual acts continued to be used without any consideration of the modern medical notion of sexual orientation. Initially, therefore, the influence of these new views did not appear to go beyond the small circles of intellectuals and members of the secularized liberal bourgeoisie.

Forensic Medicine and Psychiatry

As a concept, "sexuality" is historically contingent: in its modern sense it came to prominence in the course of the nineteenth century when science turned its efforts increasingly to determining, classifying, and explaining sexual desires that were considered as deviant. In medicine in general and psychiatry in particular, the prime focus was on the criminal and pathological aspects of human sexuality. Building on the Enlightenment suspicion of the pursuit of erotic pleasures for their own sake, already in the first half of the nineteenth century a growing body of medical or pseudo-medical works spelled out the morbid aspects of sexuality. Although sodomy had been decriminalized in several European countries during and after the French Revolution, new offenses against morality, such as public indecency, as well as ages of consent for sexual contacts were introduced. In Prussia and Austria, the death penalty for sodomy had been dropped at the end of the eighteenth century, but sodomy continued to be a criminal offense, punishable by forced labor and imprisonment. In the Habsburg Empire, the minimum and maximum penalty for "vice against nature" was raised in 1852. Homosexual behavior was made punishable again in all German states when in 1871 the Prussian penal code was adopted in the German Empire. In Britain it wasn't until 1861 that capital punishment for sodomy was replaced by a prison term from ten years to life. Whereas earlier the punishable acts were generally restricted to anal penetration, in the second half of the nineteenth century in Britain (through the Labouchère Amendment of the 1885 Criminal Law Amendment Act), as well as in Germany and Austria, other homosexual behaviors, so-called "acts similar to cohabitation," were also criminalized.[1]

1. Haberda 1927, 163–64; Weeks 1983, 1–22; Sievert 1984, 14–16; Hutter 1993; Brunner and Sulzenbacher 1998, 29–31, 37–39, 57; Sommer 1998, 43–57.

The greater demand for law enforcement in sexual matters during the second half of the nineteenth century—besides homosexuality and public indecency, prostitution and pornography were also criminalized in several countries—may be understood as a reaction to the challenges of growing urbanization, which awakened public awareness of sexual deviance. The concentration of a segmented population in big cities increased the numbers of prostitutes and also made it easier for sodomites to find each other and to realize that they were not alone in the world. Escaping the censorship that had existed in more encapsulated traditional communities, previously isolated individuals, who might have felt themselves to be unique, now discovered that in the crowded cities there were others like themselves. Innovations in urban infrastructure increased the number of opportunities for anonymous encounters. Specialized meeting places—public toilets, parks, theaters, certain bars, brothels, bathhouses, swimming pools, and railway stations—came into existence and thus fostered an emergent subculture. However, the more numerous sexual encounters in public also led to confrontations with the police, courts, and moral reformers, who considered such activity a disturbance of the social order and demanded stricter law enforcement.

As a result of the growing persecution of offenses against public decency, physicians, in their role of forensic experts in courts, were increasingly confronted with sexual deviance. Before the 1860s, medical interest in disorderly sexual conduct was intrinsically linked to forensic medicine that focused on criminal acts such as rape and sodomy. In general, experts in forensic medicine confined themselves to a physical diagnosis to furnish evidence of sexual offenses. For instance, since the seventeenth and eighteenth centuries, they were called on by judges in cases of sodomy to examine the anus of defendants in order to determine whether they had engaged in anal intercourse. The French professor in forensic medicine Ambroise Tardieu (1818–1879) also paid attention to the genitals of "active" sodomites. In his *Étude médico-légale sur les attentats aux moeurs* (1857), he claimed that pederasts arrested by the Paris police possessed penises shaped like those of dogs. The forensic doctors were only interested in the physical symptoms of sexual misbehavior, and their explanation of it was social rather than biological: it would be the result of moral failure, unfavorable living conditions, bad habits, and imitation (Hekma 1987, 50–57; Müller 1991, 91–110).

However, in the first half of the nineteenth century, some physicians began to reflect on the connections between sexual deviance and mental illness. Was lewdness a cause or a result of insanity? Or was it a form of insanity in itself? In his dissertation *Ueber die Beziehungen des Sexualsystems zur Psyche überhaupt und zum Kretinismus im besonderen* (1826), the German psychiatrist Johan Häussler considered sexual deviance as one of the causes of insanity, but he did not yet see it as a disease in itself. Various medical authorities assumed that committing "unnatural acts" could lead to physical weakness and insanity (as was thought to be the case with onanism). Thus it was believed that certain behaviors caused pathology. Around the middle of the century, however, the causal link between specific acts and morbidity was reversed in some medical analyses. In their treatment of sodomy, the French physician Claude-François Michéa (1815–1882) in 1849 and the German forensic medical authority Johann Ludwig Casper (1796–1864) in 1852 shifted the focus from the physiological characteristics of the sodomitical act to the biological disposition of the offender. Michéa and Casper were the first to assert that a preference for members of the same sex was often innate and involved femininity in men. Whereas Michéa referred to feminine tendencies that were probably caused by a rudimentary "masculine uterus," Casper explained same-sex love, which did not require anal penetration and was often confined to embraces and mutual masturbation, as a "hermaphroditism of the soul." Casper's approach set the tone for psychiatrists who began to explain sexual acts that were not aimed at procreation as symptoms of mental diseases. In fact, the phrenologists, who located various mental characteristics in different parts of the brain, had been the first to maintain that the sexual instinct was a function not of the sex organs but of the cerebellum (Lynch 1985; Shortland 1987).

Whereas earlier medical interest had focused on masturbation, prostitution, and venereal diseases, in the 1860s prominent psychiatrists became concerned with other sexual behaviors that were usually considered immoral and sometimes officially illegal. In the first half of the nineteenth century, sexual disorders only figured marginally in psychiatric classifications. Nymphomania and satyriasis, considered as physical disorders of the genitals, as well as masturbation were merely mentioned as causal factors of insanity. The famous French psychiatrist Jean-Étienne Esquirol (1772–1840), however, broke new ground in the 1810s by coining *erotomania* as a form of monomania. Erotomania, the mental fixation on love, was conceptualized as a mental disturbance in itself (Rosario 1997, 50). In 1844 the German psychiatrist Heinrich von Kaan published his *Psychopathia sexualis*, one of the first psychiatric classifications of sexual disorders. Associating the primitive with the pathological, he distinguished six modifications of the *nisus sexualis* (sexual instinct): pederasty, tribady, bestiality, the violation of human cadavers and statues, and masturbation. Masturbation was the perversion par excellence because fantasy played a central role and because, according to Kaan, it was the cause of the other derangements. (In later psychiatric taxonomies, masturbation would generally not be considered a perversion in itself, but rather it was seen as a symptom of or a causal factor in the development of morbid sexuality.) For Kaan, perversions were still ubiquitous bad habits, fostered by individual and social conditions; he did not yet consider the offender as a fundamentally different, pathological type of person. Kaan's taxonomy was followed by that of Michéa five years later. In his "Des déviations maladives de l'appétit vénérien," published in *Union Médicale* (1849), Michéa classified sexual disorders into four kinds: Greek or same-sex love, bestiality, the attraction to an inanimate object (later named fetishism), and the attraction to human corpses (necrophilia).

Psychiatric interest in the broader aspects of sexual deviance was in part triggered by the forensic preoccupation with criminal acts. The forensic specialists in somatic medicine were only concerned with the physical proof of sexual crimes, whereas psychiatrists, from the 1860s on, began to focus on the psychological makeup of the offenders.[2] Forensic psychiatrists, called upon in courts to determine the limits of legal responsibility, insisted that the diagnosis of mental illness should not be left to lawyers or common sense, but only to specialists in mental medicine. Whereas physicians initially believed that mental and nervous disorders were the *result* of "unnatural" acts, psychiatrists assumed that they were the *cause* of sexual aberrations (cf. Hekma 1987, 49–64). More and more, such disorders were viewed, not just as forms of immoral behavior, but as symptoms of an underlying morbid condition. This new psychiatric explanation was connected to a fundamental change in the meaning of sexuality as well as in the medical understanding of insanity.

In the first half of the century, the term *sexuality* mainly referred to the fact that an individual belonged to either the male or female sex. Sex difference was explained from anatomical variation: the decisive benchmarks for the evaluation of sexual behavior were the genitals and the secondary sexual characteristics. During the nineteenth century, the emphasis in medical characterizations shifted from anatomical features to the sexual instinct and psychology. Gradually, sexuality was used in the modern sense to indicate a desire for the opposite sex (or the same sex), an attraction that was based on a physical and psychological polarization and the matching of male and female elements.[3] Not only the body, but also the personality began to be understood as being completely saturated with sex and sexuality. Sex became a complicated whole of bodily characteristics, attitudes, and character features, and sexuality a complex of behaviors, experiences,

2. On the development of forensic psychiatry in the nineteenth century, see Güse and Schmacke 1976, vol. II; Foucault 1978; Smith 1981; and Harris 1989.

3. Cf. Van Ussel 1975, 37–38; Davidson 1987; Nye 1989; Nye 1991, 400; Mason 1994, 208).

feelings, desires, and fantasies. The differences between males and females were conceptualized as binary oppositions, in a physical as well as in a psychological sense. This model, which assumed a continuum between physical and psychological sexual features on one side and sexual object-choice on the other, offered both a precondition and an explanation of sexual desire. Masculinity and femininity were metaphorically presented as electric or magnetic poles, charged by inescapable mutual attraction (Mak 1997, 244).

New conceptions of mental illness facilitated the inclusion of sexual deviance in medical psychology. The replacement of the term *insanity*— *Wahnsinn* in German—by *psychosis* reflected a change in psychiatry's understanding of mental disorder. In the older Lockean and Condillacian tradition, insanity was mainly associated with intellectual shortcomings, a condition of total irrationality or diminished intelligence; but in the second half of the nineteenth century, mental illness was broadened to include disorders of the emotions, the instincts, and the will (Berrios 1995, 388). Referring to forms of partial insanity that left intellectual judgment largely intact, the diagnoses of *manie sans délire*, monomania, moral insanity, and psychopathy all indicated a growing awareness of the inadequacy of the traditional rationalistic definitions of insanity. These disorders controverted traditional opinion that to be insane was to have lost one's reason. The British ethnologist and physician James Cowles Prichard (1786–1848), who introduced the concept of moral insanity, defined it as "madness consisting in a morbid perversion of the natural feelings, affections, inclinations, temper, habits, moral dispositions, and natural impulses, without any remarkable disorder or defect of the interest or knowing and reasoning faculties, and particularly without any insane illusion or hallucinations" (cited by Sass and Herpertz 1995, 635). Prichard's understanding of moral insanity, followed later by the concept of psychopathy, facilitated psychiatry's annexation of sexual abnormalcy. Moral insanity and psychopathy were conceptualized as basically antisocial disorders that included various deviant behaviors. Prichard admitted that the boundary between the normal and the abnormal was extremely difficult to establish. Partial insanity attracted attention of psychiatrists, in large part because of legal reasons, its relevance to morality and crime. Moral insanity and psychopathy, they argued, selectively damaged the moral faculties: those afflicted lacked insight into ethical and social values. At the same time, the morally insane and psychopaths showed a heightened intensity of instincts together with an inability to control their drives. Reflex theory, postulating that nervous connections running via the spine automatically regulated all bodily organs (including the brain) quite independently of human will, became the dominant somatic model of mental and nervous disease. Both the disease categories of moral insanity and psychopathy are good examples of how cultural evaluations could determine psychiatric definitions: their core component, a disordered moral and social conscience, was highly susceptible to ethical and political judgment.

The question of whether those suffering from moral insanity and psychopathy were bad or mad remained a matter of debate within and between the legal and medical professions. Although the issue of involuntarism was disputed by clerics, moral philosophers, and lawyers who were reluctant to undermine a view of individuals as self-conscious moral agents, it became crucial in the psychiatric diagnosis of mental disorder. During the last decades of the nineteenth century, the emphasis in the debate on crime and madness in psychiatry radically shifted toward deterministic explanations of antisocial behavior. These were most forcefully articulated by psychiatrists who intervened in court as expert witnesses and who based their arguments on biomedical theories. Mentally disturbed people were considered to be deprived of moral agency and responsibility. Obsessive sexual behavior began to figure prominently in forensic psychiatry. Many moral offenders appeared to suffer from particularly strong, irresistible sexual drives and thoughts, while at the same time their nervous system lacked the strength to control them. In a legal sense, they could not be held personally responsible for their leanings because their free will was impaired. "The offender is merely an automaton, the slave of what makes him act," Krafft-Ebing, the leading forensic psychiatrist in central Europe, wrote in his *Psychopathia sexualis* (Ps 1903, 386; Ps 1999, 460). In many cases, in fact, sexual misdeeds were not understood as a sin or a crime, but as a symptom of mental disease. Psychiatrists who routinely intervened in court as expert witnesses argued that mere immorality should be distinguished from sickly perversion. Called upon to deliver expert testimony in court, the main thrust of these forensic experts was that the existent legislation ignored medical knowledge of the causes of sexual crimes and that the irresponsibility of moral offenders had to be considered in jurisdiction. Certain categories of defendants should be sent to asylums and clinics, rather than to prisons.

Classifying and Explaining Perversion

In the last decades of the nineteenth century, several psychiatrists, especially in France and Germany, began to concern themselves with classifying and explaining the wide range of sexual deviancy they discovered.
Basing their arguments on deterministic theories of hereditarian degeneration and neurophysiological automatism, more and more psychiatrists sub-
scribed to the new view that in many cases irregular sexual activities were
not immoral choices, but symptoms of innate characteristics. As forms of
mental disease, sexual disorders were considered to be related to defective
moral functioning that was caused by lesions of the brain and the nervous
system. Medicine challenged the authority of both the church and the judi-
cature and advanced a paradigm change in the understanding of sexual
deviance, especially of same-sex behavior, transferring it from the realm of
sin and crime to the domain of health and illness. Around 1870 prominent
German and French psychiatrists began to shift the focus from a temporary
deviation of the norm to a pathological state of being. Caused by natural
laws, perversion, like other deformations and disorders, called for medical
observation and treatment.

After Wilhelm Griesinger (1817–1868), the leading German psychiatrist, had defined the sexual desire for one's own sex as a constitutional
nervous disease in 1868, in the following year his successor Carl von Westphal (1833–1890) published the first psychiatric study of what he coined as
conträre Sexualempfindung (contrary sexual feeling) in a German psychiatric
journal, *Archiv für Psychiatrie und Nervenkrankheiten*. An article by Krafft-
Ebing on "Certain Anomalies of the Sexual Instinct," published in the
same journal in 1877, can be considered as a direct precursor of numerous
systematic, classificatory works on sexual pathology that were published in
the 1880s, especially in France and Germany. Krafft-Ebing distinguished
between classes of sexual abnormalities that were of a temporary, quantita-

tive, and qualitative nature. The first and second group comprised abnormal periods of sexual activity (childhood or old age) as well as absence and pathological increase of the sexual drive, while the third comprised the perversions proper: abnormalities according to either the goal (all sexual behavior not aimed at coitus) or the (human or nonhuman) object of sexual desire. Nine years later, in the first edition of his *Psychopathia sexualis*, Krafft-Ebing introduced the terms *paradoxia* (the wrong time), *anesthesia* and *hyperesthesia* (the wrong amount), and *paresthesia* (the wrong aim or object) for these categories.

Increasingly, psychiatric attention became focused on what Krafft-Ebing named *paresthesia*, the perversions proper: these were not so much associated with transitory stages in life, but with a more or less immutable constitution of particular individuals. Whereas Krafft-Ebing in 1877 distinguished only three subgroups of perversions proper (lust murder including necrophilia, anthropophagy or cannibalism, and contrary sexual feeling), in the 1880s and 1890s he and his German and French colleagues created and defined new categories of perversion by collecting and publishing case histories in a more or less systematic manner. The most important category was same-sex behavior, for which concepts like *uranism*, *homosexual*, and *contrary sexual feeling* had been invented in the 1860s. The labels *uranism*, introduced by Karl Heinrich Ulrichs (1825–1895; pen name Numa Numantius) in 1864, and *homosexuality*, coined five years later by Karl Maria Kertbeny (1824–1882), were actually of a nonmedical, proto-emancipatory origin. Ulrichs, who was a lawyer, and Kertbeny, a German-Hungarian writer, defended same-sex love and advocated the abolition of the penalization of homosexuality in Germany and the Habsburg Empire (Silverstolpe 1987; Kennedy 1988; Müller 1991). Thus, the revision of moral views on homosexual behavior at the end of the nineteenth century was triggered by political activism as well as biomedical theorizing. The impetus for more intense medical investigations of contrary sexual feeling came largely from Ulrichs, a self-proclaimed homosexual. His *Forschungen über das Räthsel der mannmännlichen Liebe*, published as twelve pamphlets between 1864 and 1879, were a source of inspiration for both Westphal and Krafft-Ebing. Although he used *contrary sexual feeling* and *uranism* more frequently, Krafft-Ebing eventually popularized the term *homosexuality*, which he sharply distinguished from *sodomy* and *pederasty*, that is, anal intercourse. The term *heterosexuality*, invented by Kertbeny, was published for the first time in *Entdeckung der Seele* (1880) by Gustav Jäger (1832–1917), a German professor of zoology and anthropology.

The final decades of the nineteenth century saw an explosion of new sexual language (Hekma 1985). After *uranism*, *contrary sexual feeling*, and *homosexuality* had been coined, *exhibitionism* was introduced in 1877 by Ernest-Charles Lasègue (1816–1885) (who also created the concept *anorexia nervosa* and popularized the term *kleptomania*), *inversion of the sexual instinct* in 1878 by the Italian forensic doctor Arrigo Tamassia (in 1882 adopted by Jean-Martin Charcot [1825–1893] and Valentin Magnan [1835–1916]), the master concept *sexual perversion* in 1885 by Magnan, *fetishism* in 1887 by Alfred Binet (1857–1911), *sadism* and *masochism* in 1890 and *pedophilia* in 1896 by Krafft-Ebing, and *unisexuality* in 1896 by Marc-André Raffalovich (1864–1934).[1] These new concepts were soon picked up outside the world of psychiatry. Various other neologisms used by psychiatrists did not become current, such as *erotomania, érotisme, frottage* (nonconsensual rubbing of one's body against another person), *algolagnia* (the love of pain), *sadiques actives* and *passives* (sadists and masochists), *tyrannism* and *passivism* (sadism and masochism), *machlänomie* (masochism), *metatropism* (male masochism and female sadism), *stercoracism* and *coprolagnia* (the obsession with dirtiness and excrement), *zooerasty* and *zoophilia* (bestiality), *mixoscopia* (voyeurism), *renifleurs* (persons who are aroused by the smell of urine), *nihilistes de la chair* (fetishists), *pinceurs* (men who derive pleasure from pinching women), *frappeurs des filles* and *flagellateurs* (men who like to flog or spank women), *sanguinaires* (men who get excited by seeing women's buttocks bleeding), *piqueurs des filles* and *Mädchenstecher* (men who got sexually excited by stabbing women), and *Zopfabschneider* (men who cut off and steal women's buns of hair). The last two groups were named *sadifetishists* by Krafft-Ebing, who also used terms like *necrofetishism* (the obsession for dead bodies) and *necrosadism* (the urge to abuse corpses).

In the 1880s all leading French psychiatrists contributed to the development of sexual pathology, while after 1890 German and Austrian experts would set the tone. English, Italian, and Russian contributions to this field, though substantial, were less numerous. Jacques-Joseph Moreau de Tours's *Des aberrations du sens génésique* (1880) was the first psychiatric textbook in this new field, followed by works of Magnan (*Des anomalies, des aberrations, et des perversions sexuelles*, 1885), Julien Chevalier (*De l'inversion de l'instinct sexuel au point de vue médico-légal*, 1885), the Russian Benjamin Tarnowsky (*Die krankhaften Erscheinungen des Geschlechtssinnes*, 1886), the Italian Paolo Mantegazza (*Gli amori degli uomini*, 1886), Krafft-Ebing (*Psychopathia sexualis*, 1886), Benjamin Ball (*La folie érotique*, 1888), Binet ("Le fétichisme dans l'amour: Étude de psychologie morbide," in *Revue*

---

1. The terms *perversion* and *fetishism* had been used before in a religious context. *Perversion* used to refer to religious phenomena turning from the correct to erroneous religious beliefs (McLaren 1997, 177). *Fetishism* had been employed by anthropologists studying "primitive" forms of religion, especially animism (Nye 1993; Pettinger 1993).

philosophique, 1887), Emile Laurent (*L'amour morbide: Étude de psychologie pathologique*, 1891), and Paul-Emile Garnier (*Les fétichistes, pervertis, et invertis sexuels: Observations médico-légales*, 1896).

During the 1890s the scientific interest in sexual perversions grew rapidly, not only in psychiatry but also in the field of criminal anthropology, for which the Italian forensic expert Cesare Lombroso (1836–1909) set the tone with his theory of the born criminal. This new branch of the human sciences gained wide recognition at international conferences organized between 1885 and 1901. Moreover, several textbooks exclusively devoted to homosexuality appeared in the 1890s: Albert Moll's *Die conträre Sexualempfindung* (1891), Albert von Schrenck-Notzing's *Die Suggestionstherapie bei den krankhaften Erscheinungen des Geschlechtssinnes, mit besonderer Berücksichtigung der conträren Sexualempfindung* (1892), Chevalier's *Une maladie de personnalité: l'inversion sexuelle* (1893), Edward Carpenter's *Homogenic Love and Its Place in a Free Society* (1894), Magnus Hirschfeld's *Sappho und Socrates* (1896), Marc-André Raffalovich's *Uranisme et unisexualité: Étude sur différentes manifestations de l'instinct sexuel* (1896), Georges Saint-Paul's *Perversion et perversités sexuelles: Une enquête médicale sur l'inversion* (1896), and *Sexual Inversion* (1897) by Henry Havelock Ellis (1859–1939) and John Addington Symonds (1840–1893). In his *Untersuchungen über die Libido sexualis* (1897), Moll (1862–1939) elaborated the most comprehensive and sophisticated general theory on sexuality before Freud wrote his *Drei Abhandlungen zur Sexualtheorie* (1905) and Havelock Ellis completed his monumental *Studies in the Psychology of Sex* (1897–1928). Widely read was Auguste Forel's *Die sexuelle Frage* (1904). The most influential of the researchers using historical and anthropological material was the dermatologist Iwan Bloch (1872–1922). His *Beiträge zur Aetiologie der Psychopathia sexualis* (1902–3) and *Das Sexualleben unserer Zeit* (1906) were the first compendia of sexology that stressed the cultural dimensions of sexuality. According to Bloch, the need for varied sexual stimuli was universal and accidental, while external conditions explained the distinct forms of sexual behavior found in different cultures. The Viennese ethnologist Friedrich S. Krauss (1859–1938) also gathered ethnographic-historical data.[2]

These and many other publications made a substantial contribution to the emergence of a scientific discourse on sexuality, as a result of which by the end of the nineteenth century, perversions could be recognized and discussed. Several taxonomies were developed, but the one designed in Krafft-Ebing's *Psychopathia sexualis* eventually set the tone, not only in medical circles but also in everyday life. The first edition of this highly

2. On the relation between anthropology and sexology, see Bleys 1996 and Somerville 1998.

eclectic encyclopedia of sexual aberration appeared in 1886, soon followed by several new and expanded editions and translations in several languages. Because Krafft-Ebing regularly published fragments from new editions of the book in current medical journals, he actively furthered knowledge of his *Psychopathia sexualis* in medical circles. Early on, he had recognized the importance of the sex drive, publishing his first writing on sexual pathology in 1877, but with his much-quoted book, intended for lawyers and doctors, he became famous as one of the founding fathers of scientific sexology. By naming and classifying virtually all nonprocreative forms of sexuality, he was one of the first to synthesize medical knowledge of sexual perversion. The first edition was a rather slim book counting 110 pages and including fifty-one case histories; the twelfth edition, the last one he worked on before he died, was a volume of 437 pages, illustrated with observations from over three hundred cases. The discussions in *Psychopathia sexualis* are informed by a great deal of knowledge and opinions absorbed from others, and the author seriously revised his book several times, especially by adding new categories of sexuality and new case histories.

Krafft-Ebing distinguished perversion from perversity as well as from abnormality. Perversion was considered as a permanent constitutional disorder—be it inborn or acquired—that affected the whole personality, whereas perversity was just passing immoral conduct of normal persons. According to Krafft-Ebing, sexual behavior could be abnormal without being perverse: as long as the goal of sexual behavior was coitus, he did not consider it as perverse, though individuals might indulge in abnormal acts to heighten the pleasure accompanying coitus. He viewed the sexual drive as perverted if eccentric behavior in itself (even without intercourse) was experienced as a source of pleasure.[3] Although he also paid attention to exhibitionism, bestiality, pedophilia, necrophilia, urolagnia, coprolagnia, nymphomania, satyriasis, incest, and several other derangements, Krafft-Ebing distinguished four main perversions: sadism, masochism, fetishism, and contrary sexual feeling.

Inspired by the work of Westphal and Ulrichs, Krafft-Ebing had discussed contrary sexual feeling since 1877 in several articles. Same-sex attraction figured prominently in this group, but his understanding of contrary sexual feeling should not be confused with present-day notions of

3. Krafft-Ebing, for instance, emphasized the distinction between masochism and what he called "sexual bondage." The latter was characterized by a strong abnormal degree of dependence of one sexual partner vis-à-vis the other; such a relationship was not perverse, though, Krafft-Ebing claimed, as long as the unequal power relation did not stand in the way of the aim of sexual activity, namely intercourse. He used the term *masochism* to indicate that sexual dependence and subjection had become goals in themselves, simultaneously turning intercourse into an irrelevant act.

homosexuality. Whereas homosexuality nowadays refers to same-sex object-choice, Krafft-Ebing and most of his colleagues explained same-sex attraction, at that time often referred to as inversion, as a biological and psychological mixture of masculinity and femininity. Homosexual orientation was associated with an inverted gender identity, which also included what we now consider as transvestism and transsexuality.[4]

In the second edition of *Psychopathia sexualis*, Krafft-Ebing differentiated between inborn and acquired forms of contrary sexual feeling, but in the fourth edition (1889) he also introduced a further subdivision of both forms in four subcategories according to the degree of gender inversion; he considered these as different phases in a continuing process of degeneration.[5] Thus, acquired contrary sexual feeling was subdivided into simple reversal of sexual feeling, eviration (in men) and defemination (in women), transitory sexual metamorphosis, and sexually paranoiac metamorphosis. The subcategories of constitutional contrary sexual feeling were psychic hermaphroditism, homosexuality, effemination (in men) or viraginity (in women), and androgyny (in men) or gynandry (in women). Psychic hermaphroditism was what we would now designate as bisexuality: with the predominant same-sex desire, there were traces of heterosexual feeling; and contrary to what the term suggested, neither the body nor the psychological makeup showed any signs of inversion. Simple reversal of sexual feeling and homosexuality both referred to an exclusive desire for the same sex without any further psychical or physical inversion. In eviration and defemination as well as in effemination and viraginity, same-sex desire was accompanied by psychic characteristics of the opposite sex. Transitory sexual metamorphosis also included the physical sensation of the opposite sex while still being aware of one's biological sex, whereas the expression *sexually paranoiac metamorphosis* was used for the delusion that one belonged to the opposite sex. Both forms of sexual metamorphosis resemble what we now call transsexuality. The most extreme and rarest form of inborn contrary sexual feeling, androgyny or gynandry, was accompanied by signs of physical inversion, but Krafft-Ebing emphasized that these did not affect the genitals so much that they merged into physical hermaphroditism. In *Psychopathia sexualis*, physical hermaphroditism was not discussed; only in

4. On the changing conceptualization of same-sex desire from "inversion" to "homosexuality," see Marshall 1981 and Chauncey 1982–83. On transvestism and transsexuality, see King 1981 and Prosser 1998.

5. Krafft-Ebing's differentiation of constitutional and acquired perversion was not clearcut. Although triggered by environmental influences, the ultimate cause of acquired contrary sexual feeling was, he believed, an underlying (degenerate) predisposition. Careful examination of acquired cases had taught him that they were based on an already existing "latent" homo- or bisexual proclivity.

Krafft-Ebing's estate did I find an unpublished case history of a patient diagnosed as a pseudohermaphrodite. The twenty-six-year-old man had been hospitalized because of serious mental problems, and these were related to the infirm development of his genital organs.[6] Behavior that is now known as travesty, on the other hand, was a recurring phenomenon in Krafft-Ebing's casuistry, but he did not consider it as a syndrome in itself: it was subsumed under the wide category of contrary sexual feeling and discussed as one of the symptoms of psychical inversion. Some men with an irresistible urge to cross-dressing, however, were not diagnosed with contrary sexual feeling but with "clothing fetishism."

In the fourth edition of *Psychopathia sexualis*, Krafft-Ebing introduced fetishism. He referred to Lombroso, who had used fetishism as an explanatory model in his introduction to the Italian translation of the book, and in later editions to Binet, who actually had been the first to give *fetish* a sexual meaning. Relabeling already collected cases that had been categorized under "paradoxical acts" and assembling new ones, Krafft-Ebing expounded on the erotic obsession with certain parts of the body (especially hands and feet), physical handicaps (such as lameness), hair, shoes, nightcaps, handkerchiefs, gloves, toiletries, ladies' underwear, fur, velvet, silk, animals, wet clothes, and even rings, mourning ribbons, and roses. Fetishism sometimes assumed vast and obsessive proportions. For example, Krafft-Ebing presented the case history of a fetishist who collected hundreds of leather gloves: "In his office he always had ladies' gloves lying on his desk. Not an hour passed without him having to touch and stroke them" (*Ps* 1898, 180). He also referred to the case of a man who had been arrested because he had stolen ladies' handkerchiefs; the police found 446 of them in his house (1891h, 74–75).

In 1890 Krafft-Ebing published the first edition of his *Neue Forschungen auf dem Gebiet der Psychopathia sexualis* in which he coined *sadism* and *masochism* as the most fundamental forms of psychosexual perversion. These concepts referred to behaviors that he had earlier labeled as *active* and *passive flagellation*; men who were first diagnosed as fetishists because they were obsessed with women's hands and feet were now also relabeled as *masochists* because they desired to be punished and maltreated with those hands and feet. *Sadism* was derived from the Marquis de Sade and *masochism* from the Austrian novelist and historian Leopold von Sacher-Masoch (1836–1895), whose literary and historical work centered on the figure of the cruel woman. Between 1856 and 1870, Sacher-Masoch taught history at the University of Graz, where Krafft-Ebing was nominated professor of psychiatry in 1872. They seem not to have met each other, but Krafft-Ebing knew

6. Case history of AW (December 11 and 18, 1894), Nachlass Krafft-Ebing.

of Sacher-Masoch's literary works like "Eine galizische Geschichte" (1858) and *Venus im Pelz* (1870), and perhaps he heard rumors about the "literary champion of masochism," as he characterized Sacher-Masoch (*Ps* 1903, 142; *Ps* 1999, 164; Johnston 1972, 234; Höflechner 1975; Koschorke 1988). One of his masochistic patients who had corresponded with Sacher-Masoch gave Krafft-Ebing insight in his letters. By coining *masochism* as a sexual perversion, Krafft-Ebing foisted upon Sacher-Masoch a notoriety that was harmful to his already dubious social reputation, although Krafft-Ebing stated in *Psychopathia sexualis* that as "a man Sacher-Masoch surely does not lose the respect of his cultured fellow beings simply because he was afflicted with a sexual anomaly through no fault of his own" (*Ps* 1903, 101–2; *Ps* 1999, 120).

During the 1890s Krafft-Ebing again expanded his taxonomy, first in some articles and then also in *Psychopathia sexualis:* in 1894 he introduced *zoophilia erotica, zooerasty,* and *stercoracism* and in 1896 *pedophilia erotica* (1894c, 1894f, 1896b). The first two referred to sexual desire for or sexual intercourse with animals, but they were differentiated from *bestiality,* a term that Krafft-Ebing also used. He defined bestiality as mere perversity, immoral behavior, whereas zooerasty was a perversion, an inborn, pathological disposition. Zoophilia erotica was a form of fetishism, according to Krafft-Ebing, and it did not include actual sexual intercourse with an animal. He used the term *stercoracism* for scatology and an obsession with dirtiness. Pedophilia was a constitutional and pathological desire for children or adolescents, which was differentiated from mere immoral abuse of minors.

Given today's general understanding of heterosexuality, the way Krafft-Ebing introduced and used this term is quite remarkable.[7] It appeared for the first time in the fourth edition of *Psychopathia sexualis* under the rubric of fetishism. The author defined heterosexuality as the desire for the other sex, but at first the term did not connote normality. Employing the term in his discussion of perversions, he did not contrast heterosexuality to deviant forms of sexuality. The first heterosexuals in Krafft-Ebing's work were, in fact, fetishists. Since he tended to associate the normal sexual instinct with a built-in, unconscious procreative aim, he considered heterosexuals as perverts because their attitude toward coitus was marked by total indifference and they seemed to practice sex for other purposes (Katz 1995, 21–32). Judged by a reproductive standard, heterosexuality was a nonprocreative perversion that seemed to converge with homosexuality. However, as I will

7. I am indebted to Jonathan Ned Katz for pointing me to Krafft-Ebing's employment of the term.

explain below, in Krafft-Ebing's work heterosexuality (as well as homosexuality) increasingly began to vacillate between normalcy and perversion.

In the days of Krafft-Ebing, psychiatrists were not only concerned with labeling sexual deviancies and bracketing them as perversions, but they also tried to explain them as biological and psychological phenomena. The development of sexual pathology can be understood in the context of major currents in psychiatry. Changing views of sexuality were congruent with trends in general theories of psychopathology: they embraced both the dominant somatic etiological notions of late-nineteenth-century psychiatry, the pathology of nervous tissue and degeneration theory, as well as the attempt to escape the limitations of the somatic model by elaborating a psychological understanding of mental disorders.

In explaining sexual perversion, several psychiatrists tried to integrate it with current biomedical thinking. When it appeared to be difficult to explain sexual disorders as defects of the reproductive organs, the nervous system and the brain came into view as possible sites of explanation. In the last decades of the nineteenth century, psychiatry was characterized by a growing and pervasive emphasis on heredity as key factor in the etiology of mental illness. Although many psychiatrists continued to believe that perversion was sometimes acquired through bad environmental agents, seduction, and corrupt habit formation like masturbation, they increasingly stressed that sexual disorders, like many mental diseases in general, were inborn. Following the dominant somatic approach in psychiatry that situated mental disorders in the nervous system and particularly in the cerebral organs—"mental diseases are brain diseases" was Wilhelm Griesinger's famous dictum—many psychiatrists assumed that not only physical traits were hereditary, but intellectual and moral traits as well. In a popular lecture for the Volksbildungsverein in Vienna, Krafft-Ebing explained that cultural and moral progress depended on the organic development of the nervous system, especially that of the brain, and the heredity of intellectual qualities:

> The intellectual and moral progress of mankind is an accomplishment of the brain and the reason for this particular progression is based on the fact that the higher stage of development of one generation becomes an inborn disposition of the following generations. Heredity is the natural law which causes this process. We inherit from our ancestors not just our physical traits but also our moral and intellectual abilities. . . . Because culture and morality are always the product of a given stage of development of the brain's structure and capacities, it is clear that adequately

comprehending specific later cultural advances is as impossible to primitive man as having a proper understanding of lower forms of culture and morality is impossible to us today. Although it would be possible to train a young native from the South Seas Islands and turn him outwardly, in terms of his behavior, into a European, it would be as little possible to turn his appetite for human flesh into revulsion within his short life span and to arouse in him the shame which is inborn in civilized man, as it would be possible for us to experience the beauty of the artifacts in our art museums if we were to rely on the sensibility of our own primitive predisposition. (1892h, 6–7)

From the 1860s and 1870s on, psychiatrists increasingly began to draw upon physiological explanations. Especially in Germany and France, materialist definitions of insanity were used to free mental medicine from metaphysics, philosophical speculation, and religion. Neurophysiologists were convinced that the mind could be reduced to brain functions. Neurological research on the cerebrospinal axis posited a continuous but hierarchical view of nervous functioning that ranged from the lower reflexive levels of the nervous system to the highest mental operations of the cerebrum. Medical speculation on the hierarchical structure of the nervous system became increasingly tied up with an evolutionary conception of the development of the mind: mental faculties like reason, memory, imagination, and will were viewed as the latest acquisitions in the evolutionary history of man that set him apart from the rest of the animal world.

In addition to the pathology of nervous tissue and Darwinism, the theory of hereditary degeneracy played an important part in psychiatric explanations of mental illness in general and sexual perversion in particular. It was argued that while reproductive heterosexuality was the result of evolutionary progress, sexual disorders showed that natural processes could also move backward in a process of devolution; nature was capable of producing monsters or "stepchildren of nature," as the British psychiatrist Henry Maudsley (1835–1918) and Krafft-Ebing put it more mildly (Maudsley 1874, 43; 1867d, 777; Ps 1887, vi, 139). Like his French colleagues, Krafft-Ebing was deeply influenced by the French psychiatrist Benedict Auguste Morel (1809–1873). Two years before Darwin published his Origin of Species, Morel, in his Traité des dégénérescences physiques, intellectuelles et morales de l'espèce humaine (1857), had devised a theory of retrograde evolution to explain several pathological phenomena from the influence of environment as well as heredity. He believed that the extraordinary demands of modern civilization on the nervous system were responsible for the rise of mental disturbances. His theory of hereditary degeneration, which translated the Christian doctrine of man's regression after original sin into a biological metaphor, was the medical counterpart to Lamarckian rather than Darwinian biology. In Lamarck's as well as Morel's view, there was no clear distinction between innate and acquired characteristics. Heredity and environment were not seen as competing alternatives; both theories purported to explain how these factors interacted. Lamarck's theory of evolution, which in France was more popular than that of Darwin, held that environment and somatic change could affect the reproductive cells; characteristics thus acquired could be transmitted to future generations.

Adapting the Lamarckian idea of the inheritance of acquired characteristics, Morel explained how physical and mental disorders could result over several generations from behavioral accommodation to a pathogenic environment. His theory, synthesizing heredity, the environment, and racial decline, presented a dismal countercurrent to the predominantly optimistic outlook that the Darwinian emphasis on natural selection seemed to propagate. Families, races, or cultures were presumed to follow the pattern of growth, maturity, and decay seen in organisms. Acquired disorders could be inherited from "tainted" relatives, and once mental illness had a hold, it followed its inevitable course in the "neuropathic family": it was handed on to the descendants and caused deterioration over the generations until the line died out.

In the second half of the nineteenth century, the theory of degeneration found widespread acceptance as a biomedical, philosophical, and cultural framework. Linking pathology and cultural malaise, degeneration theory provided explanations in psychiatry, criminal anthropology, and cultural theory.[8] Projecting the stigmata of deviance onto lower stages in the evolution of mankind, the idea of degeneracy suggested a logical relationship between normality and progress, and between abnormality and decay. The French psychiatrist Magnan, a colleague of the famous Charcot, sealed the inclusion of degeneration theory in psychiatry by purging it from its religious overtones, which still haunted the work of Morel. He believed that sexual disturbances could be ascribed to differing lapses and instabilities in various nervous centers, and he was one of the first attempting to identify particular perversions with particular degenerative stages of the nervous system (Lanteri-Laura 1979, 51–52).

Although degenerate sexuality was often associated with the primitive, common belief also held that it was generated by the advance of civilization. Cultural and intellectual achievement was often bought at the price of mental health and sexual modesty. Krafft-Ebing asserted that the "savage races" lacked shame and modesty and that morality had only become pos-

---

8. Wettley and Leibbrand 1959; Gilman and Chamberlain 1985; Gay 1986, 329–90; Kershner 1986; Pick 1989.

sible with the advent of (Christian) civilization, but at the same time he stressed that highly developed cultures facilitated sexual excess and that the uncivilized were free of perversion.

> The episodes of moral decay always coincide with the progression of ef-feminacy, lewdness and luxuriance of nations. These phenomena can only be ascribed to the higher and more stringent demands that circum-stances place upon the nervous system. Exaggerated tension of the ner-vous system stimulates sensuality, leads the individual as well as the masses to excesses. . . . Greece, the Roman Empire, and France under Louis XIV and XV, are striking examples of this assertion. In such periods of civic and moral decline the most monstrous excesses of sexual life may be observed. . . . Large cities are hotbeds in which neuroses and low morality are bred; see the history of Babylon, Nineveh and Rome, and the mysteries of modern metropolitan life. It is a remarkable fact that among savages and half-civilized races, sexual intemperance is not ob-served. . . . (Ps 1903, 6–7; Ps 1999, 9)

In artificial industrial society, which had forced individuals out of stable communities, the harmony between intellectual and moral faculties was lost. The analysis of degeneration was embedded in a critique of the in-creasingly frantic conditions of modern civilization, stressing the vast range of novel stimuli that produced nervous exhaustion, fatigue, and mental dis-turbances: materialism, luxury, urbanization, agitation; the absence of reli-gion; unhealthy work, capitalist competitiveness; excessive leisure, food, and drink; immoral habits, lewdness; the use of alcohol, tobacco, opium, hashish; and the influence of other intoxicants. The corruption of civilized life was an impetus to degeneration, which in turn functioned as a breeding ground for more social evils. Crime, mental retardation, madness, nervous disorders, sexual perversion, alcoholism, prostitution, suicide, the declining birth rate, and sometimes even political agitation were all treated as effects of widespread moral decline.

Degeneration was associated with the lack of inhibitory control of the "higher" faculties over the more primitive levels of the central nervous sys-tem. Not only epilepsy, but also abuse of alcohol, morphine, and immoral-ity were striking examples of neurophysical disinhibition. Degeneration was largely understood as a failure of the will to command the senses; in-creasingly, modern man appeared less governed by moral laws and had be-come more and more a slave of his physical desires. "Being insusceptible to ethical feelings, if not their absence altogether, is to be understood as a mental disorder which is characteristic of a whole group of degenerative mental pathologies," Krafft-Ebing wrote.

In general it can be assumed that the unconscious dimension plays a larger role in their minds than it does in the minds of normal people. Morel describes these individuals correctly, at least with respect to that what was handed down to them through heredity, as instinctive people. Their obsessions, their impulsive acts, and their strange mental associations justify such an understanding. (1897e, 359–60)

The popularization of the theory of degeneration, like that of Darwinism, contributed strongly to the spread of the alarming idea that civilization was nothing more than a thin veneer and that civilized man might still "go ape" (Kershner 1986, 420; cf. Harris 1991, 41). In this respect, degeneration theory was nonetheless ambivalent. On the one hand, the sexuality of perverts, the lower classes, and also that of children was a constant reminder of the savage condition to which civilization could revert; but on the other hand, perversion was associated with corruption, decadent luxury, and "unnatural" sensibility in modern society and culture. In his book *Entartung* (1892), the physician and culture critic Max Nordau (1849–1923) argued that many of the leading artists and writers of the day who broke with tradition were degenerates and suffered from sexual psychopathy.

The Psychology of Sexual Desire

Whereas the first historians of sexology, often psychiatrists themselves, emphasized that superstitious beliefs and cruel practices had been replaced by sound medical science and humanitarian treatments, more recent historical work has associated medical theories of sexuality with social, political, and moral control. Not only has psychiatric interference with sexual deviance often been characterized as the climax of the medicalization of sexuality; it has also been considered as a typical expression of conservative bourgeois morality and Victorian hypocrisy. As the eager reception of degeneration theory by psychiatrists illustrates, there are elements that would substantiate such a judgment, although one should be careful not to evaluate past psychiatric ideas and practices according to contemporary scientific and moral standards. Psychiatrists often relied uncritically on conventional standards of sexual conduct in their diagnosis of perversion, thereby equating immorality or mere nonconformity to mental disorder. Uncontrollable sensuality was pictured as a severe threat to civilization; in the medical view, the history of mankind was a constant struggle between animal lust and moral behavior.

On the first pages of *Psychopathia sexualis*, Krafft-Ebing expounded how difficult it was to keep the sex drive under restraint. He believed that morality had only been developed after a long and difficult struggle against the bestial instincts (1892h, 6). Christianity, law, and education had all helped to bridle man's animal lust, yet notwithstanding the efforts of these cultural institutions, individual man was always in danger of sinking into the mire of everyday sensuality. "Love unbridled is a volcano that scorches and consumes all around it; it is an abyss that swallows up everything—honor, substance and health" (*Ps* 1903, 2; *Ps* 1999, 6). Echoing ethnographic and historical works on sexuality and marriage, Krafft-Ebing stressed that the rise of civilization had only been possible after the sexual instinct had been

suppressed and refined. Christianity's introduction of the feeling of modesty and shame was the major indicator of the transition from the primitive
to the civilized. He saw a progressive development of mankind from a primitive, lawless promiscuity through matriarchy to patriarchy and monogamous matrimony, which proved the maturation of human society. The sexual role division in the Western nuclear family marked the apex of the
evolutionary development of humanity during which sex differences had
progressively increased.

    Like other psychiatrists, Krafft-Ebing indeed surrounded various sexual
behaviors with an aura of pathology, echoing nineteenth-century stereotypical thinking on issues like masturbation, masculinity, and femininity.
Time and again, he stressed that masturbation and child sexuality were major factors in the etiology of perversion. He also strongly endorsed the belief
that women, though completely swayed by their reproductive organs,
lacked intense sexual feeling and, contrary to males, were inclined to chas-
tity, love, and monogamy. "If it were otherwise," Krafft-Ebing wrote, "the
whole world would be a brothel, and marriage and family inconceivable
concepts" (Ps 1903, 13; cf. Ps 1999, 15).[1] Yet male sexuality, aimed at a
release of built-up tension, was considered more difficult to control, and
men were basically viewed as polygamous. Like other doctors, Krafft-Ebing
upheld the double standard: "The unfaithfulness of the wife, as compared
with that of the husband, is morally of much wider bearing, and should
always meet with severer punishment at the hands of law" (Ps 1903, 14; Ps
1999, 16). Although he did not favor prostitution, he tacitly took it for
granted that males found sexual gratification with prostitutes. To demand
sexual abstinence of men before marriage, he contended, was not a realistic
option (1902b). Prostitution was basically a necessary evil; it was not seen
as unusual at all for bourgeois men to hire the services of lower-class prostitutes. Significantly, Krafft-Ebing was not the only physician who sometimes
encouraged male homosexuals to visit a prostitute in order to practice "normal" intercourse.

    The early psychiatric theories were nonetheless all but static or coher-
ent on these issues: they tended to be riddled with ambiguities and contradictions, and therefore they cannot be merely regarded as a medical or
moral disqualification of lust and sexual aberration. Differences among the
various national sexological traditions are relevant here. In France, psychiatry's interference with sexuality was motivated by concerns about the
decreasing fertility rate, effeminacy, the hegemony of heterosexuality, the
family ethic, and the proper roles of men and women. In Germany, Austria,

---

1. On nineteenth-century attitudes toward women's sexuality, cf. Degler 1973 and Gay
1986; on masturbation, see Barker-Benfield 1973, Hall 1992, and Laqueur 1992.

and Britain, the development of sexology in the last decade of the nineteenth century was closely connected with efforts to abolish laws outlawing
homosexual behavior, as is exemplified by the work of Krafft-Ebing, Hirschfeld, and Havelock Ellis. Ironically, this difference in national sexological
traditions—the French one being somewhat more conservative—can be
explained by the fact that disorderly sexual conduct, such as homosexuality, was not punishable in France, while German, Austrian, and British
legal codes laid down penalties for it. The traditional orientation of medical research of sexuality in France was not so much a response to the legal
situation or efforts at sexual reform but to fears of male impotence, depopulation, and national decline (Nye 1991; 1993; & 1999; Verplaetse 1999).

Although psychiatry gained unprecedented cultural prominence in late-
nineteenth-century Paris, by 1900 Germany (Berlin) and Austria (Vienna)
had replaced France as the center of the medical research of sexuality. The
emerging new science of sexology—the term *Sexualwissenschaft* was introduced in 1906 by Iwan Bloch—contributed important theoretical innovations.[2] First, there was a change in emphasis from a somatic to a psychological interpretive framework, psychiatry being increasingly caught between
neurology and psychology. Psychiatry's predominantly forensic focus and
preference for physiological explanations were gradually replaced by considerable broader concerns, addressing more general psychological issues of
human sexuality. Among other things, this meant that sexuality was more
and more seen as disconnected from reproduction. This conceptual break-
through, based on a new psychological style of reasoning, was introduced
by French psychiatrists like Binet and even more in the work of German
and Austrian experts, while it can also be traced in the writings of the
British Havelock Ellis. Most French doctors, however, still adhered to
physiological and anatomical explanations, conceptualizing sexuality as an
undifferentiated procreative instinct embedded in the biological sex of
men and women. Also, French specialists on sexual deviance tended to
classify all perversions under a single nosological entity, be it inversion
(Charcot and Magnan) or fetishism (Binet), whereas central European psychiatrists, like Krafft-Ebing, in generally isolated the numerous disorders in
various subclassifications. The second important innovation was a shift
away from attempts at classifying disease categories within clear boundaries
toward efforts aimed at a tentative understanding of normal sexuality in
the context of perversions as extremes on a graded scale of health and illness, normal and abnormal, and masculinity and femininity. Finally, after

2. The term *sexology* is in fact of American origin. It was coined by Elizabeth Willard,
author of *Sexology as the Philosophy of Life* (1867) (Bullough 1994, 26). The term was not used
in French until 1933 (Nye 1991, 401).

1900 some scholars began to consider the impact of cultural differences in explaining various forms of sexual behavior.

Krafft-Ebing's sexual pathology provides a case in point. Influenced by degenerationist thinking, his biological approach to sexuality has often been contrasted with Freud's psychological one. However, in *Psychopathia sexualis* there is a striking inconsistency between, on the one hand, physiological explanations situating the sexual drive in the nervous system and in a "psychosexual center" in the brain and, on the other hand, the author's clinical descriptions and specifications of perversion. Although the case histories frequently refer to physical examinations of patients, including craniometry and sometimes anatomies of the brain if they had died while under medical supervision, these were not very relevant for Krafft-Ebing's classification and definition of perversion. Around 1890, when the terms *fetishism, sadism,* and *masochism* were introduced, his focus shifted from a physiological to a more psychological understanding (Hauser 1994).

According to Krafft-Ebing, the sexual instinct is a function of the cerebral cortex. He postulated the existence of cerebral centers, which determined an individual's sexual personality, thus considering perversions like sadism, masochism, fetishism, and homosexuality as "cerebral neuroses." At the same time, however, he had to admit that no definite region of the cortex had yet been identified as the exclusive seat of this instinct and that distinct cerebral lesions associated with sexual pathologies had not been found either. In the field of sexual pathology, convincing scientific explanations that connected physiological disorders with deviant desires and behaviors were absent. The French psychiatrist Magnan was in fact the only one who set up a classification of sexual perversion on an neuroanatomical basis by locating various disorders in different areas of the nervous system (Rosario 1997, 86). Magnan's classification was not very successful though; in general, anatomical and physiological models failed to have a serious impact on clinical descriptions of sexual disturbances. In clinical practice there was only proof of the *psychological* existence of what Krafft-Ebing—following the French psychiatrist Moreau de Tours—dubbed *sens génital* (genital sense). Krafft-Ebing understood this "sixth sense" in a functional way.

The search for lesions in the central nervous system did not prove to be successful, so psychiatrists often resorted to functional explanations. These enabled them to stay committed to a physiological interpretation of mental disorders, without having to localize them anatomically. In his case histories, Krafft-Ebing often referred to examinations of his patients' genitals as well as the standard physical stigmata of degeneration, such as an aberrant skull, a cleft lip, misshapen ears, deformed teeth, or a neuropathic eye. However, such references to physical abnormalities were of secondary importance: psychological characteristics were in fact considered decisive in diagnosing perversion. Perversions were functional disorders of the instinct, and they expressed themselves in large measure as psychological phenomena. The seat of the sexual instinct was everywhere and nowhere, or, to be more precise, it was located in the personality (Davidson 1990). Therefore, a proper diagnosis of perversion was not primarily determined by bodily characteristics or actual behavior, but by individual character, personal history, and inner feelings: perception, emotional life, dreams, and fantasies. What is crucial, Krafft-Ebing wrote, is the association of the abnormal act with its "psychological motive," the "abnormalities of thought and feeling," even if people were not aware of this; discussing sexual desire, he—as well as some of his clients—frequently used the psychological terms *unconscious* and *latent* (*Ps* 1903, 355; *Ps* 1999, 420).

Most typical of Krafft-Ebing's psychological understanding of sexuality was his explanations of contrary sexual feeling, masochism, and fetishism. The first proved that biological sex did not determine "psychosexual personality" and sexual preference; in many case histories of homosexual men, Krafft-Ebing noted that despite their effeminate feelings and preferences, their physical appearance was masculine. This challenged the view that urnings were anatomically distinctive. Although physicians might believe that there were underlying physical causes of perversion, the conceptualization of homosexuality as a form of contrary sexual *feeling* indicates that the psychological experience of sex and sexual desire was considered crucial in the psychiatric diagnosis of its symptoms. Echoing Westphal, who had characterized homosexuality as "an inborn inversion of the sexual feeling *while being conscious of its pathological nature*," Krafft-Ebing stressed that this disorder dominated the way of thinking and feeling completely (Mak 1997, 217; italics added). In establishing his detailed subclassification of levels of contrary sexual feeling, he relied on mental features in particular, namely the degree of homosexual sensibility that was present and the psychic characteristics of the opposite sex. Only the most extreme and rarest forms of contrary sexual feeling—sexually paranoiac metamorphosis and androgyny or gynandry—were accompanied by signs of physical inversion, and even these never merged into physical hermaphroditism.

In Krafft-Ebing's definition of masochism, the differentiation of outward behavior versus mental experience and imagination was essential. Masochism differed from mere flagellation, he emphasized; masochists did not desire to experience actual physical pain, but they derived pleasure from the inner feeling of being dominated and abused. This perversion was all about imagination and fantasy. Often, Krafft-Ebing concluded in his descriptions of what he identified as "ideal" or "symbolic" masochism, fantasies were not realized, or only symbolically. He used this as an argument to reject the term *algolagnia*, meaning the love of physical pain. The last term was introduced by Schrenck-Notzing (1862–1929) in 1892 and used by Albert Eulenburg (1840–1917), who published a series of studies on sadism and masochism.

Individual fetishes could only be accounted for if one considered the psychological mechanism of association: the lust these individuals had experienced on a specific occasion had become fixed in their imagination. In his explanation of fetishism, Krafft-Ebing tended to follow Binet, who asserted that the major forms of sexual pathology were psychologically acquired by exposure to certain accidental events. Although in Binet's view, a certain hereditary disposition was a necessary precondition, it alone could not explain which object—certain parts of the body (hands and feet in particular), physical handicaps, hair, shoes, boots, nightcaps, handkerchiefs, gloves, toiletries, ladies' underwear, fur, velvet, or silk—was selected as the sexual one. According to Binet, the sexual desire for a partner of the same sex, for an animal, or for a masochistic scene could also be viewed as forms of fetishism. Emphasizing early childhood experiences, he argued that chance events especially determined the major forms of sexual pathology of which fetishism was the model. Schrenck-Notzing also argued that extraneous influences and education were actually the most significant etiological factors in the genesis of perversion. Rejecting degeneration theory—in which perverts found a welcome excuse for their leanings, according to Schrenck-Notzing—he claimed that he could cure perverts, especially homosexuals, by hypnotism and suggestion therapy. Although Krafft-Ebing endorsed the associationist theory only in part, feeling it was only relevant for the specific choice of fetish, he also believed in the power of suggestion in treating perversion.

However, Krafft-Ebing was of the opinion that Binet and Schrenck-Notzing were wrong to assume that all perversions were caused by psychological association. In his view, contrary sexual feeling, sadism, and masochism could not be explained by it, and he also continued to stress degeneration as a necessary precondition of fetishism. For him, the underlying causes of all perversions remained degeneration and heredity. Nevertheless, Krafft-Ebing, like Binet and others, shifted the medical discussion away from explaining sexuality as a series of interrelated physiological events toward a more psychological understanding. Perversion was not so much rooted in physical as in so-called functional disorders. In this new psychiatric mode of reasoning, perversions were disorders of a natural urge that could not be located in physiology, in specific tissue or an organ (Davidson 1990). Stressing the impact of sexuality on human feeling, thinking, and behavior, Krafft-Ebing asserted that the "unconscious life of the soul" strongly affected the functions of the body (1889c, 1186). Thus, prior to Freud, psychiatrists already began to view human sexuality as distinct from the instinctual sexuality of animals, and they established the idea that sexual disorders could result from unconscious psychological causes.

The development of a psychological conception of sexuality in Krafft-Ebing's work shows how a new understanding of normal sexuality evolved from the psychiatric analysis of the abnormal. At first he highlighted the psychological dimension of sexuality in his discussion of masturbation and the perversions. The difference between masturbation and normal coitus, Krafft-Ebing explained in 1875, was that the first involved nonphysiological stimuli, such as fantasies—he frequently used the expression *psychical onanism* for indulging in sexual fantasy—whereas the second was a purely physiological act, comparable to an automatic reflex (1875b, 427). Next, Krafft-Ebing based his diagnosis of the main perversions—sadism, masochism, fetishism, and contrary sexual feeling—on inner feelings, subjective experiences, and character traits rather than on physical characteristics and outward behavior. It was the psychological attitude behind outward appearance and behavior that counted as the defining criterion of contrary sexual feeling. Although some urnings might show some physical characteristics of the opposite sex, the decisive feature of contrary sexual feeling was psychical inversion. Some of them might be able to perform intercourse with a woman, Krafft-Ebing noticed, but only by using a "psychical trick," that is, by fantasizing about men (*Ps* 1903, 19; *Ps* 1999, 654). Neither did the satisfaction of sadistic and masochistic desires depend on physical stimuli: perception was crucial. In this connection, Krafft-Ebing spoke of "psychic lust," also because of the central role of fantasy in the sexual experience of sadists and masochists. Many masochists pointed out that it was often difficult to connect psychological and physical experiences. Following Binet, Krafft-Ebing used the idea of psychological association to explain why fetishists were obsessed with a particular object or body part: the close connection between sexual arousal and the fetish had become fixed in the imagination.

Thus the psychical dimension of sexuality first appeared as a typical constituent of perversion: certain mental stimuli prevented the spontaneous physiological process from taking its course. Later, however, Krafft-Ebing also drew attention to the decisive role of the mind in the development of normal sexuality. Not only did he point out that the sense of pleasure depended on "a psychical performance of the organ of consciousness (the cerebral cortex)," he also used the expression *psychologically dissatisfied* to refer to the lack of sexual fulfillment that some people experienced (1891b, 95). In an article on sexual anesthesia, for example, Krafft-Ebing presented the case history of Mr. X, a twenty-nine-year-old businessman, whose problem was that he wanted to marry while having no sexual feelings. He had no trouble with his potency, however; he told Krafft-Ebing that he regularly visited brothels, but this was, as he stated, only for physical release, satisfying a purely physical impulse, just like other people ate when they were hungry. What worried him though was that he never experienced any emotion during the act or feeling toward his partner, "whom he experienced as a lifeless object, as 'a piece of wood.'" Women were a matter of indifference to him, although he did not hate them; nude women did not excite him: they were simply "an instrument for his coarser sensual needs." How a man could fall in love with a woman or be jealous about her, he did not understand: "X experiences his malfunction as painful. . . . He believes that it is a mental failure, for spinally he is all right, always potent" (1899g, 179–80). This case history, like others, clearly showed that normal sexual functioning was considered as more than just the physical ability to have intercourse. Sexual satisfaction was not just the result of "the operation of a spinal reflex," Krafft-Ebing noted in another article, "but a course of events which is complicated by psychocerebral processes. If this were not so, coitus for a man would merely be a masturbatory act in a women's body" (1894b, 93).

It is remarkable that Krafft-Ebing diagnosed this patient as suffering from sexual anesthesia, because from a purely physical perspective he did not lack the sexual urge. Other cases of anesthesia also show that the problem was not so much impotency as the missing of the psychic impulse to engage in a sexual relation. The sexual instinct was not only important for reproduction, Krafft-Ebing stressed, but also for the full psychological development of individuals and for engaging in a love bond, the glue of marriage. Again and again, he noticed that patients suffering from sexual anesthesia tended to be unsociable and emotionally underdeveloped: "The area of social, altruistic feelings, which are rooted in the sexual instinct, is always substantially injured. Individuals with such a sexual malfunction can only be rational persons, they are never men of feeling" (1899g, 175). From the social perspective, Krafft-Ebing pointed out, sexual relations depended on a psychic mechanism. In his view, the criterion of true love was "the mental satisfaction derived from the sexual act" (Ps 1903, 19; Ps 1999, 21). Only if physical pleasure and spiritual fulfillment went hand and hand could sexual intercourse be truly satisfying:

> Where the body of the beloved person is made the sole object of love, . . .
> or if sexual pleasure alone is sought without regard to the communion of
> soul and mind, true love does not exist. Neither is it found among the

disciples of Plato, who love the soul only and despise sexual enjoyment. (*Ps* 1903, 19; *Ps* 1999, 20–21)

Next to the psychologization of sexuality, there was another way in which Krafft-Ebing's approach foreshadowed Freud's. Whereas the differentiation of healthy and pathological sexuality was the basic assumption in his work (reproduction being the touchstone), in his discussion of the main perversions, he at the same time subverted the barriers between the normal and the abnormal. Despite the effort to distinguish perversion from normalcy, there is a tendency in *Psychopathia sexualis* to undercut distinctions between divergent desires and to make various forms of normal and abnormal sexuality more or less equivalent and exchangeable, thus abolishing a clear boundary between health and perversion. Sadism, masochism, and fetishism were not only disease categories, but also terms that described extremes on a graded scale of health and illness and that explained aspects of normal sexuality. He explained that sadism and masochism were inherent in normal male and female sexuality, the former being of an active and aggressive nature, the latter passive and submissive. They were the most extreme forms of sexual hyperesthesia: sadism, at bottom, was a quantitative extension of the normal sexual psychology of males, while masochism was an exaggeration of the female sexual nature. It followed that sadism was essentially a male disorder and masochism a female one. However, most of his cases were of male masochists, and therefore he assumed that masochism in males was related to inversion.

Similarly, in Krafft-Ebing's view, fetishism could not be distinguished from normal sexuality in absolute terms; again the distinction was largely a quantitative one, rather than a qualitative one. Fetishism, in a sense, was part and parcel of normal sexuality because the individual character of sexual attraction and, by extension, monogamous love was grounded in a distinct preference for particular physical and mental characteristics of one's partner. In fact, so-called physiological fetishism was what held together the institution of marriage. This was in line with Binet's assertion that it was sometimes difficult to differentiate between normal and pathological fetishism. Fetishism was only true perversion when the sexual impulse was focused, not on a person as a whole, but exclusively on a single feature or object. Fetishists displayed exaggerated sexual behavior, a kind of "hypertrophy" in the normal level of genital excitement that was caused by the disruption of a healthy balance between the natural passions and artificial psychological stimuli (Nye 1989, 42). Nevertheless, Binet argued that all love was to some extent fetishistic, thus indicating that it was a general tendency at the heart of sexual attraction. Echoing this view, Krafft-Ebing discussed fetishism not only as a perversion, but also in the context of the general psychological laws of sexual life. Apart from serving as the glue of love, fetishism also played an important role in the process of evolution. Fetishism involved certain aesthetic preferences, and therefore it favored the selection of the fittest and the transmission of physical and mental virtues.

Krafft-Ebing went back on making hard and fast distinctions between normal and abnormal sexualities, holding that—in the fashion of modern physiology—one could only measure quantitative differences along a scale of infinite variations. "The elements which constitute psychopathology are the same as those of healthy life, only the conditions under which they develop are different," he wrote in his *Lehrbuch der Psychiatrie auf klinischer Grundlage* (1897e, 25). As a consequence, perversions did not form a wholly distinct class, an isolated group of monstrous phenomena, but they tended to be considered merely as variations within a wide range of natural possibilities. Ordinary sexuality appeared to have features of perverted desire. In addition, the barriers between masculinity and femininity diffused in psychiatric theory. Inversion—spanning the gulf between the masculine, the actively aspiring, and the feminine, the passively receptive— occupied a major place in Krafft-Ebing's sexual pathology. The extensive medical discussion of several forms of physical and especially mental inversion highlighted the chance character of sex differentiation and signaled that exclusive masculinity and femininity might be mere abstractions (cf. Storr 1998).

Krafft-Ebing and many of his colleagues had identified contrary sexual feeling with degeneration because it manifested an abnormal, inverted physiology or psychology that was interpreted as a countercurrent in the normal evolutionary process of increasing sexual differentiation. However, when in the mid-1890s the concept of sexual intermediacy was grounded in contemporary embryological research and in evolutionary theories, this view was reconsidered. The first stressed that the early state of the human embryo was characterized by sexual indifference, and the second suggested that primitive forms of life lacked sexual differentiation. Echoing Ernst Haeckel's law of recapitulation, man appeared to be of a bisexual origin from a phylogenetic as well as an ontogenetic perspective. Many biologists assumed that male and female physical characteristics developed through a gradual process of differentiation from an initial period of sexual neutrality or potential hermaphroditism. In evolution as well as in the development of the embryo, there was a continuing differentiation of and struggle between male and female elements. To be sure, increasing evidence of the common origin of male and female sex from a sexually undifferentiated condition was not necessarily accompanied by an egalitarian conception of the biological worth and significance of the two sexes. In fact, nineteenth-century biomedical science fostered the belief that masculinity was a sign of higher development and femininity of lower development. In the evolutionary perspective of the era, the masculine mind was more advanced than the female.

In the mid-1890s, Krafft-Ebing began to show an increasing interest in a "bisexual" hypothesis to explain homosexuality and referred to the work of the American physicians James G. Kiernan (1852–1923), G. Frank Lydston (1857–1923), and the French researcher Julien Chevalier (cf. 1895c). They argued for a biogenetic explanation of homosexuality by stressing the original bisexuality of our forebears. Whereas Kiernan designated homosexuality as an atavistic phenomenon, which could be explained phylogenetically as one of the various kinds of hermaphroditism that were reversions to the evolutionary ancestors of the human species, Lydston argued it was a throwback to an early ontogenetic, embryonic stage of sexual indeterminacy. Embracing both explanations, Chevalier maintained that the initial bisexual potential of the embryo and the hermaphroditism of the evolutionary ancestors of the human species both explained homosexuality. Krafft-Ebing accepted two premises, stressed in particular by Chevalier: first, that proceeding from the original bisexuality of the embryo, an ontogenic struggle goes on during human development, with one sex conquering the other under normal circumstances; and, second, that inverted sexuality is a developmental disturbance in the present state of monosexual evolution, not an atavism in the sense of Lombroso's well-known theories. Such disturbances, he reasoned, could occur either in the anatomical development of the organism, resulting in physical hermaphroditism, or independently in the corresponding psychical centers, resulting in contrary sexual feeling. Notwithstanding his predominantly psychological approach, Krafft-Ebing adhered to a biogenetic explanation of contrary sexual feeling as well. In doing so, he slightly distanced himself from degeneration theory, which posited, after all, that abnormal biological phenomena were closely connected to social and cultural developments in modern civilization.

The biogenetic theory conflicted with the degenerational one. Although Darwinism had often been used to prove that heterosexuality was a natural norm for higher forms of life and that perversions like homosexuality were necessarily abnormal, evolution theory could also be invoked to undermine the conventional differentiation between male and female. Darwin viewed masculinity and femininity not as static properties, but as malleable functions that depended on the contribution any given trait made to the survival and reproductive success of the organism. Ulrichs, who between 1864 and 1879 published a dozen brochures on uranism, referred to Darwin to prove that homosexuality as a psychophysical intermediacy—a "migration of the soul": a woman's soul in a man's body and vice versa—was natural, a notion that was elaborated by Magnus Hirschfeld. Ulrichs postulated that a double sexual germ was present in each embryo. The explanations of same-sex behavior by Ulrichs and various psychiatrists problematized the traditional natural-unnatural dualism: the love of urnings was like the love between a man and a woman, because in both cases a male and female element attracted each other. Explanations of homosexuality as a form of inversion demonstrate how, in the nineteenth century, sexual attraction was not conceivable without a physical or psychological polarization and matching of male and female elements. Ulrichs, as well as Benkert, played a prominent part in the "invention" of not only homosexuality, but also heterosexuality. They defended same-sex love by comparing it with the love between man and woman and their sexual desire for each other.

Hirschfeld, leader of the first homosexual rights movement in Germany and founder of the first sexological journals, *Jahrbuch für sexuelle Zwischenstufen* and *Zeitschrift für Sexualwissenschaft,* was even more profoundly indebted to Darwinian notions of evolution than his predecessors. Whereas Darwin envisioned a gradual transformation of life-forms over time, Hirschfeld applied this notion synchronically rather than diachronically. Differentiating between, successively, anomalies in the sex glands, the genitals, secondary sexual and psychological characteristics, and sexual orientation, Hirschfeld espoused the view that there was a seamless continuum of human sexual types in nature ranging between fully male and fully female. Under the rubric of sexual intermediacy, he subsumed various biological and psychological fusions of manliness and femininity that in the twentieth century would gradually be reclassified as radically separate phenomena, such as homosexuality, hermaphroditism, androgyny, transvestism, and transsexuality. He defined homosexuality as a form of sexual orientation that was accompanied by developmental anomalies in secondary sexual as well as psychological characteristics.

It will be clear from my discussion of the scientific debate on sexuality that Freud was not a radical pioneer but that he built on psychiatric theories of sexuality formulated by others in the 1880s and 1890s (cf. Ellenberger 1970; Sulloway 1979). Psychiatric theories opened up a new continent of knowledge, not only because they treated sexual abnormality as disease instead of as sin or crime, but even more because they made clear that a proper understanding of the nature of sexuality carried substantial significance for the existence of the individual as well as society at large and therefore deserved serious study. Krafft-Ebing claimed in his *Lehrbuch der Psychiatrie* that life is marked by two basic instincts, that of self-preservation (which manifested itself in appetite) and that of sexuality

(1897e, 75). In his biogenetic explanation of sadism and masochism, which he borrowed from Kiernan, he connected sexuality and appetite. Kiernan had argued that reproduction by cannibalism was the primal form of the sexual impulse, and from this Krafft-Ebing concluded that an instinctive urge to victimize or be the victim might be explained under the same rubric. In the preface of *Psychopathia sexualis*, he quoted Friedrich Schiller's dictum that love and hunger govern human life. Although Krafft-Ebing pointed to the potential threat the sexual instinct posed to civilization, at the same time he drew attention to its constructive role in culture and society:

> Sexual life is no doubt the one mighty factor in the individual and social relations of man that discloses his powers of activity, of acquiring property, of establishing a home, and of awakening altruistic sentiments toward a person of the opposite sex, toward his own children, as well as toward the whole human race. Sexual feeling is really the root of all ethics, and probably also of aestheticism and religion. (*Ps* 1903, 1–2; cf. *Ps* 1999, 5–6)

Krafft-Ebing thus viewed sexuality not merely as a blind biological force. Foreshadowing Freud's theory on the origins of culture, he postulated that the sexual drive itself contained the seeds of civilized life and that human civilization had in fact emerged from the realm of brute instinct to which nature still consigned animals. In subjective experience, the sexual act was not only accompanied by sensual pleasure, but also by responses of a social and ethical nature. Krafft-Ebing considered love as a social bond that was inherently sexual, and he tended to value the longing for physical and psychological union with a partner as a purpose in itself. "Ethical surroundings are necessary in order to elevate love to its true and pure form; sensuality, however, will ever remain its principal basis. Platonic love is a platitude, a misnomer for 'kindred spirits'" (*Ps* 1903, 12; *Ps* 1999, 14).

Although Krafft-Ebing opposed feminism and did not speak in favor of political equality of the sexes per se, in his historical scheme of the development of human sexuality, the emergence of moral consciousness out of natural instinct is tied to the social, religious, and legal equality of women. Female modesty, he argued, secured the ethical dimension of human sexuality. Contrary to the promiscuous male, woman is selective in her choice of sexual partners; as a result, her sexual behavior provided the basic foundation of marriage, the institution that warranted the advancement of human sexuality from the primordial violence that characterized sexual behavior before the rise of civilization. The Christian world was superior to other cultures, especially the world of Islam, Krafft-Ebing claimed, because

Christianity recognized woman as the peer of man and had consolidated monogamy both morally and legally.

Stressing that both love without sexuality and sexual pleasure without love were incomplete, Krafft-Ebing clearly conveyed the modern ideal of romantic love. It was his appreciation of the relational aspect of sexuality that contributed to his changing view of homosexuality. At the end of his life, he was inclined to think that homosexuality was the equivalent of heterosexuality and therefore not a disease. In this way he echoed Ulrichs and Benkert, who had defended same-sex love by comparing it with the love between man and woman and their sexual desire for each other. His discussion of same-sex love indicates that procreation was not anymore considered to be an absolute, unshakable norm—notably, he did not mention contraception in his discussion of perversion. While he still focused on heterosexual intercourse as the norm, at the same time he implicitly acknowledged that reproduction was not the only, perhaps not even the most important goal of coitus: instead, affection appeared as the major purpose. The implicit shift in his thinking from reproduction to affection as the main purpose of sexuality might help explain the fact that in the twentieth century, the heterosexual-homosexual dichotomy has become the dominant categorization of sexual orientation.

Krafft-Ebing's thinking was in line with other sexologists who in the 1890s increasingly questioned the assumed exclusive naturalness of the reproductive instinct; more and more, primacy was assigned to the satisfaction of desire. The German sexologist Albert Moll, who corresponded with Krafft-Ebing on a regular basis (even lending him case histories) and who edited *Psychopathia sexualis* in the 1920s, broke new ground by positing two major instincts as basic for what he called the *libido sexualis*: discharge (*Detumescenztrieb*) and attraction (*Contrectationstrieb*). The first referred to the sexual act proper, the second to social needs. In his *Untersuchungen über die Libido sexualis* (1897), which in many respects followed Krafft-Ebing's reasoning directly, Moll explicitly detached the sexual impulse from reproduction. He compared normal and abnormal sexual forms side by side. The new biogenetic theory, which was inspired by American scientists such as Kiernan and Lydston, held that perversions were components of a more general sexual instinct and could be explained by developmental disturbances. Reproductive heterosexuality lost its naturalness and became increasingly understood as the result of a developmental synthesis of component impulses. According to the German psychologist and philosopher Max Dessoir (1867–1947), sexuality during puberty was still undifferentiated and indefinite. He concluded that not only homosexuality but also heterosexuality was acquired in culture. Thus it became more and more difficult to tell the difference between compelling perverted appetites and natural instincts.

When idiosyncratic desire became dissociated from reproduction and widely divergent fancies became sexualized, a new way of distinguishing the normal from the abnormal was required. Accepting sexuality, not just procreation, as a fact of life and a vital physical force, a new domain of knowledge appeared, one inhabited by desiring individuals. Moll, in his *Die konträre Sexualempfindung* (1891), and Havelock Ellis, in his *Studies in the Psychology of Sex* (1897–1928), began to question the dangers of masturbation: whereas earlier physicians had viewed child sexuality as abnormal, they began to recognize the relative normalcy of infantile sexual manifestations. Psychiatrists also discussed the question whether sexual abstinence and dissatisfaction were harmful to one's physical and mental health (cf. Hill 1994). Krafft-Ebing was of the opinion that in general they were not necessarily so for normal, healthy people, but at the same time he indicated that for both men and women a satisfying sexual relationship was desirable, especially for their psychic well-being. Married women who did not experience orgasm in sexual intercourse, he contended, ran a considerable risk of developing nervousness, neurasthenia, and hysteria (1888e). In his view, not only sexual hyperesthesia, but also sexual anesthesia, the absence of sensuality, was pathological, in men as well as in women. Moreover, he argued that enforced sexual abstinence was not advisable for neuropathic individuals, especially males, because it might result in a serious aggravation of their nervous and mental disorders (1888d). Max Marcuse (1877–1963), who was an editor of two sexological journals—*Sexual-Probleme* and the *Zeitschrift für Sexualwissenschaft und Sexualpolitik*—took this argument one step further. Marcuse, who openly criticized the concept of sexuality as an instinct aimed at reproduction, voiced the opinion that abstinence could lead to nervous disorders in otherwise healthy people. Considering sexuality a universal human need that should find fulfillment, he began to favor contraception.

Havelock Ellis, who among British doctors wrote most insightfully on sexual matters, held that sexuality in itself was neither a threat to moral character nor a drain on vital energies. In his *Studies in the Psychology of Sex*, he distinguished himself as a sexual reformer rather than as a medical scientist. His ideas on sexuality were related to his criticism of both traditional Christianity and Victorian bourgeois morality. His branch of utopian socialism not only aspired for an economic reorganization of society, but also for a reform of cultural and personal life, of family, marriage, and sexuality. His *Studies in the Psychology of Sex* were not an exclusively medical work. Apart from biomedical writings, he drew on a variety of sources: anthropology, literature, and not least the self-disclosures of individuals about their own sexual experiences. Like that of Iwan Bloch, Havelock Ellis's approach was characterized by cultural relativism, to describe the variety in sexual behaviors, and biological determinism, to explain the complex natural process that presumably underlay the diversity of sexual experiences. For him, sexuality was a pivotal force in human life, not only because it served the propagation of the human race, but also, at the level of the individual, because it was a key to a fulfilling life.

Havelock Ellis, who has been characterized as a central figure in the emergence of a modern sexual ethos, believed that modern society inhibited the full development of an essential and basically healthy human nature, and he stressed the importance of sex for interpersonal relations (Robinson 1976). As a "sexual enthusiast," Havelock Ellis distanced himself from other nineteenth-century medical theories on sexuality by arguing that not so much the sexual arousal, the stimulation of sexual desire, begged for an explanation; impotence and frigidity, rather than satyriasis and nymphomania, posed problems. He argued that sexual activity hinges upon tumescence (arousal) and detumescence (release), and that arousal was not an automatic occurrence but had to be pursued in a conscious and artful manner. Analyzing the rituals of courtship, Havelock Ellis endeavored to explain the whole of sexual psychology, normal as well as deviations. He contended that sexual deviations like homosexuality, fetishism, exhibitionism, urolagnia, and coprolagnia could be understood as various manifestations of a single psychological process. All sexual deviations involved an imitation of both the actions and the emotions of normal heterosexual courtship and intercourse. Thus he explained, like Krafft-Ebing, sadism and masochism as "emotional residues of animal courtship" that could still be observed in man's tendency to domination and woman's delight in submission. Stressing the inborn nature of homosexuality and criticizing doctors who viewed it as a disease, Havelock Ellis called homosexuality only a statistical abnormality. He also criticized medical theories that linked masturbation with serious mental and physical disorders, although he did not condone it because "autoerotism," as he named it, tended to divorce the physical and affective dimensions of sexuality. He was far from advocating uninhibited sexual abandon: affection, intense emotional attraction, and intimate relationships formed the proper context for sexual activity (Robinson 1976, 33).

The changing meaning of heterosexuality, not only in the work of Havelock Ellis, but also in that of Krafft-Ebing and Moll, underlined the shift from a conception of the sexual impulse as a reproductive instinct toward a view of sexuality that emphasized erotic desire and pleasure in the context of the love bond and personal fulfillment, irrespective of the reproductive potential. Defined as the desire for the other sex, the term at first did not signify normalcy but was employed in discussions of perversion. The normal sexual instinct was associated with a built-in, unconscious procreative aim. Not only perverts but also heterosexuals seemed to enjoy sex for other purposes than reproduction; because they digressed from the reproductive norm, they were considered perverts. Judged by a reproductive standard, heterosexuality was a nonprocreative perversion that seemed to converge with homosexuality. However, repeatedly referring to the bipolar sexual attraction between males and females, Krafft-Ebing, Moll, and Havelock Ellis—while still stressing that propagation was the biological goal of sexual behavior—began to suggest that heterosexual desire, the sensual pleasure of men and women, free from any conscious tie to reproduction, was an essential element of their intimacy. "Voluptuous feelings accompanying the sexual act are of no mean importance for the physical, psychical, and social well-being of individuals," Krafft-Ebing added (1891b, 100). From this it was only a small step to Freud's lusting "libido" and "pleasure principle," according to which the sexual desire's only built-in aim is its own satisfaction. Freud's theory on sexuality would play an important role in stabilizing, publicizing, and normalizing the new heterosexual ideal (Katz 1995).

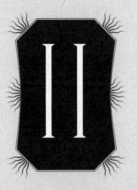

II

Extending the Boundaries of Psychiatry

THROUGHOUT HIS PROFESSIONAL CAREER, KRAFFT-EBING'S PSYCHIATRIC
views of sexuality, as described in part 1, were far from static and coherent.
He never claimed to have the final word, and his scientific approach to
sexuality, as it crystallized in the 1890s, was in several ways ambivalent.
His first efforts to arrive at a better understanding of sexuality, dating from
the late 1870s, were predominantly motivated by a forensic and somatic
orientation, but later on his focus shifted toward a more comprehensive
clinical and psychological interpretive framework. Furthermore, he gradually moved away from his earlier efforts at classifying the various categories
of sexual deviancy or disease, trying to grasp them within relatively fixed
boundaries, toward a much more tentative understanding of normal sexuality in the context of perversions as extremes on a graded scale of health
and illness, normal and abnormal. His changing views of sexuality were
congruent with his general theories of psychopathology, which were rather
idiosyncratic: his work is a bricolage of elements taken from biological
models of mental illness, pathological-anatomical approaches, and degeneration theory, while it also tried to escape the limitations of the dominant
somatic etiological notion of late-nineteenth-century psychiatry by elaborating a psychological understanding of mental disorders.

The vastly divergent, at times even contradictory, tendencies in Krafft-
Ebing's work can be explained by looking at his general career in psychiatry
and the changing institutional setting of his psychiatric practice, as well as
by considering the changes in the social background of his patients and
the way he assembled his case histories. Krafft-Ebing was one of the most
prominent psychiatrists in central Europe before Emil Kraepelin and Sigmund Freud, each in their own way, set the tone for psychiatry. Although
today Krafft-Ebing is known in particular as the author of *Psychopathia sexualis*, he worked in many branches of psychiatry and wrote several leading

textbooks. As a professor of psychiatry at the Universities of Strassburg (1872–73), Graz (1873–89), and Vienna (1889–1902), he was actively engaged in the process that caused the main institutional locus of medical psychiatry to shift from the asylum to the university, as a result of which psychiatry became more or less recognized as an academic discipline in medical faculties. Yet he also moved beyond the institutional confines of psychiatry in other ways, by advancing its moral role in society and by building his own private practice.[1]

1. For the facts on Krafft-Ebing's life and professional career, I depend for a large part on Hauser 1992 and the obituaries that appeared after Krafft-Ebing's death: Dornblüth 1902; Pagel 1902; Schüle 1902; Allerhand 1903; Eulenburg 1903; Fuchs 1903; Karplus 1903; Kornfeld 1903; Moll 1903a & 1903b; Söldner 1903; Sterz 1903; *Grazer Tagesblatt*, December 24, 1902; *Tagespost* 332 (1902); *Jahrbuch für sexuelle Zwischenstufen* 5 (1903): 1292–97. Also helpful were Fuchs 1902 & 1921; Wagner-Jauregg 1902, 1903, & 1908; Fischer 1935; Walter 1983; and Salvetti 1984.

Professional Struggles

Richard von Krafft-Ebing was born in 1840 in Mannheim, Germany. Since the Catholic Krafft-Ebing family had been ennobled around 1800 by the Austrian emperor, from birth his title was *Freiherr*, or baron. His father was a district administrator of the Grand Duchy of Baden. Richard went to school and studied medicine in Heidelberg, where his maternal grandfather, Carl Joseph Anton Mittermaier (1787–1867), was a prominent professor of criminal law. During his studies, Krafft-Ebing lived in his grandfather's house, an intellectually stimulating and enlightened environment. After passing his examinations early in 1863, which permitted him to practice as a physician, he was granted a doctoral degree later that same year. His dissertation, which was published by the renowned publishing house of Ferdinand Enke, dealt with a topic that touched on psychiatry: sensory deliria (*Die Sinnesdelirien*).[1] The book was based on research in the Illenau asylum near Baden-Baden as well as on his personal experiences with hallucinations (during his training in the ward of internal medicine in Heidelberg, he had acquired typhoid, which caused serious fevers) (1864, 9).

During the summer of 1863, Krafft-Ebing attended lectures by the famous Wilhelm Griesinger (1817–1868) in Zurich on nervous and mental illness that included clinical demonstrations at the university clinic Burghölzi. The young Krafft-Ebing was deeply impressed by Griesinger and decided to specialize in psychiatry. His grandfather, who was interested in forensic psychiatry, may also have pushed him in this direction. Not only did Mittermaier pave the way for his grandson to publish in the medico-legal journal *Friedreichs Blätter für gerichtliche Medizin*—for which Krafft-

---

1. Mittermaier probably introduced Krafft-Ebing to this leading publishing house of medical works. Enke also published several other works by Krafft-Ebing, including his textbooks and seventeen editions of *Psychopathia sexualis*. (Letter of Krafft-Ebing to Ferdinand Enke [July 24, 1865], Verlagsverträge, Archiv Ferdinand Enke Verlag).

Ebing wrote the annual review on forensic psychiatric literature beginning in 1866—his grandfather also helped him to obtain his first post in psychiatry. Mittermaier was a good friend of Christian R. W. Roller (1802–1878), medical director of the Illenau asylum and a leading figure in German psychiatry at that time. After having served as a volunteer for three months, Krafft-Ebing got an appointment as junior physician in this institution early in 1864. Before he started his training in psychiatry in Illenau, he made an instructional tour to Vienna, where he attended lectures of leading physicians of the renowned Vienna school of scientific medicine. He also visited Prague, where he gained some experience in obstetrics, and Berlin, where he attended lectures of Rudolf Virchow (1821–1902), one of the leading medical scientists in Germany.

Krafft-Ebing started his career in psychiatry in an asylum in which the idealist "moral" approach to mental disease, dating from the early nineteenth century, was still in vogue. Roller, one of the leading asylum psychiatrists in Germany at that time, was strongly committed to the idea that psychiatric diseases were "diseases of the soul" that could not be reduced to organic disorders of the brain and nervous system. According to Roller, psychiatry was a medical discipline unlike the others. He believed that mental patients should be removed from the daily social environment that had caused their insanity and be isolated in a special therapeutic setting, in a mental asylum, which functioned as a refuge, offering a special, healing atmosphere. Illenau was situated in the countryside far away from towns, with its staff living on the premises. The daily life of its patients consisted of a meticulous regime of work, religious activities, special diets, sport, and leisure activities, among which music figured prominently. One anecdote about Krafft-Ebing tells how he frequently played the piano and improvised songs, in an attempt to cheer up the patients. All activities at Illenau, in fact, had a therapeutical purpose (Schüle 1902, 313). The asylum enjoyed fame for its sophisticated facilities and the humanitarian treatment of patients; in the early 1860s, it was one of the first German asylums to introduce the nonrestraint principle, which was developed in the 1830s in England.

Krafft-Ebing's training period at the Illenau asylum proved to be profoundly formative, both in terms of his approach to patients and scientifically.[2] Although Roller strongly opposed the new medical psychiatry being developed at German universities beginning in the 1860s, his junior staff welcomed the innovative scientific ideas in mental medicine (especially

2. For Krafft-Ebing's early views on psychiatric care, see his report of his two-day visit to Gheel in Belgium in November 1866 (1867c). Gheel was famous because in this village patients lived in the community and were not hospitalized.

those of Griesinger and Morel), Darwinian biology, and the new science of experimental psychology as developed by Gustav Fechner (1801–1887) and Wilhelm Wundt (1832–1920). Krafft-Ebing used his daily interaction with patients for research, and while at Illenau he published articles on forensic psychiatry, dementia paralytica, epilepsy, transitory insanity, the connection between physical brain damage and mental disease, and the therapeutical use of electricity. For the remainder of his life, Krafft-Ebing would stay in close contact with Illenau and especially with two colleagues who became good friends: Heinrich Schüle (1840–1916), who was later director of the asylum, and Wilhelm Erb (1840–1921), who became a leading neurologist.[3] Early in 1869, after leaving Illenau, Krafft-Ebing set up practice as a nerve doctor in Baden-Baden, specializing in electrotherapy. In the same year he undertook an instructional tour through Italy and France (Krafft-Ebing 2000). During the Franco-Prussian War of 1870–71, he served at a medical station in a military camp in Rastatt, where he treated soldiers suffering from typhus (1871a). After his discharge from the army, he was put in charge of an electrotherapeutic institute in Baden-Baden.

When Krafft-Ebing started his career in the 1860s, a psychiatrist had generally little professional status; as a standard specialization, psychiatry was not well established until the end of the century. It was definitely one of the least attractive specialties within medicine for an aspiring young physician. Working in asylums, most psychiatrists—or alienists, as they were often called in the nineteenth century—were marginal figures at best, within the field of medicine as well as in society at large. At mid-century, the professional situation of asylum psychiatry was even troubling. Mental asylums provided few posts and offered hardly any prospects for a scientific career. Moreover, asylum conditions deteriorated in the second half of the century (in many respects Illenau was the exception that proved the rule). Hailed as sources of cure in the first decades of the nineteenth century, the public asylums were silting up with ever-expanding numbers of chronically ill patients. The majority of the patients of public mental institutions were drawn from the ranks of the poor and selected for essentially negative social reasons, rather than on the basis of sound medical criteria; the asylum thus began to be a last resort for paupers, beggars, the disabled, the elderly, demented patients, and those who were a nuisance or a danger to society. Cure rates were low, and the often underfunded and overcrowded asylums had increasingly less in common with ordinary hospitals, which by the 1870s, as therapeutic institutions, began to target the

3. Letters of Heinrich Schüle and Wilhelm Erb to Krafft-Ebing, Nachlass Krafft-Ebing. For the history on Illenau, see Kohl 1997.

growing group of middle-class patients, especially with the improvement of hygienic conditions and anesthetic techniques.

By that time, however, public opinion no longer considered asylums as hospitals to cure but as custodial institutions. Psychiatrists came to realize that this carried with it unintended and unwelcome professional consequences. Not only were they secluded in remote, monotonous, and oppressive institutions and thus consigned to an ignominious backwater of the medical profession, but they were also vulnerable to the accusation of locking people up on arbitrary grounds. Perceived as those in charge of removing the insane from society, alienists emerged in popular opinion more as guardians of law and order than as doctors who cured patients, even though it was invariably stressed that hospitalization was for the lunatic's own good (1890g, 1806). As long as their main institutional locus was the mental asylum, psychiatrists did little more than act as caretakers, and they could not escape the conclusion that the mental asylum had failed as a hospital. Moreover, to scientifically motivated psychiatrists, the asylum hardly proved to be a stimulating environment for their own intellectual growth.

From the birth of psychiatry around 1800, it had been a central problem for the new profession to define its expertise as a medical field. During the first half of the nineteenth century, the special character of psychiatry was justified by its emphasis on "moral treatment." This, however, did not require somatic treatment of the insane, and it was not a truly specific medical expertise. In fact, philosophers, jurists, and the clergy could and did claim to be at least as good as medical men in the practice of moral treatment (Goldstein 1987). Psychiatry's dominion included many issues fraught with explosive religious and moral implications, and this made it close to impossible for psychiatrists to carve out their own niche and gain authority as medical men. Even in the middle of the century, psychiatrists still had substantial difficulties in convincing other scholars and the public that, as physicians, they had exclusive and scientific insight into the nature of insanity. The classification of the varieties of insanity remained subject to imprecision, uncertainty, and disagreement because it generally could only be based on more or less fleeting symptoms that were exceedingly difficult to measure according to the exact standards of positivist science.

For quite some time, psychiatry's social and intellectual position was, put mildly, a vulnerable one. Alienists longed to be recognized not just as "moral entrepreneurs" in mental asylums, but as doctors and scientists. They sought to establish closer ties with the rest of the medical profession by trying to push psychiatry as an academic discipline and a natural science. By the late 1860s, it became clear that their attempts had not been altogether in vain, as the first university chairs for psychiatry were established in Germany and Austria. When Griesinger started his psychiatric clinic in the Charité Hospital in Berlin in 1865, he set the tone of university psychiatry in central Europe. Between 1866 and 1882, similar clinics were opened in Göttingen, Zurich, Vienna, Heidelberg, Munich, Strassburg, Graz, Leipzig, and Bonn. Directed by professors of psychiatry, these clinics were dedicated to research and teaching. Patients were selected on the basis of medical criteria. The new psychiatric clinics were not just hospital wards to treat patients but also teaching facilities: patients were shown to medical students and discussed on ward rounds, and they were demonstrated in lectures. In their search for knowledge of the causes of mental disorders, physicians followed the example of laboratory medicine: brain anatomy, neurophysiology, and biochemistry would lead psychiatry out of the obsolescence of the asylum and onto the road of medical status and progress. The story of psychiatry's rise as an academic discipline is closely connected, as will be discussed below, to the growing popularity of biological psychiatry during the second half of the nineteenth century (Shorter 1997, 71–81).

Krafft-Ebing, who following his dissertation had published numerous articles and some monographs, was one of those psychiatrists hoping to find a position at a university. In the 1869 annual report of the local Medical Officer of Health in Baden, he was characterized as "an ambitious man thoroughly educated in the sciences" and as someone who "takes a great interest in forensic medicine and psychiatry and hopes one day to lecture on these subjects at a university" (cited in Hauser 1992, 32). Just when Krafft-Ebing was applying at the University of Leipzig in 1872, he was nominated adjunct professor of psychiatry at the University of Strassburg. Strassburg had been conquered from France in the Franco-Prussian War, and the German authorities attempted to turn this university into a showcase of German science. However, because of the poor clinical and teaching facilities, and perhaps also because Krafft-Ebing—who admired French culture and science—disagreed with the highly nationalist Prussian policies, he left Strassburg within a year to become medical superintendent of Feldhof, the newly established mental asylum of the Austrian province of Styria, situated a few miles from Graz.[4] This position comprised a professorship in psychiatry at the University of Graz as well.

Upon his arrival in Graz, Krafft-Ebing's professional élan was again se-

4. Krafft-Ebing's psychiatric interests (sexual pathology, forensic issues, and hypnotism) as well as his theoretical frame (degeneration theory combined with psychological approaches) were heavily influenced by French examples. His Francophile leanings had been fostered by the cultural climate in Baden, which was geared toward France rather than Prussia (Hauser 1992, 320–21).

verely challenged. As an adjunct professor, his position in the university's medical faculty was weak. Moreover, teaching psychiatry to medical students proved no easy task. Krafft-Ebing felt that medical students should be exposed to both psychiatric theory and clinical practice. Clinical teaching in Feldhof was inconvenient for several reasons: the asylum was located outside of town, quite a distance from the university; there were only chronic patients, who could hardly be cured; and he faced serious internal opposition to using patients in his teaching because others felt that the presence of strangers could upset them and aggravate their illness, as would be the risk of public examinations and demonstrations of their cases.[5] Apart from teaching facilities in the asylum, Krafft-Ebing needed a psychiatric clinic at the university, so that he could demonstrate patients to his students, preferably "fresh and curable cases," as he phrased it in a letter to the provincial administration. Much to his disappointment, he was only granted a small observation ward.[6]

There were substantial differences between the asylum in Illenau and the large and overcrowded asylum in Feldhof. Designed for 320 patients, it held 400 in 1879, Krafft-Ebing reported, and three years later there were 516 inmates (1879, 3; Laehr 1882, 64; cf. Laehr and Lewald 1899, 105). Whereas Illenau's medical staff could work in relative independence of government interference, Feldhof directly fell under the Department of Health in Vienna and the provincial government of Styria, which in the asylum was represented by a nonmedical administrator. Although Krafft-Ebing insisted that the management of asylums should be in medical hands, as medical director he continued to be dependent on government officials who often applied nonmedical criteria for the admission of patients (1881). In Feldhof he was faced with generally poor, uneducated, chronic, and sometimes violent patients who were difficult to treat and who included criminals suffering from mental derangements.

In a very critical account of the conditions in which the insane lived in Styria, published as a brochure in 1879, Krafft-Ebing presented a dismal picture of the asylum. After expressing his indignation about the inhuman treatment the insane received from their relatives outside the asylum, he asserted not only that Feldhof was too small to admit all patients from Styria, but also that it had not lived up to expectations. Therapeutic facilities were lacking, the staff was forced to resort to outdated methods like

5. Letters of the medizinischen Fakultät der k. k. Universität Graz to the Ministerium für Cultus und Unterricht (March 17, 1881) and of Krafft-Ebing to the medizinischen Fakultät der k. k. Universität Graz (October 10, 1881), Archiv Karl Franzens Universität Graz.
6. Letters of Krafft-Ebing to the Landes-Ausschuss des Herzogthums Steiermark (April 8, 1873) and the Professoren Collegium der medizinischen Fakultät der k. k. Universität Graz (October 22, 1873), Archiv Karl Franzens Universität Graz.

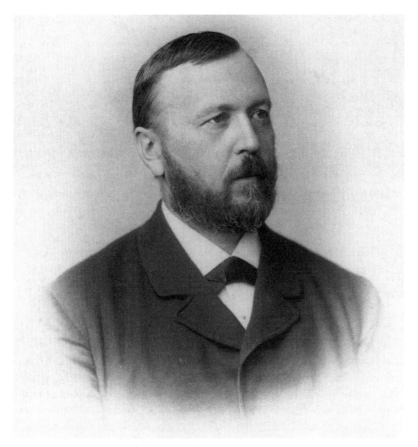

Figure 5. Krafft-Ebing around 1880. (Krafft-Ebing Family Archive, Graz, Austria)

restraint and isolation cells, and the physical health of the patients left much to be desired. All hope of curing patients had vanished, Krafft-Ebing continued: the wards were filled with numerous restless and raving patients, and only 20 percent of those admitted to Feldhof could look forward to an improvement of their condition. Many patients stayed on in the asylum until their, often premature, death. In such an institution, psychiatry had become more akin to routine custodial care than to a gratifying professional and scientific calling. Krafft-Ebing also complained about the bad location of the asylum and its poor architectural structure, which was unsuited for its medical purpose.

> Leaving aside whether or not public opinion is right in claiming that a lunatic asylum should never have been built on this place outside Graz— exposed to storms as well as the heat of the sun, with poor connecting

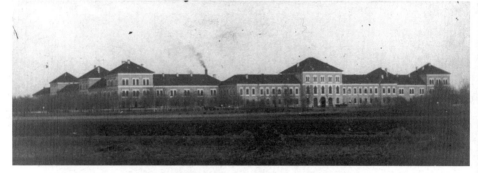

Figure 6. The mental asylum Feldhof near Graz, where Krafft-Ebing became medical superintendent in 1872. (Krafft-Ebing Family Archive, Graz, Austria)

roads to the town, and without a park, it cannot be denied from a technical point of view that the very simple architectural design of this asylum might indeed facilitate the care of massive numbers of chronic, mostly incurable patients; yet is hardly appropriate for a hospital with the aim to cure people. (1879, 15)

The best solution, Krafft-Ebing concluded, would be the construction of a new mental hospital in Graz, which should include a university clinic and admit patients on a voluntary basis as well. Whereas admission to an asylum was subject to legal regulations and usually involved time-consuming bureaucratic procedures, in clinics only medical criteria would be applied.

Confronted with authorities and lay management who were reluctant to accept medical expertise as the crucial factor in the running of a mental asylum, Krafft-Ebing's efforts to reform Feldhof failed. Disillusioned with the prospects of a large public asylum, Krafft-Ebing withdrew from asylum management and turned his full attention to the university. Since 1874 he had been in charge of a small clinical ward for the observation of psychiatric patients in the old mental asylum of Graz. What he wanted was a larger psychiatric and nervous clinic within the general hospital of the university, close to the other medical departments and dedicated exclusively to the medical treatment of potentially curable patients (1890b, 17). He felt that it was important that this clinic admitted patients whom he would be allowed to use as illustration material in lectures for medical students who did not specialize in psychiatry. As prospective general practitioners, these students should be trained in the early diagnosis of mental illness.[7] With an eye to his teaching, research, and writing, as well as to being able to

7. Letter of Krafft-Ebing to the Professoren Collegium der medizinischen Fakultät der k.k. Universität Graz (October 22, 1873), Archiv Karl Franzens Universität Graz.

design effective methods of treatment, Krafft-Ebing needed a wider variety and a higher turnover of more acute patients than the asylum could provide for. What he wanted was, as he put it, good "usable patient-material" (1890b, 9). This was especially important for demonstrations so as to make his lectures more concrete and attractive for medical students, for whom courses in psychiatry were not compulsory, and to convince a nonmedical audience of the social importance of psychiatry. Apparently, he presented many patients in his lectures and courses; in 1890 he reported that to this end he had called upon some three thousand of them in the previous seventeen years (1890b, 33).

After his resignation as medical superintendent of Feldhof in 1880, Krafft-Ebing focused his activities on teaching and research. He had already established a reputation in the academic world with a series of publications on various subjects. Within psychiatric circles, his work on temporary mental derangements, including the so-called *Dämmerzustand* (a mental state between dreaming and being awake) and *Zwangsvorstellung* (irresistible thoughts, later conceptualized as obsessive-compulsive disorder), was considered innovative (1864; 1865; 1867b; 1868a). Even more important were his numerous publications on legal issues: he tackled questions involving, for instance, criminal acts under the influence of alcohol, the legal responsibility of hysterical patients, the self-accusations of the mentally ill, the validity of legal testimony in different psychopathological conditions, and dubious mental states in civil law.[8] He was a pioneer and leading expert in the field of forensic psychiatry, and his *Lehrbuch der gerichtlichen Psychopathologie* (1875) was the first textbook in the German-speaking world to separate psychiatry from the rest of medicine as far as legal matters were concerned.

Throughout, his writings in this area show that he sought to broaden the field of psychiatry. Again and again, he argued that the current legal stipulations for distinguishing between offenders responsible for their actions and those who were not were far too formal and narrow. Usually, judges only accepted the diagnosis of lasting intellectual impairment as a valid symptom of insanity. According to Krafft-Ebing, this juridical conception of mental illness, and hence that of legal irresponsibility, was outdated: modern psychiatry showed that mental illness could be of a transitory nature and that it also included disordered emotions and deficient moral consciousness, which, apparently, left reason intact. Affective disorders figured prominently in his work:

8. 1865; 1867a; 1867b; 1868a; 1868b; 1868d; 1869e; 1871b; 1872a; 1872b; 1872c; 1873a; 1873b; 1873d; 1873e; & 1875c. He also wrote reviews for the main German psychiatric journals, covering virtually all the contemporary forensic literature.

Deluded by the idea that only those people are insane who talk madly, one has simply ignored the expressions of disturbed feeling. Being ignorant of the insights of modern psychology that the imagination of man essentially depends on the quality of his feeling and that the motives of his will and actions are primarily determined by his feeling, one has completely failed to understand how disturbed feelings can make human action unfree. (1867b, 9–10)

In addition, many mental disruptions were caused by, for example, dreaming, sleepwalking, somnambulism, hallucinations, intoxications, alcohol, fevers, or epilepsy, and these could not be taken for insanity as such but were nevertheless highly relevant from a forensic viewpoint. The same applied to several cases of pelvic disorders caused by gynecological lesions, menstruation, excessive masturbation, and sexual excitement without orgasm, which, Krafft-Ebing believed, could produce delusions. Essentially, he tried to convince his readers that there were many mental conditions that suspended the powers of the free will but that were very difficult to identify as pathological by laypersons. Echoing the physiological conception of disease, he pointed out that modern medical science demonstrated that there was no clear boundary between the normal and pathological. All these arguments served one clear message: since deranged emotions and impulses could drive man to commit criminal acts and since there was good reason to speak of diminished criminal responsibility in such cases, the psychiatrist should have more say in jurisdiction vis-à-vis lawyers and others such as police authorities, clergymen, and educators.

These forensic considerations also inspired his best-selling *Psychopathia sexualis*, which procured him fame—although not uncontested—inside as well as outside the medical world. Especially in the field of homosexuality, Krafft-Ebing was confronted not only with lawyers, but also with forensic experts in somatic medicine, who were responsible for furnishing physical proof of "unnatural vice." Their investigation was generally restricted to a physical examination, and they in fact supported the prevailing juridical approach. Psychiatrists like Krafft-Ebing, however, focused on the personality of the offender and cast doubts on the current interpretation of the law. By the turn of the century, the somatic experts in forensic medicine had lost some of their authority in Austrian courts, while the psychiatric viewpoint was partly acknowledged. From 1901 on, homosexual offenders could be cleared of charges if a psychiatrist diagnosed a "psychopathological condition" and concluded that the offense had been committed under the influence of an "irresistible urge" (Hacker 1987, 29; cf. Müller 1991, 109–10).

With his three-volume *Lehrbuch der Psychiatrie auf klinischer Grundlage*

(1879–80), partly based on hundreds of observations, Krafft-Ebing established his reputation as a leader in clinical psychiatry. It became a standard textbook in psychiatry and would remain so for two decades until it was replaced by that of Emil Kraepelin.[9] Over the years, seven editions came out as well as translations in English, French, Italian, and Hungarian. Like other nineteenth-century psychiatrists, Krafft-Ebing was eager to contribute to a valid classification of psychiatric diseases. The basic psychiatric disorders, according to Krafft-Ebing, could be divided into three categories: emotional disturbances (feelings and dispositions, including strong variations therein), mental derangements (involving the mind, memory, imagination), and those of a psychomotoric nature (drives and will). Beyond these groups, his classification of the psychoses was based on a series of dichotomies. He differentiated between psychoses with and without intellectual retardation as well as between those with or without lesions of the brain (organic versus so-called functional psychoses or psychoneuroses). The functional psychoses were subdivided into degenerative and non-degenerative as well as into melancholia (defined as "a painful inhibition of psychological functions") and mania ("an exalted facilitation of psychological functions") (1872d; cf. Berrios 1995, 392).

Krafft-Ebing was a highly organized and efficient author, digesting vast amounts of literature—German as well as English, French, and Italian—and using and reusing the same material for different purposes. His published work amounts to hundreds of articles and about ninety books (including numerous reeditions and translations). He published on a wide variety of subjects, including forensic issues, the classification and causes of mental disorders, alcoholism, moral insanity, sexual perversions, melancholia, paranoia, epilepsy, paralysis, multiple sclerosis, peripheral nerve lesions, obsessive behavior, tabes, neurosyphilis, hysteria, neurasthenia and nervousness, the psychiatric implications of menstruation, the therapeutic use of electricity and hypnosis, administrative and legal issues of psychiatric treatment, and the teaching of psychiatry at the university (Hauser 1992, 388–453). At the end of his career, several of his articles were collected in four volumes under the title *Arbeiten aus dem Gesammtgebiet der Psychiatrie und Neuropathologie* (1897–99). Translations of his works into English, Italian, French, Hungarian, Russian, Swedish, Dutch, Spanish, and Japanese contributed to his international reputation. He was on many editorial boards and contributed on a regular basis to prestigious journals like the forensic *Friedreichs Blätter für gerichtliche Medizin*, the *Allgemeine Zeitschrift für Psychiatrie* (the official organ of German asylum psychiatrists), and the

9. Carl Gustav Jung (1875–1961) recalled in 1925 that Krafft-Ebing's textbook had inspired him to become a psychiatrist (McGuire 1989, 7).

academic *Jahrbücher für Psychiatrie und Neurologie*, the journal of the Austrian Verein für Psychiatrie und Neurologie. He also contributed on a regular basis to *Der Irrenfreund* and some Vienna-based medical journals.

In 1882 Krafft-Ebing, who was in a relatively powerless academic position as *Extraordinarius*, acquired a full professorship, and five years later neurology was added to his chair.[10] At the same time, the small psychiatric observation clinic was extended with a ward for nervous disorders (Fossel 1913, 17; Hauser 1992, 87). His struggle for clinical psychiatric wards in the university's general hospital—which he won in 1886 only after having threatened to leave Graz for a professorship in Freiburg—was not only a strategic move to strengthen his position in academia, but also of importance for the configuration of psychiatry as a promising medical specialty.[11] Three years later, in 1889, Krafft-Ebing moved to the more prestigious University of Vienna, which had two chairs of psychiatry. He first succeeded Max Leidesdorf (1818–1889) on what was named the first chair of psychiatry; in 1892, after the death of Theodor Meynert (1833–1892), he obtained one of the most prestigious positions in psychiatry when he was elected to the second chair while also receiving the honorary title of *Hofrath*. The first chair was linked to a provincial mental asylum, the Niederösterreichischen Landesirrenanstalt, the second to a smaller psychiatric clinic in Vienna's general hospital. Whereas the asylum mainly hospitalized chronic patients and its supervision included many administrative tasks, the clinic in the hospital, which carried more academic prestige, only admitted a limited number of more acute patients with mental as well as neurological disorders.[12] In 1892 Krafft-Ebing also succeeded Meynert as president of the Verein für Psychiatrie und forensische Psychologie (renamed Verein für Psychiatrie und Neurologie in 1894), the most important professional organization for psychiatrists in Austria. Unlike Meynert, who was obstinate and antagonized people, Krafft-Ebing was a diplomatic chairman who enlisted people's support; under his leadership, the membership of the society tripled, from 50 to 150 members. From 1895 until 1901, Sigmund Freud was a member of the administrative committee. Although Krafft-Ebing dismissed Freud's seduction theory at a 1896 meeting of the society as a "scientific fairy tale" and although he felt that Freud generally did not empirically

10. Letter of the Ministerium für Cultus und Unterricht Z. 7008 to the Dekanat der medizinischen Fakultät der k. k. Universität Graz (May 5, 1882), Archiv Karl Franzens Universität Graz.

11. Wagner-Jauregg 1902, 318; Wagner-Jauregg, Festrede zur Enthüllung der von Krafft-Ebing-Büste. Manuskript. Obersteinerbibliothek des neurologischen Instituts, Universität von Wien, 5.

12. For the development of psychiatry in Vienna in the 1880s and 1890s, see Lesky 1965, 183–91, 373–405; Berner et al. 1983; Hirschmüller 1989 & 1991; and Gröger, Gabriel, and Kasper 1997.

validate his theories with a sufficient number of cases, the two men must have been on good professional terms. Freud owned Krafft-Ebing's textbooks and regularly received autographed copies of his works on sexual pathology; moreover, Krafft-Ebing actively supported Freud's application for a professorship at the University of Vienna.[13]

Krafft-Ebing established himself firmly at the university in Vienna, like earlier in Graz, but he was nevertheless engaged in a continuous struggle with the medical faculty and university administrators over lack of resources, poor facilities, and the establishment of psychiatry as a medical specialty, fully integrated into the curriculum.[14] He complained that psychiatry was merely an optional specialization and not an obligatory subject in the curriculum of the medical faculty—only between 5 and 10 percent of all medical students took his courses (1890h). In his view, it was a scandal that the majority of general practitioners, who in Austria were authorized to commit individuals to a mental asylum, had not received any training in the diagnosis of mental illness.

> If citizens were only digesting, breathing, moving machines, one could be satisfied with such a state of affairs. However, they are feeling, thinking, and acting beings who, moreover, bear responsibility for their actions. Their psychical functions are a valuable asset for the state and their development, maintenance, and recovery, if disturbed, should belong to the most important interests of society. (1890h, 776)

The lack of psychiatric knowledge among physicians in general was all the more deplorable, Krafft-Ebing asserted, because many admissions to mental asylums could be prevented if general practitioners were able to diagnose the first symptoms of arising insanity; in an early stage, many mental illnesses were still curable. Moreover, a course in psychiatry would make doctors more attentive to the many people in modern society who had lost their mental balance and who were in imminent danger of becoming mentally ill. The study of psychiatry was useful, Krafft-Ebing admonished his students,

> since it will sharpen your experience and knowledge with regard to all those individuals in today's society who, to be true, are not considered to be mentally ill, but who nevertheless may not be considered as men-

---

13. Hauser 1992, 147–61; for Krafft-Ebing's influence on Freud, see also Sulloway 1979; Swales 1983; and Gay 1988, 136–40.

14. Exhibiten-Protokoll 1872/1873–1888/1889, medizinischen Fakultät der k. k. Universität Graz, Archiv Karl Franzens Universität Graz; Med. Pers. Akt Krafft-Ebing, Archiv Universität von Wien; Personalakt Krafft-Ebing, Allgemeines Verwaltungsarchiv des Österreichischen Staatsarchivs. See also Krafft-Ebing 1889a; 1890b, 20–22, 28; 1890h; 1890i; Wagner-Jauregg 1902, 319.

tally well-balanced. They display various malfunctions in their mental and moral personality and they are misguided and odd in their way of acting, feeling, and thinking. (1890g, 1803)

For medical students who did not specialize in psychiatry, it was particularly important to be confronted with mild and acute cases of mental and nervous illness, such as the neurotics, neurasthenics, hysterics, and hypochondriacs who were admitted to his psychiatric clinic. However, the clinic of Vienna's general hospital was in fact no more than an observation ward for incoming patients that lacked the space, tranquillity, and stability necessary to examine the progression of acute mental disorders, to experiment with new treatments, and to teach medical students. In Vienna, as in Graz, the pressure of nonmedical regulations for admitting, transferring, and discharging growing numbers of (chronic) patients placed great strains on the orderly functioning of the university clinic in which research and teaching had to be priorities (1890i; 1896c, 29).

The desire to escape the constraints and frustrations of institutional psychiatry must have driven Krafft-Ebing to further broaden and diversify his professional territory. At the Universities of Graz and Vienna, he tried to push the boundaries of psychiatry into the direction of neurology, partly because the anatomy and physiology of the nervous system were promising fields that were part of established medical science. Some neurologists tried to establish their professional identity by setting themselves apart from psychiatrists; American neurologists had succeeded in doing so as early as 1875, but in central Europe the two medical specialties were closely connected. Krafft-Ebing asserted that psychiatry was a branch of neurology and that psychiatric clinics should be linked up with neurological clinics rather than with asylums (1890b, 29). This clearly served the purpose of distancing himself from the lunatic asylum while strengthening his ties with mainstream medicine.

Already in 1869, after his training in psychiatry at Illenau, Krafft-Ebing had established himself as a "nerve doctor" in Baden-Baden, and during the rest of his career, he would be engaged with organic nervous disorders, especially tabes dorsalis, a paralysis of the legs often accompanied by mental derangement, and general paralysis—at that time also known as, respectively, progressive paralysis, tabes cerebralis, paralytic madness, and dementia paralytica. From the middle of the nineteenth century on, physicians postulated that these diseases were late manifestations of syphilis, an assumption that was definitively proved in 1905 when the syphilitic spirochetes was discovered and then found in tabetic and paralytic patients. In fact, neurosyphilis was the only psychiatric disease that eventually proved to be a successful target for bacteriological research. Under Krafft-Ebing's supervision, one of his assistants, Josef Adolf Hirschl (1865–1914), experimentally tested the causal link between syphilis and general paralysis. Nine patients who suffered from general paralysis were injected with the fluid from the sores of known syphilitics. Because during the subsequent six months the patients showed no reaction to the injection, Krafft-Ebing and Hirschl concluded that they already had syphilis. Although this experiment was controversial from an ethical point of view, which is why Hirschl's name was not made public, Krafft-Ebing presented these results in 1897 at one of the plenary sessions of the twelfth International Congress of Medicine in Moscow—a definite sign of the international prestige he enjoyed (1900a; cf. Benedikt 1906, 395).

The alliance with neurology was a means to raise not only the scientific level of psychiatry but also its social prestige as it attracted more patients from the middle and upper classes who feared being associated with the insane. By advertising psychiatric care as involving "nerves" and by posing as "nerve doctors," psychiatrists met the needs of this lucrative clientele, who at all costs wished to avoid confinement in a mental asylum, primarily geared as it was to housing the incurably and chronically insane of the pauper classes. Social prejudices concerning asylum psychiatry entailed that physicians in private practices and "nervous" clinics often used face-saving organic diagnoses to avoid the odium of mental disease. Hearing that one suffered from a physical disorder of the nerves was far more acceptable than learning that one was mentally deranged (Shorter 1992, 216–17; 1997, 113). Nervous diseases were not supposed to be part of institutional psychiatry. In the last three decades of the nineteenth century, numerous private "nervous" clinics and sanatoriums were established in central Europe for well-paying middle- and upper-class patients. These offered a variety of physical treatments such as massages, rest cures, and various other therapies (including electro-, light, hydro-, and dietary therapies). Although they would never advertise this, many of these establishments also admitted psychiatric patients, as long as they were controllable and kept quiet.[15]

Krafft-Ebing had an active role in this expansion of psychiatric care. Along with his clinical work, he developed a private practice, and in 1886 he founded the sanatorium Mariagrün in a suburb of Graz for an exclusive, wealthy clientele suffering from a variety of psychosomatic complaints and relatively mild nervous disorders, especially neurasthenia. Nervous diseases not only referred to somatic disorders of the central and peripheral nervous system, but also to neurosis, "nervousness," or "weak" and "tired" nerves.

15. Shorter 1990, 183; on the role of private institutions in the development of psychiatry, see Ackerknecht 1986; Shorter 1989; cf. Berger 1892.

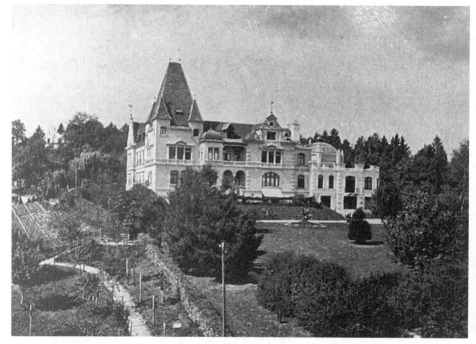

Figure 7. The sanatorium Mariagrün founded in 1886 by Krafft-Ebing. (Krafft-Ebing Family Archive, Graz, Austria)

Publishing scientific as well as popular works on neurasthenia, Krafft-Ebing played an important part in the introduction of this new and fashionable, but also rather vague disease category in central Europe. Neurasthenia, conceptualized as an exhaustion of the energy of the central nervous system, had been coined as a clinical entity by the American neurologist George M. Beard (1839–1883) in 1869, and his main works on the subject were translated into German in the early 1880s. The explanation of neurasthenia resembled the energy model that also defined the understanding of nonprocreative sexual activities. It was widely believed that the supply of vital force in humans was finite and that an overburdening of the mental faculties would tax the body in other processes. According to Beard and other doctors, the overexpenditure of nervous energy was caused by the demands of modern urbanized society in which an increasing proportion of the population was engaged in sedentary brain work rather than supposedly healthy physical labor. Krafft-Ebing also explained neurasthenia in terms of a disturbance of the balance between the accumulation and the expenditure of nerve force.

Neurasthenia was posited as a functional nervous disease, and it occu-

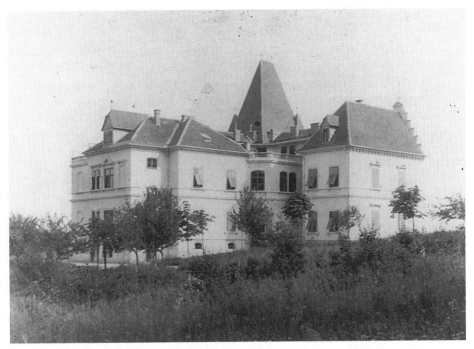

Figure 8. The sanatorium Mariagrün. (Krafft-Ebing Family Archive, Graz, Austria)

pied a broad borderland between mental health and insanity.[16] Krafft-Ebing diagnosed many of his private patients as suffering from neurasthenia; their treatment was important for the prevention of more serious nervous and mental disorders, he maintained, because these could emerge from affected nerves. These patients were not (yet) insane and should not be hospitalized in asylums but treated in other (semi-)medical institutions. In the commercial brochure Krafft-Ebing published together with Anton Stichl and his former assistant Hugo Gugl, who were in charge of Mariagrün, the sanatorium was advertised as a comfortable place to stay, "far removed from the hassles of the world" for "all those fellow men who have been shaken in their nervous powers by the pressures of life." They explicitly stressed that "mentally disturbed patients" were excluded.[17] Most of the middle- and upper-class patients treated between 1887 and 1891 in Mariagrün were diagnosed with neurasthenia (nearly 60 percent), followed by hysteria (nearly 25 percent), morphinism (morphine addiction; nearly 10 percent),

16. On the conceptualization of neurasthenia, see Gosling 1987 and Shorter 1992, 222–27; for a social history of nervousness in Germany, see Radkau 1998.

17. Gugl, Krafft-Ebing, and Stichl 1886, 3–4; cf. Laehr and Lewald 1899, 106; Hauser 1992, 118, 126.

and spinal disease (about 5 percent) (Gugl and Stichl 1892, 15–16). They
were offered a peaceful and pleasant environment, rest cures, copious diets,
facilities for entertainment, physical therapies such as massages, and a variety of different baths. Implicitly these well-paying patients were permitted
to be demanding with the staff. Whereas in asylums and clinical wards
Krafft-Ebing mainly treated lower-class patients with more or less serious
mental derangements, the sanatorium as well as his private practice catered
to men and women from the higher ranks of society for whom hospitalization was not desirable. Among them were several members of the German,
Austrian, and Hungarian aristocracy and other wealthy patients from all
over Europe; they provided Krafft-Ebing the reputation of a "society doctor."[18] Although he also advocated the establishment of public institutions
for nervous patients of the lower classes, he must have been clear-minded
enough to see that here was a profitable market to be exploited (1895a,
128; Karplus 1903, 21). This clientele was not only more interesting and
more rewarding than the generally poor asylum population, but it also gave
him the possibility of uplifting the social prestige of psychiatry.

Krafft-Ebing ventured beyond the asylum and the clinic to seek a new
clientele as well as to enlarge the audience for the new medical specialty,
not only among medical students and physicians but also among the lay
public. In various ways—in lectures, demonstrations, writings—he tried to
popularize psychiatry. Being a good lecturer and often demonstrating patients, Krafft-Ebing's courses in Vienna attracted a large audience, consisting of medical students as well as others (Söldner 1903, 224; Stekel
1950, 80). His contemporaries have characterized his lectures as "showy,"
"glamorous," and "highly sensational," as theater performances rather than
academic lectures (Stransky 1938, 195–96; Szeps-Zuckerkandl 1939, 165–
66). In this respect he resembled the famous French neurologist Jean-
Martin Charcot, whose clinical lectures on hysteria in Paris were also
public happenings.[19] On occasion, Krafft-Ebing's more or less public activities—such as lectures, spectacular demonstrations of hypnosis, and his

18. Thus Krafft-Ebing was, for example, consulted by Paul, duke of Mecklenburg (Autograph 213/61–3, Österreichische Nationalbibliothek, Vienna). He advised his friend and colleague Bernhard von Gudden, who treated King Ludwig II of Bavaria until they both drowned
in the Starnberg lake (Szeps-Zuckerkandl 1939, 129). Krafft-Ebing was also rumored to have
treated Crown Prince Rudolf of Austria and his mother, Empress Elisabeth. Evidence for this
is lacking, however; early in 1889, a month after Rudolf's suicide, the Habsburg court issued
a statement explicitly denying that Krafft-Ebing had treated Elisabeth for neurasthenia (Johnston 1972, 232; Morton 1980, 290). Elisabeth's youngest sister Sophie as well as Kaiser Wilhelm's mother-in-law, Adelheid von Schleswig-Holstein, were among the many aristocratic
patients in the sanatorium Mariagrün (Krafft-Ebing 2000, 160).

19. Charcot's calling card in Krafft-Ebing's estate suggests that they met when Krafft-
Ebing visited Paris.

treatment of high-placed patients—were covered by the press. Moritz
Benedikt (1835–1920), a professor of electrotherapy in Vienna who dis-
qualified Krafft-Ebing's scientific stature, noted slightingly that Krafft-
Ebing, dealing with "fashionable" topics like neurasthenia, sexual perversions, and hypnosis, had a fine nose for "worldly success" and was endowed
with "journalistic talent" (Benedikt 1894, 75–76).[20]

Krafft-Ebing also sought to advance the moral authority of his specialty
in the wider community. He believed that as a psychiatrist he had a moral
task to fulfill in society. Especially in the fields of forensic psychiatry and
sexual pathology, he posed as an enlightened moral entrepreneur: ignorance and prejudice should make way for a scientific and humanitarian approach. Deeply influenced by his grandfather Mittermaier, who advocated
reforms in jurisdiction, punishment, and the prison system, the forensic
field had been an incentive for Krafft-Ebing to specialize in psychiatry after
his medical studies. Again and again, he insisted that jurisdiction and punishment had to be geared toward a medical diagnosis and that criminals
who couldn't be held responsible for their actions should be treated medically rather than being punished. Especially in the field of sexual perversion, he began to take a stand against what he viewed as ignorance and
prejudice about moral offenders, whom as a forensic expert he came to
know so well. Only those who were aware of the immorality of their actions
and who could control their leanings were considered to be responsible
and punishable in a legal sense. Stressing the significance of the distinction
between immoral perversity and sickly perversion, Krafft-Ebing repeatedly
insisted that only professional psychiatrists were qualified to diagnose mental illness in court. Echoing the concept of moral insanity, he pointed out
that acts covered by the law were often behaviors of a pathological nature
over which moral offenders had hardly any control. Although individuals
who suffered from moral insanity were a danger to society, they should not
be considered as criminals but as sick persons, as "stepchildren of nature"
in need of compassion. In a popular lecture on the development of morality, he asserted that it was the task of science to save "moral idiots" who
suffered from a defective development of their brain, from scorn:

> Science shows that such moral monsters are stepchildren of nature, un-
> fortunate creatures, against whom society has to protect itself, to be sure,
> but who should merely be rendered harmless and who should not be

20. Benedikt, who said of Krafft-Ebing that "scientifically and critically he was incapable
to the point of feeblemindedness," seems to have been one of Krafft-Ebing's most explicit
enemies at the University of Vienna (Benedikt 1906, 392). Benedikt, who felt underestimated
by many of his colleagues, criticized Krafft-Ebing because of his supposedly lenient views on
homosexuality, his experiments on paralytic patients, and his hypnotic demonstrations. These
attacks were partly motivated by professional envy. On Benedikt, see Ellenberger 1993.

made to suffer for their social incapacity and their sexuality, for which they cannot be held responsible. (1892h, 8)

As a member of the liberal intelligentsia, Krafft-Ebing, although not politically active in a strict sense, generally felt obliged to raise his voice against social evils on behalf of mental and moral health. Together with Max Nordau (1849–1923), among others, he contributed to a manifesto denouncing anti-Semitism—*Freiheit, Liebe, Menschlichkeit. Ein Manifest des Geistes von hervorragenden Zeitgenossen*—published in 1893, in which he denounced the increasing class antagonisms and ethnic conflicts as a "spiritual epidemic." He also supported the pacifist movement of Bertha von Suttner (1843–1914), expressed his aversion to the rising nationalism, and expounded the ideal of an international legal order that would ban war (1892h, 16–18; Stekel 1950, 62). Addressing a wide nonmedical audience from time to time, Krafft-Ebing also revealed himself as a cultural critic. Like many others in fin de siècle Europe, he believed that mental and nervous diseases were increasing and that these were typical for modern industrialized and urbanized society (1884a). At the same time he took a strong stand against the widespread distrust of natural science. When asked to give a lecture on the history of the plague in Vienna for the Volksbildungsverein, he dealt with the panic that had broken out after three people involved in laboratory experiments with animals involving the plague had been infected and died. Criticism of science was also voiced in the Austrian parliament. Krafft-Ebing, however, pleaded for scientific research even though certain risks could not be ruled out; laboratory experimentation, he argued, was the only way to suppress this contagious disease that had claimed thousands of lives in the past (1899b).

Although Krafft-Ebing was at the apex of his career while in Vienna, he never felt at home in this city as he had earlier in Graz. The academic climate in Vienna was spoiled by power struggles and intrigues, and Krafft-Ebing, not one to make enemies easily, was engaged in an uphill struggle for years. Notwithstanding his aversion to divisions and dissension, he seems to have antagonized some of his colleagues in the medical faculty as well as some government officials. Partly due to his outspoken views on forensic issues and also on sexual perversions—views that were often considered too lenient—he was passed over for a position on Austria's Supreme Medical Council (Benedikt 1906, 392; Wagner-Jauregg 1950). At the end of the nineteenth century, forensic experts were increasingly emphasizing the extent to which mentally disturbed defendants posed a danger to society instead of pointing to illness as an extenuating circumstance.

In a letter to a friend, written early in 1894, Krafft-Ebing expressed his frustration with Vienna as well as with the clinic and hospital where he practiced. He complained bitterly about

Vienna with its soot, dust, wind, lack of walks for me and my family, its miserable clinic which sneers at every human feeling and the bureau-cratic spirit which rules the hospital, not to mention the Jewishness with which one is confronted everywhere. . . . For the next ten years there is no hope for the clinics here. Not only money, but also many other things are lacking. . . . [O]ne's feeling and fair aspiration have to be blunted to endure the miserable conditions of my clinic, the stain on Vienna. Ethi-cal sacrifices are the most difficult to make, for one sacrifices a large part of one's own moral substance.[21]

Weighed down by many time-consuming administrative duties, badly equipped wards, and high numbers of incurable patients, Krafft-Ebing re-tired early in 1902 at the age of sixty-one (Fuchs 1902, 264). After cele-brating his thirtieth anniversary as a professor of psychiatry at the Univer-sity of Vienna, he returned to Graz to devote himself to writing and his work for the sanatorium.[22] However, his lifestyle had never been a healthy one: he was overweight and overworked, always making long hours late at night, while drinking large amounts of black coffee.[23] During his last term at the University of Vienna, he suffered from chronic pains due to migraine and neuralgia.[24] All this had taken its toll over the years. At the end of the first year of his retirement, Krafft-Ebing died at the age of sixty-two. Just before his death, he managed to reedit the twelfth edition of *Psychopathia sexualis* and the seventh edition of his psychiatric textbook. He also com-pleted a substantial monograph on menstrual psychosis.

In his obituaries, written by close friends, students, and colleagues, Krafft-Ebing is depicted as a serious, hardworking man with a strong sense of duty. All noted his aristocratic appearance and complaisant character. Obviously he strongly believed in good manners and bourgeois respectabil-ity, and in his association with other scholars he was very diplomatic. As his friend Heinrich Schüle wrote: "He did not easily open himself up to others and associate with people; he was formal and reserved by nature" (Schüle 1902, 327). He was attacked several times, but unlike many of his

21. Letter of Krafft-Ebing to an unidentified friend (February 26, 1894), autograph 469/16–2, Österreichische Nationalbibliothek, Vienna. Krafft-Ebing's anti-Semitic statement is surprising in the light of his firm rejection of racism.
22. Akademisches Jubiläum des Hofrathes Freiherrn von Krafft-Ebing 1902–3, 1–2; Fest-schrift Freiherr von Krafft-Ebing 1902.
23. Communication by Marion Krafft-Ebing, granddaughter of Richard von Krafft-Ebing.
24. Letter of Krafft-Ebing to an unidentified friend (October 23, 1902), autograph 146/38–1, 2, Österreichische Nationalbibliothek, Vienna.

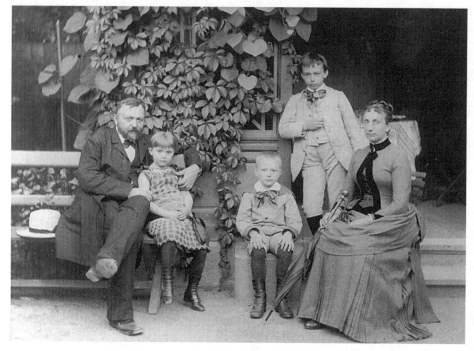

Figure 9. Krafft-Ebing with his wife, two sons, and daughter around 1884. (Krafft-Ebing Family Archive, Graz, Austria)

colleagues, he tried to avoid personal polemic. Apparently Krafft-Ebing was not able to cope with the highly competitive academic climate and the ruthless plotting and scheming by some of his colleagues. Moreover, his successor Julius Wagner-Jauregg clearly suggested that Krafft-Ebing's complaisance bordered on the naive:

> He was . . . extremely dignified by nature, and this was not always to his advantage. He was very peace-loving. In his entire life, he never wrote a polemic article and in his professional as well as in his private life he avoided any controversy or fight. He was perfectly honest, without any distrust. He did not even harbor the degree of suspicion which is part of the common insight into human nature, . . . and his goodness was often taken advantage of.[25]

At the same time he had few close friends; as a dedicated father to his family, he seems to have confined all intimacy to his wife—since 1874 he

25. *Grazer Tagesblatt*, December 24, 1902.

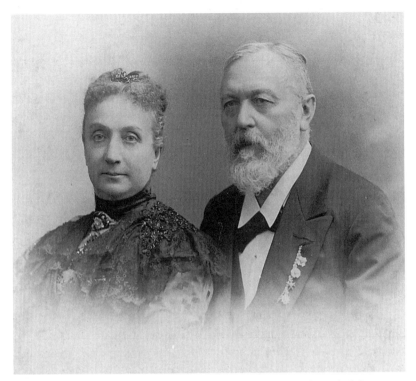

Figure 10. Krafft-Ebing and his wife, Marie Louise Kissling, at the end of their lives. (Krafft-Ebing Family Archive, Graz, Austria)

was married to Marie Louise Kissling (1846–1903)—and their three children (Fuchs 1921, 183). Although he was often praised for his kindness toward his students and patients, one cannot escape the impression that he was rather distant, reticent, even stiff and uncreatively formal—an impression that is reinforced by the arid style of his writings. There may be some truth in Emil Kraepelin's characterization of Krafft-Ebing. Kraepelin, who visited Krafft-Ebing in Graz in the summer of 1888 (right after meeting the flamboyant and impulsive Meynert), wrote about him in his memoirs:

A bigger contrast than that between him and Meynert is hardly possible. He was well-educated and, without doubt, very experienced, but in general he came across as an unimaginative, almost parochial man. His views were not surprising at all and although their sophistication was obvious, they did not attest to a superior intelligence. He told me that he often finished his book manuscripts long before the publisher's deadline, and this struck me as very characteristic of the man; he was orderly and systematic, but without special flair. (Kraepelin 1983, 58)

Psychiatry's Panacea:
Degeneration Theory

For psychiatry to be a distinct branch of modern medical science, it was necessary to emphasize the somatic mechanisms underlying mental disorders. Krafft-Ebing was deeply influenced by Wilhelm Griesinger, who promoted psychiatry as a natural science at the university. Griesinger's materialism was more methodological than ontological: his contention that mental diseases were brain diseases was intended as a heuristic rule for psychiatric research. In clinical practice Griesinger still followed the anthropological approach of asylum psychiatry in which body and soul were viewed as one. However, for most of his contemporaries and immediate successors, the significance of Griesinger's establishment of psychiatry on a neuropathological basis far outweighed the importance of his clinical program for a psychological investigation of psychopathology (Güse and Schmacke 1976, vol. 1; Verwey 1985). At the beginning of his career, Krafft-Ebing also strongly embraced the then new anatomical and physiological approach in psychiatry that situated mental disorders in the nervous system, in the cerebral organs in particular. "Physiology has also expanded its blessing into the field of psychiatry," he introduced his dissertation on the sensory deliria, published in 1864; "where once preconceived opinions and fruitless metaphysical views prevailed, now facts are collected by means of plain empirical research in order to construct a solid structure in the future" (1864, v).

Thus Krafft-Ebing self-confidently expressed the general theoretical postulate for which Griesinger had set the tone and that became popular in psychiatry in the 1860s and 1870s. The somatic-pathological approach was especially strong in Germany and Austria, where a new generation of psychiatrists working at universities and conducting laboratory research into the physical causes of mental disease rejected the philosophically and theologically inspired psychiatry of the Romantic period for its overly theoretical emphasis and its lack of effective therapies. Like other psychiatrists, Krafft-Ebing tried to gain scientific legitimacy through identification with the more fashionable natural sciences. Typically, in his inaugurals at Strassburg and Vienna as well as in his *Lehrbuch der Psychiatrie*, he presented an overview of the history of psychiatry as a progression from metaphysical and philosophical speculation to the sound method of natural science (1873c; 1889a; 1897e, 41). Apart from gaining scientific legitimacy at the university, the biomedical approach to mental disorders was also important in the forensic context. In general, courts tended to accept only "real" physical disorders as a valid ground for deciding that defendants were not responsible. Forensic psychiatrists put forward somatic explanations of mental illness especially to stress that the abnormal psychical condition of offenders was rooted in the body and that it was permanent rather than passing (Güse and Schmacke 1976, 208–17).

The behavioral symptoms of the insane mind—the sole basis for commonly used classifications of insanity—were to be considered as the symptoms of a diseased brain. Mind was a function of the brain, and disordered emotions, reason, or willpower could be localized in separate areas of the cerebral organs and the nervous system. Referring to brain anatomy and the latest results of neurophysiology and following current research into the pathology of blood vessels in the nervous tissue, Krafft-Ebing believed that the ultimate cause of all mental disorders were lesions of the brain (Schüle 1902, 308; Salvetti 1984). In his *Lehrbuch der Psychiatrie*, again and again he echoed Griesinger's dictum that mental diseases were brain diseases. There is no doubt, he contended, that mental disturbances are "manifestations of changes in the organ, which under normal conditions brings about psychical processes. . . . [M]ental disorders are diffuse malfunctions of the cerebral cortex" (1897e, 17).

However, already in 1869 Krafft-Ebing had admitted that the natural scientific approach did not always live up to its expectations. Apparently, he remarked in an article on hereditary insanity published in that year, organic disorders causing mental illness were in most cases so minute that the lesions escaped scientific observation and could only be hypothesized (1869a, 441). Thus, autopsy findings in melancholic patients, Krafft-Ebing reported five years later in a book about melancholia, did not offer any proof that lesions could be identified at a specific anatomical site. Melancholia belonged to the group of so-called psychoneuroses, he asserted, and these had to be construed as functional rather than structural disorders. Psychoneuroses were mental illnesses caused by real changes in brain function, supposedly caused by subtle affections of the finest texture of nervous tissue or by delicate chemical processes, but in which no organic lesion could be proved with the microscope (1874, 64). Even more striking is that in his psychiatric textbook, in which he so strongly favored the natural scientific approach, Krafft-Ebing acknowledged at the same time that the results of laboratory research were scarce and that in clinical practice it was hardly possible "to connect clinical pictures of mental diseases to uniform pathological anatomical findings" (1897e, 42).

Medicine's appropriation of mental disorders as part of its rightful and "natural" sphere of involvement and the scientific credibility of psychiatry required Krafft-Ebing's commitment to positivism and a conception of mental illness as an organic disease of the brain or the nervous system. However, the belief in the somatic basis of insanity was hardly confirmed by contemporary anatomical and physiological evidence. Apart from neurological disorders like dementia paralytica (neurosyphilis), epilepsy, muscular atrophies, and spinal affections, the findings yielded by anatomical and physiological research in the field of psychiatry were disappointing (Scull 1989, 24; cf. Shorter 1997, 69–112; Jacyna 1982). Postmortem examinations had consistently failed to document gross or microscopic lesions in the brains of the insane, an embarrassment that forced physicians to posit functional rather than structural lesions. Neuropathology did not prove that every form of mental and behavioral disorder was rooted in an organic substratum, and it did not offer a perspective in regard to therapy. No matter how enthusiastically psychiatrists like Krafft-Ebing welcomed the natural scientific approach, there was no denying that the gap between anatomical and neurophysiological research, on the one hand, and clinical observation, on the other, was, at least for the time being, unbridgeable. "We have too little knowledge," Krafft-Ebing thus admitted, "of the anatomical processes underlying the clinical symptoms of insanity, not to mention the anatomical variations" (1897e, 275).

As a consequence, the scientific identity of psychiatry, despite its connections with neurology, continued to be an issue of concern in the last decades of the century. There were many or even too many contradictory classifications, and the physical processes underlying mental disorders generally remained obscure while natural scientific approaches to insanity yielded little to improve its treatment. The failure of the somatic model to localize mental disorders left the doctors with mere symptom descriptions that were idiosyncratic: new terms were introduced time and again, and one and the same term was given varied applications. Even worse, psychiatry remained burdened with therapeutic impotence. This was all the more embarrassing for psychiatrists because they longed to be recognized not just as "moral entrepreneurs" in mental asylums, but also as medical scientists. As a result of the scientific revolution in medicine, the gap between psychiatrists and other physicians widened in the final third of the nineteenth century: the latter were able to affiliate themselves successfully with natural scientists. Although the modern physician's power to cure was only slightly better than that of the traditional doctor, public confidence in the physician as a man of science increased, mainly because of improvements in diagnosis and his increasingly specialist and technical physiological knowledge. Whereas medicine in general, by relying more and more on experimental physiology, began to meet the new standards of natural science, surgery reaped the benefits of new antiseptic and anesthetic techniques, and bacteriology brought a new understanding of contagious diseases, psychiatrists could hardly boast comparable etiological or therapeutic innovations. It was at this point that degeneration gained importance as a diagnostic orientation in psychiatry.

Krafft-Ebing's doubts about the possibility of locating mental diseases in the body did not affect his belief that many psychological disorders were congenital and that degeneration was the underlying cause. On the contrary, the very lack of empirical evidence for the physical causes of insanity made him stress the importance of degeneration as an explanation. During his Illenau years, he had embraced not only Griesinger's work but also that of Morel. In a paper published in 1869, Krafft-Ebing claimed that he had studied in detail the family trees of many hundreds of patients, and in other articles he pointed to heredity as an important predisposing cause of (moral) insanity as well as criminality (1869a, 443; 1868b; 1871b; 1872a; cf. Schüle 1902, 309). As the leading apostle of degeneration theory in central Europe, he stressed the role of heredity in the etiology of mental illness until the end of his career. Krafft-Ebing claimed that mental disorders could be inherited from "tainted" relatives and that many forms of insanity were basically degeneracy. Adopting Morel's preoccupation with the "neuropathic family" and the so-called anthropological method, the compilation of family trees, he introduced this viewpoint in clinical practice. He understood heredity to be pivotal in the anamnesis of many of his patients. Therefore, their family history had to be carefully investigated in order to establish if psychiatric and neurological derangements, somatic illnesses, crimes and deviant behaviors, eccentricity, genius, addictions, or stress could be found among relatives in both past and present (1897e, 159). Virtually all of Krafft-Ebing's case descriptions begin with a listing of the patient's diseased and eccentric relatives. A case history from *Psychopathia sexualis*, that of a twenty-eight-year-old employee who was diagnosed with acquired contrary sexual feeling, may serve as an example:

> He came from a highly respected patrician family in central Germany, in which nervousness and insanity have frequently occurred. His great-grandfather on his father's side and his sister died insane; his grand-

mother died of apoplexy; his father's brother died insane, and a daughter of the latter died of cerebral tuberculosis. His maternal grandmother was melancholic for years; his maternal grandfather was insane. A maternal uncle took his own life in an attack of insanity. The patient's father was very nervous. An elder brother was very neurasthenic, and had anomalies in his sex life; another was the subject of case 155 [and hospitalized in a psychiatric clinic on his wedding day after having exposed his genitals and masturbated before the assembled guests]; a third was eccentric in conduct, and was said to be subject to fixed ideas. A sister suffered from convulsions, and another died from convulsions as a small child. The patient was constitutionally predisposed, for at an early age he had been peculiar, irritable, irascible, and had impressed those around him as being abnormal. (Ps 1891, 244; cf. Ps 1999, 596)

Krafft-Ebing was not alone in stressing the importance of heredity. In late-nineteenth-century psychiatry in general, especially in France, degeneration was a central organizing concept. Jacques-Joseph Moreau de Tours—who between 1840 and 1860 endeavored to establish insanity as an organic phenomenon and to certify it as an exclusively medical problem—was one of the first to posit hereditarianism as a scientific explanation of lunacy. The theory of hereditary degeneration gained acceptance particularly among the generation of psychiatrists who began their internships in the 1860s. Not surprisingly, in the 1870s and 1880s hereditarianism became the main diagnostic orientation of French psychiatry. It has been argued that psychiatrists had pragmatic motives for embracing the theory of degeneration, as they considered it a means to solve certain professional difficulties as well as to expand their territory (Dowbiggin 1991). When the belief that insanity was an organic disease was hardly confirmed by contemporary anatomical and physiological evidence, degeneracy theory became even more important—not so much because heredity offered a more precise understanding or better treatment of mental disease, but because it was an alternative means to win scientific legitimacy. Based on Lamarck's theory of biological evolution, it appeared to substantiate the somatic model of mental illness necessary for the legitimation of psychiatrists' claims to scientific expertise.

In asylum psychiatry, the varieties of insanity were usually classified according to psychological symptoms recorded at the moment a patient was admitted. Morel proposed to identify mental illness on the basis of etiology or underlying causes. Since he believed that heredity was the cause of many different symptoms, he argued that several mild as well as serious disorders ought to be combined in one nosological category called hereditary madness. Thus Morel's work offered a naturalist model of mental pathology that seemed to make sense of clinical data in fashionable biological terms. The concept of hereditary degeneracy opened up the possibility of going beyond a mere description and grouping together of psychological symptoms and explaining both the etiology and the nature of mental illness "objectively" by reference to a hidden but fundamental biological cause; after all, heredity was grounded in reproduction, an essentially organic and unconscious process. Since the behavior of one generation might be reflected in the genetic inheritance of the offspring, degeneration was simultaneously symptom and cause in the Lamarckian model. Degeneration offered both a theory to explain disease and could be used as a diagnostic label.

The theory was so attractive for psychiatrists because it gave them a unifying, established scientific concept that could be used to bring various aspects—including constitution, pathological behavior, mental symptoms, moral influences, and social conditions—under one rubric. Thus in Krafft-Ebing's model of disease, a multitude of widely divergent causes could be responsible for mental disorders. In his psychiatric textbook, he expanded on the importance of the differentiation between predisposing and immediate, often accidental causes, and argued that only the expert, the psychiatrist, was able to sequence the multiple factors and thus establish a hierarchy of necessary and sufficient causes (1897e, 134–97). Besides internal, individual predisposing causes of mental disease such as heredity, neuropathic constitution, and education, numerous environmental and behavioral factors (which could only be certified statistically) were held responsible for triggering mental illness: modern civilization, unfavorable social conditions, nationality, climate, season, particular life phases, sex, profession, marital status, social class, and excessive religious experiences. The immediate causes could have a material as well as a nonmaterial character. In addition to physical breakdowns of the brain or the nervous system, resulting from injuries, and certain diseases and intoxicants like alcohol, cocaine, opium, lead, and mercury, Krafft-Ebing mentioned various emotional and moral influences as well as bad habits, especially in the sexual sphere. Because the ultimate causes of mental disease were all but obvious to Krafft-Ebing, his own terminology was quite vague. Characteristically, in his discussion of the etiology of mental disease, he used terms like "predisposing and accidental factors," "predisposing causal moments," "causal factors," "causal moments," and the "ultimate, indeed decisive link in the chain of causes" (1865, 31; 1868a, 110; 1897e, 134). All these expressions evaded a clear monocausal explanation. Moreover, physiological explanations overlapped with psychological, behavioral, and environmental ones. Hereditary taint could be manifest as well as latent, and the label of degeneration included constitutional and acquired disorders. To make things even more complicated, Krafft-Ebing asserted that in the transmission of hereditary derangements from parents to children, more often than not their form changed.

Like other psychiatrists who followed Morel, Krafft-Ebing thus adopted an inexact and extremely flexible interpretation of hereditary madness. Basically, the theory started from the assumption that there were causal relations between physical processes, mental traits, and environmental factors, but there was no definite answer to the question of what was cause and what effect. Distinctions among biological, psychological, social, and moral pathologies were left unarticulated or they were ambiguous. It was virtually impossible to disentangle the complex interaction of body, mind, and environment in hereditary degeneration theory. Not only were bodily as well as mental characteristics said to be hereditary; the theory also authorized a vague form of psychosomatic interaction: bodily operations affected mental states and vice versa. Besides, environmental influences and bad habits were believed to affect mental structures. These factors could destabilize the finely tuned nervous system and brain and find expression in uncontrollability, disinhibition, and automatism, symptoms that were considered to be characteristic of mental illness. Thus, in their etiology, psychiatrists could still prioritize "moral" events, such as loss or grief, religious or political excitement, and sexual excess, without necessarily contradicting a somatic view of insanity. Despite the argument that neither sin nor personal moral failure caused mental disease, their naturalist explanations did not rule out individual lifestyle as leading to mental disorder. The theory of degeneration appended an extra somatic qualification to these customary explanations: a hereditary predisposition was a necessary precondition if social, moral, or psychological forces in the individual's environment were to induce insanity. In this way heredity became the single most significant etiological factor in accounting for madness.

The attractiveness of the concept of hereditary degeneration for psychiatrists in the days of Krafft-Ebing may well be specifically accounted for by its vagueness and indeterminacy. When they found it well near impossible to demonstrate that there was a single physiological cause in each individual case of madness, the idea that many psychological and behavioral disorders could be traced to an underlying, invisible constitution must have been a tempting alternative. It is difficult to escape the impression that psychiatrists consciously or unconsciously capitalized on the imprecision of degeneration theory in order to divert attention away from the lack of empirical evidence of the somatic basis of mental illness and their ignorance of which particular lesion or physiological process caused insanity. On the one hand, the hereditarian explanation of mental disorder tied them securely to the anchor of somaticism, which by and large justified their special medical competence to treat the insane, but, on the other hand, it allowed enormous scope for the consideration of moral, social, and psychological phenomena. Despite the effort made to produce classifications based on the malfunctioning of the nervous system and the organs of the brain, psychological and behavioral symptoms—volitional incapacities, delusions, moral and emotional derangements—still largely guided their analysis of the characteristics of the mentally ill.

Although degeneration theory lacked a convincing empirical basis and was beset by contradictions, it offered psychiatrists an appealing cognitive model. It served them quite well in masking the scientific imprecision of their discipline, especially the failure to find organic or physical changes and lesions that would explain mental disturbances. Promoting their professional authority as scientific experts was all the more important because psychiatrists were still facing nonmedical competition from philanthropes, clerics, lawyers, philosophers, and others who claimed to possess legitimate knowledge regarding the treatment of the insane (Goldstein 1987). Furthermore, psychiatrists used degeneration theory to rationalize the low cure rates in mental asylums and to exempt themselves from responsibility for this therapeutic failure. It was no surprise that there were so few cures, thus their argument ran, because asylums were full of chronic, long-term patients of whom it could be assumed that they had reached the end of a long and irreversible pathological process: all the neurological taint of their ancestors had accumulated itself in them and therefore it was only natural that they were doomed to madness. Their incurability derived from their fundamental hereditary weaknesses, caused by their ancestors' unwillingness to refrain from depraved and unhealthy conduct. Already early in his career, Krafft-Ebing published an article on the possible cure of lunatics whose ancestors suffered from mental disorders (1869a). Relying on nearly three hundred case histories of patients from the Illenau asylum, he argued that only those who had not displayed any manifest symptoms of hereditary taint at birth could look forward to an improvement in their condition or even full recovery. Most of the patients did not show any sign of improvement, though, and they all seemed beyond the pale of efficacious medical treatment. The determinism inherent in degeneration theory entailed a profound therapeutic skepticism. Yet this could not keep Krafft-Ebing from treating his patients with all kinds of therapies available at the time, including hydro- and electrotherapy, other physical therapies, traitement moral, hypnosis, morphine and other medications (1891g).

Degeneration theory not only catered to the specific professional needs of late-nineteenth-century psychiatry; it also served a larger and more covert political purpose. It signaled a crisis in the social optimism that had characterized both liberalism and positivist science. Suggesting that the seeds of inevitable decay lay dormant in each human being, degeneration became a dominant cultural idea that articulated anxieties in society at large. The broad social acceptance of hereditarianism signified a turn away from environmentalism and optimistic notions of social reform. In the second half of the nineteenth century, it undermined Enlightenment faith in benevolent nature and its discoverable, rational laws, the belief that ill health and social ills would be eliminated, and the idea that individuals and society could be perfected. Degeneration theory, stressing the hereditarian catchphrase "abnormal variations," was based on an almost totally negative determinism: forces outside of and antedating the lives of individuals would fundamentally shape them in ways beyond their control. Here disease was destiny; the struggle was more for survival and less for perfection.

From the perspective of degeneration theory, insanity was not a more or less temporary affliction of consciousness and rational thought, but a constitutional deviation of the instincts. Emotional derangements, altered moods, and even patterns of behavioral deviance were widely advanced as legitimate diseases in themselves. The concepts of heredity and degeneration served to clothe these borderland ills in a somatic garb. The postulation of a continuum of various mild and serious derangements enabled psychiatrists to extend the boundaries of mental pathology by adding to their patients a substantial number of people who behaved and thought erratically yet who were rarely believed to be completely mad. Among the victims of degeneration were persons who had unimpaired intellectual capacities but who showed a disturbance of their feelings and impulses and, consequently, perversity in morals. So-called psychopaths, upsetting the order of society with their alcoholism, kleptomania, sexual perversions, suicidal tendencies, crime, and violence, were considered the prime examples of degeneration. Exemplifying both moral and physical degeneration, such individuals were believed to be mentally ill and antisocial. Krafft-Ebing came up with a wide definition of degenerates: they not only included people with serious mental disorders, sufferers from moral insanity, psychopaths, and debauchees, but also people with exceptional character traits, eccentrics, misanthropes, political scatterbrains, ardent social reformers, religious fanatics, and genial but monomaniac and otherworldly scholars and artists (1868b, 208; 1869a, 446–47).

Degeneration theory strengthened the association of mental disorders with social evils. Whereas in the first half of the nineteenth century, psychiatrists had posed as agents of a humanitarian mission aimed at alleviating the lot of the most pitiable human beings who in the past had been unjustly and brutally maltreated, now, with regard to these social problems, they set up for protecting the moral order of bourgeois society. Especially in France, the increased public presence of psychiatrists, who were largely supported by the state, was symptomatic of the more influential moral and political role of medical professionals in society (Nye 1984). They were not regarded simply as doctors healing the sick, but they also embodied certain moral and social ideals and aspirations. Indicating that prevention was better than cure, some psychiatrists began to place an emphasis on the hygienic rather than the curative aspect of their work. The control of the supposedly increasing incidence of mental disorders was not only a medical but also a social problem. The analyses of psychiatrists simultaneously covered issues of mind and body as well as of society and morality. Some of them felt that they had an important role to play as guardians of health and morality in society at large.

Especially in his works on neurasthenia and neurosyphilis, Krafft-Ebing stressed the pathogenic impact of modern society (1884a; 1885b; 1892d; 1894g; 1895a; 1895b; 1898a; 1900a). Although the two diseases were very different in terms of their etiology, he understood them both as typically modern, dramatically growing diseases in which social and cultural factors were prominently involved.[1] According to Krafft-Ebing, there were many drawbacks to the progress of civilization. Since the French Revolution, and the instability and loss of security it had brought, modern society was afflicted by an increasing nervousness and a growing prevalence of syphilis— he did not even hesitate to speak of "a moral and physical bankruptcy" (1884a, 8). Modern man's peace of mind was severely disturbed by rapid economic and social change, individualism, raising ambitions and ruthless competition, the mechanization and high pace of labor, the increasing intellectual demands of office work, the way children were overburdened by curricular demands in schools, the continuing political conflicts in parliamentary democracies, social agitation and political turmoil, class antagonism, and women's emancipation. In addition, he felt that the overconsumption of meat, coffee, tea, alcohol, and tobacco weakened the nervous system. In spite of his clinical experiments suggesting that syphilis was the necessary cause for general paralysis, Krafft-Ebing continued to highlight cultural factors in the explanation of this fatal neurological disease. For him, Hirschl's discovery of the connection between syphilis and dementia paralytica confirmed the relationship between disease and immorality in modern society. "If one would try to summarize the etiology of paralysis in

1. In light of new and ever-changing diagnostic labels, it is probably impossible to determine whether psychiatric disorders had indeed increased in the nineteenth century, but there is evidence that organic brain and nervous diseases such as neurosyphilis (paralysis and tabes) and alcoholic dementia, and possibly also what is now diagnosed as schizophrenia, had become more prevalent (Shorter 1990, 181–82; 1997, 53–64).

two words," Krafft-Ebing concluded in his Moscow lecture, "thus they should run as follows: syphilization and civilization" (1900a, 15). To account for the increase of psychological and nervous complaints as well as sexual dissoluteness, the man who hated Vienna particularly blamed hectic big cities and their titillating amusements, their "horror plays, adultery comedies, trapeze artists, nerve-shattering music [that of Richard Wagner especially], loud color patterns, strong wines, cigars, liqueurs, gambling dens, exciting press reports on crimes and accidents" (1884a, 18). All but hiding his critique of modern urban life, he wrote:

> Whoever observes for the first time the commotion of the modern metropolis, marked by its pursuit of money and enjoyment and its unleashing of savage passions, while abandoning physical and mental rest, sleep, family life and bliss, will—if his nerves are still healthy—feel most uncomfortable and yearn for the peace and quiet of his rustic family life. (1884a, 16–17)

Along the same line, Krafft-Ebing argued that psychiatrists could play an important role in the field of social hygiene. He claimed that mental and nervous diseases might be prevented by promoting healthy lifestyles and marriages, a sound physical and moral education, and long holidays in the countryside. Keeping "tainted" individuals from procreation might also serve this same end—already in 1873 he suggested, albeit with caution, the possibility of legal regulations in this field (1873c, 390; cf. 1890g, 1803–4).

The theory of hereditary degeneracy, postulating that deviant behaviors and mental disorders tended to go from bad to worse, provided a scientific language for talking about social and political problems. For late-nineteenth-century Europeans, it summed up the terrible human costs of modernization and it expressed deep conservative and liberal fears of the disorder of "mass society," of the "dangerous" classes in big cities, of recurring revolution and class struggle, and of democracy and socialism. "No sooner has the French Revolution afforded the third estate with its rights and social position," Krafft-Ebing worried aloud, "than a fourth stands up for its fancied rights, often not in a very parliamentary manner, but by means of dynamite, fire, and murder" (1885b, 6). The diagnosis of mental instability and even insanity was never far away when he considered socialism and revolutionary movements: "Leaders of revolutions fall ill frequently, as was demonstrated by the Commune of Paris. This can be explained by the fact that often eccentric, problematic figures suffering from a hereditary defect are heading such movements" (1897e, 139; cf. 1884d; 1892j).

Krafft-Ebing was not alone in medicalizing social and political issues. Poverty and antisocial tendencies were increasingly viewed in hereditarian

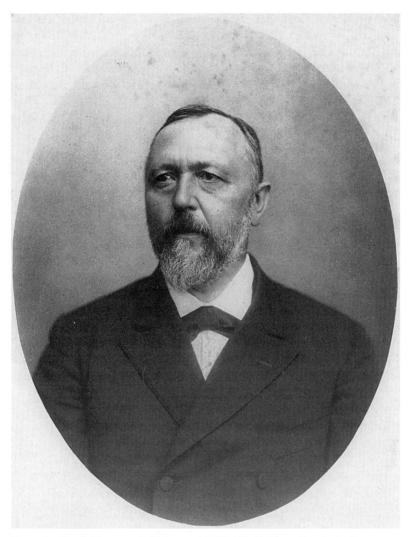

Figure 11. Krafft-Ebing, probably around 1890. (Krafft-Ebing Family Archive, Graz, Austria)

terms. Labeling the poverty-stricken as atavistic misfits in an otherwise evolving world, physicians and social theorists conferred the stigma of moral incapacity on those concerned. If poverty was a product of an inevitable biological process, it was decreed by a natural order unresponsive to human intervention. Society was viewed as an organism, as a body that could suffer from illness, and its supposed degeneration was discussed as a scientific, medical-biological fact. The liberal Enlightenment concept of human nature that stressed the fundamental commonalties shared by all

men was superseded by increasing emphasis on inborn differences and "natural" hierarchy. The theory of hereditary degeneracy, like Darwinism, indeed insisted on the primacy of the body as the definer of behavior and
mental capacities, and it provided an overarching biological rationale for
pathologizing a wide variety of social problems. The ultimate effect of the
degeneration message was to naturalize social and political issues.

Professional Controversies

Historians of psychiatry, and of psychoanalysis in particular, have viewed Krafft-Ebing as a typical representative of the Viennese school of medicine, which emphasized a somatic approach to mental illness. Influenced by degenerationist thinking and biological theories aimed at providing a cerebrospinal topography of mental pathology, he indeed presented himself as a "materialist" psychiatrist, even though he frequently highlighted cultural and social factors in his explanations of mental disorders. In practice, however, both the natural scientific approach and the concept of hereditary degeneracy seem to have had less relevance for his treatment of patients than might be suggested by the overall materialist theoretical framework of his thinking and writing.

When Krafft-Ebing was nominated to succeed Max Leidesdorff as professor of psychiatry in Vienna, it was met with protests by Theodor Meynert, the famous brain anatomist who since 1875 occupied the other psychiatric chair at the University of Vienna and who advocated a strictly natural scientific approach in psychiatry. He considered Krafft-Ebing a traditional psychiatrist who was not in tune with the latest scientific developments.[1] The very definition of psychiatry was at stake. Krafft-Ebing's approach, characterized as "clinical-psychological" by Meynert's colleagues who elected Krafft-Ebing, differed substantially from the materialism of Meynert and other leading German psychiatrists such as Paul Flechsig (1847–1929) in Leipzig, Eduard Hitzig (1838–1907) in Halle, and Karl Wernicke (1848–1905) in Breslau, Meynert's own preference for the chair

1. Letter of Theodor Meynert to the Ministerium für Cultus und Unterricht (June 5, 1888); Theodor Meynert, Promemoria anlässlich des Referats über die Wiederbesetzung der psychiatrischen Klinik in den wiener Landesirrenanstalt (January 12, 1889), Allgemeines Verwaltungsarchiv des Österreichischen Staatsarchivs, Vienna, ad 12984/89.

in psychiatry.[2] Vienna's medical school gave priority to basic scientific research over curing patients—therapeutic nihilism was its parole—and Meynert, who set the tone for other German university psychiatrists, studied psychiatric illness in the laboratory with the microscope. Rejecting psychiatry's preoccupation with labeling symptoms, he displayed little interest in clinical practice, let alone living patients. For him and his students, scientific psychiatry was basically brain anatomy and physiological experimentation, and their work consisted of, for instance, comparing samples of dissected brains of deceased patients anatomically and histologically with brain slices of laboratory animals. They conceived the brain in terms of a complicated mechanistic reactor to the external world and explained the etiology of insanity largely by reference to the anatomical localization of discrete cerebral lesions (Marx 1970). Meynert assumed that conscious mental activity was not inherently different from automatic reflex action. The materialist model, on which this research was based, was mechanistic and reductionist in the sense that it sought to explain every symptom of mental disease in terms of cerebral structure and neurological physiology.

On the whole, Krafft-Ebing's approach to mental illness cannot be characterized as materialist in this reductionist sense. Whereas Meynert and his students defined all psychological functions in terms of neurological mechanisms, Krafft-Ebing's psychiatric practice focused on clinical description and analysis of behavioral and psychological symptoms of mental illness. He was far from denying the importance of anatomy and physiology for psychiatry, since without a firm basis in these laboratory sciences, psychiatry would become alienated from scientific medicine, but he opposed reductionism. In contrast to Meynert, Krafft-Ebing basically viewed brain anatomy and neurophysiology as auxiliary sciences. In his writings he referred to dissections a few times, but he hardly conducted anatomical and physiological research himself, also because of a handicap of his eye that made microscopic observation difficult for him (Kornfeld 1903, 24). As discussed already, Krafft-Ebing realized early on that biological psychiatry fell short of its high expectations. Therefore, his materialism was methodological rather than ontological, and his positivism was colored by the view that psychiatry was a moral and cultural enterprise, instead of a strictly scientific undertaking. Psychiatric symptoms were not, he insisted,

> mathematic variables, physical phenomena, or chemical secretions. On the contrary, appearing as feelings, perceptions, and aspirations, they form a class of their own. Moreover, they are not directly tangible, but they can only be investigated indirectly by examining the expressions

2. Notice of the commission on "die Wiederbesetzung der Lehrkanzel für Psychiatrie," Allgemeines Verwaltungsarchiv des Österreichischen Staatsarchivs, Vienna, 12984/89 Z 759.

and actions of the subject under observation. These psychical expressions are mirrored in the consciousness of the observer who can only properly assess them on the basis of logical reasoning. (1889a, 818)

In his 1902 valedictory lecture to his students, he stressed that this way of understanding patients made psychiatry a specialty that differed from the rest of medical science. He told his audience that "only in psychiatry you have the opportunity to learn about the whole man, whereas any other clinical field deals only with a part of man."[3] On several occasions Krafft-Ebing stressed that psychiatry was more than just a medical specialty; its object was the human body as well as the mind, and therefore it overlapped with anthropology, psychology, pedagogy, the social sciences, the humanities, and even with theology and philosophy (1897e, 21; 1890b, 22–23).

Yet in a methodical sense, Krafft-Ebing was much less idealistic and in this respect he even counts as a decidedly "unphilosophical" psychiatrist (Schüle 1902, 329). In his statistical model of disease explanation, the labeling and classification of mental pathologies started with the collection of individual cases. Given his view of medicine as an art as well as a natural science, he relied heavily on experience and induction. He emphasized repeatedly that psychiatry, for the time being, could claim to be no more than a descriptive science and that a lot of empirical material had to be assembled before the fairly young academic discipline could be raised to the level of an explanatory science (1897e, 41; 1889a, 817). Much of his work, consisting for a large part of case histories and forensic reports, is indeed descriptive and has an unsophisticated, pragmatic character.

Krafft-Ebing's clinical psychiatry militated against a rigid somatic interpretation of mental disorder, also because he recoiled from the moral implications of materialist explanations. Meynert's neurophysiological automatism led to the conclusion that large portions of brain function were outside of personal control. From a moral perspective, the materialist model, though widely accepted in theory, could not provide an adequate description of some "higher" mental processes that were considered fundamental for humankind. There was no place for the sense of moral progress that was attributed to willpower and judgment by Christians and liberals alike. The belief in the power of the will, enabling man to free the self from the domination of determinist forces, was a way of coping with otherwise insuperable moral problems presented by biological materialism. Consequently, many psychiatrists hedged physiological determinism by defining willpower, imagination, and moral judgment as supraphysical states of consciousness.

3. *Neues Wiener Journal*, (undated) 1902, Nachlass Krafft-Ebing.

The tension between the dominant theoretical conception of mental illness as an organic disease and clinical practice that focused on psychological symptoms and remedies was widespread in late-nineteenth-century psychiatry (Berrios and Porter 1995, 152, 549). Krafft-Ebing was not alone in supplementing his natural scientific model with clinical observations. Apart from the fundamental theoretical and philosophical differences concerning the ultimate causation of mental disease, there was also a more continuous and pragmatic tradition of psychiatry (Verwey 1985). Before 1850 German psychiatry was divided between *Psychiker* and *Somatiker*, and from the 1860s on there had been a division between advocates of scientific medicine and those who favored anthropological-philosophical models. Yet in their actual treatment of patients, many psychiatrists tended to be eclectic and practical. For many there was no contradiction between a somatic approach to mental disturbances and a willingness to consider their psychological and subjective aspects. They might focus on clinical observation and description, or they might refer to degeneration theory, in both cases without immediately seeking answers to fundamental questions on the ultimate cause of insanity or the nature of the body-mind relationship. In daily practice, the approach in clinical psychiatry was multifaceted and sometimes even inconsistent. Psychiatric insights were based on a combination of clinical experience, introspection, empathy, and commonsense psychology.

Although Krafft-Ebing was deeply influenced by the scientific approach in medicine, he developed a psychiatry that was not primarily based on brain anatomy and neurophysiology but on extensive clinical observations. To a large extent, history would put him in the right. Meynert's reductionism turned out to be a dead-end street in psychiatry (Shorter 1997, 99–109). Kraepelin, who would set the tone in the early twentieth century, developed a clinical psychiatry that was based on the same methodological materialism as advocated by Krafft-Ebing. The latter's approach also shows some resemblance to the hermeneutic, psychologically oriented psychiatry that would be developed by Eugen Bleuler (1857–1939), Ludwig Binswanger (1881–1966), and Karl Jaspers (1883–1969) (Schmitt 1983). Krafft-Ebing's clinical method focused not so much on the specific characteristics of a particular illness as on very detailed histories of individuals. "Psychiatry never deals with disease entities, but always with diseased persons," he wrote in his psychiatric textbook, and therefore its approach could only be "strictly individualistic" (1897e, 243). The most valuable method was in fact a "historical-genetic" and "anthropological" diagnosis.

Like other clinical psychiatrists, Krafft-Ebing tried to escape from the dilemma between latent organic causes and manifest psychological symptoms by analyzing individual histories of the mentally ill in order to discover the process of a disease. The intelligibility of a mental illness depended on the proper description of its symptoms as well as of its progression. Already in the 1860s, when he worked together with Heinrich Schüle in the Illenau asylum, Krafft-Ebing had developed an individualizing case history method (Schüle 1902, 307–8). The psychiatrist should consider "the complete mental and physical makeup of the individual because often the mental disorder is the result of the previous conditions of life and personal development" (1897e, 135). Emphasizing the importance of minute observation and the inductive method, he laid down a standard for writing up psychiatric case histories. Apart from the patient's name, age, occupation, admission date, and date of consultation, information should be listed about physique, physiognomy, ancestry, family medical and mental health history, prenatal conditions, childhood and puberty history, onset and development of mental disorders, and especially about the subjective condition: moods, imaginative powers, dreams, fantasies, perceptivity, intellectual capacities, decisiveness, and moral awareness. No piece of information about the patient was, in Krafft-Ebing's view, irrelevant. The case history analysis sought to present a coherent and interlinked picture that ran from physical appearance, cerebral defects, and presence or absence of a hereditary predisposition, to the history of childhood illnesses and traumatic episodes, intellectual capacities and defects, and the affective and moral makeup (1897e, 238–42). The very essence of psychiatric knowledge consisted of understanding the individual in all his aspects. Much of Krafft-Ebing's work was descriptive and consisted primarily of case histories and, in the field of sexual pathology, as we will see in part 3, also of autobiographies written by his patients. Whereas other psychiatrists used case studies to illustrate their classification of symptoms and their theories, for Krafft-Ebing case descriptions constituted the core of his work. In his career, he collected more than twenty thousand of them.[4]

4. Richard von Krafft-Ebing, Manuskript Nr. 854, Institut für die Geschichte der Medizin der Universität von Wien; cf. Fuchs 1902, 11; Sterz 1903, 62–63.

Alternatives: Psychological Therapies

The strictly mechanistic and reductionist model of brain function advocated by Meynert and his students left no room for a psychological approach in psychiatry. Krafft-Ebing's methodological materialism, by contrast, did not exclude psychology; for him psychological and neuropathological research complemented each other. As long as there were simply no tools or mechanisms by which to measure physiological brain deterioration in the living, abnormal behavior and psychological symptoms remained the only available indications of mental disorder. Although Krafft-Ebing opposed psychiatrists' concern with philosophical questions like the existence and quality of the soul, and although he argued that psychiatry should be an integral part of medicine, as a clinician and a forensic expert he stressed the importance of the psychological aspects of mental disease as well as of its treatment. A psychosis was not merely a disease of the brain, but it affected the personality of the patient. Therefore, his treatment had to be "psychical and individualistic" (1897e, 20).

The years between 1860 and 1900 have been characterized as the era of "brain mythology" in psychiatry, indicating that explanations of mental illness focused on anatomical anomalies or physiological lesions in the brain. However, by the 1880s a new psychological paradigm began to gain support among psychiatrists. More than anything else it was, ironically enough, the expansion of the psychiatric field in the direction of organic nervous diseases—which itself was a logical consequence of psychiatry's orientation toward somatic medicine and neurology—that more or less forced psychiatrists to draw opposite conclusions on what they had been looking for all along. Their growing interest in a number of nervous illnesses—some of them with a long history, such as hysteria, others newly discovered, such as neurosis and neurasthenia—involved a recognition of the importance, if not complete autonomy, of psychological symptoms and remedies (Micale 1990, 92; Micale 1995; Shorter 1992).

Under the influence of the scientific approach of psychiatry, which implied that both mental and neurological diseases had to be explained somatically, the basic differentiation between psychotic and nervous disorders faded in the second half of the nineteenth century, even though the former were considered far graver than the latter. A new differentiation, however, was introduced in the 1880s between, on the one hand, mental and nervous diseases that could be demonstrated to be organic in nature and, on the other hand, the so-called functional mental and nervous disorders for which no organic pathology had yet been found (though physical causes were often implicitly assumed). The psychiatric interpretation of a lesion as functional was consistent with its physiological definition as non-localized, meaning anatomically independent of a specific organ. Functional psychoses like melancholia, mania, paranoia, delusions, and hallucinations constituted a remaining group of the organic psychoses (dementia, imbecility, intoxications), in the same way as neuroses—and also disorders like hysteria and neurasthenia as well as sexual perversions—were conceived as a remaining functional group within neuropathology (Shorter 1992, 215; Verwey 1995).

It was the differentiation between structural and functional disorders that made psychiatrists like Krafft-Ebing stress the importance of psychological symptoms and remedies in clinical practice. As far as functional disorders were concerned, the neurological reflex model was played down and psychological symptoms on the sensory side—especially irrational, intuitive, and unconscious aspects of mental life—were upgraded. Although Krafft-Ebing seemed strongly committed to the somatical model, his case histories testify to his sensitivity to the psychological evolution of various mental disorders and their connection to certain personality types. Furthermore, in the therapeutic context, the psychological approach gained ground. From 1886 on, Krafft-Ebing and his assistants began to use hypnosis and the so-called "psychical therapy," not only in the treatment of neurotic, neurasthenic, and hysteric patients in his sanatorium, but also when treating the perverts who consulted him in his private practice.

Hypnosis, inducing a state resembling sleep or one of modified consciousness, had already been introduced in medicine by Franz Anton Mesmer (1734–1815) in the late eighteenth century. Since the mid-1870s, sensational public performances by lay hypnotists were popular among the general public in Austria, as in other parts of Europe, and hypnotism drew considerable press coverage. Because these performances tended to be associated with charlatanry and moneymaking, hypnosis became a controversial practice among doctors. In 1880 the stage performances of the Danish magnetic artist and hypnotist Carl Hansen (1833–1897), which attracted large crowds, caused a lively debate about hypnosis in Austrian medical newspapers (Shorter 1992, 153–54). The Ministry of Health of Lower Austria, which commissioned medical experts to write a forensic report on hypnosis, prohibited Hansen—who was not a medical doctor—to do his demonstrations in Vienna because his techniques were considered hazardous to the health of his subjects. However, many physicians were not opposed to hypnotism as such. It seems that in the 1880s more and more patients began to ask for this treatment, which perhaps explains why hypnotism unexpectedly began to attract serious attention from prominent medical men. As far as their private practices were concerned, psychiatrists tended to propagate views and offer therapies that would strike resonance with their patients, and necessarily so, because it was a competitive world and patients were always free to consult other doctors.

French psychiatrists had set the fashion in applying hypnosis in mental medicine. Quite soon two competing schools evolved, a psychological one, centered around Hippolyte Bernheim (1840–1919) and Ambroise-Auguste Liébeault (1823–1904) at the university of Nancy, and a neurological one, led by Jean-Martin Charcot of the Salpêtrière in Paris.[1] Charcot linked responsivity to hypnosis to hysteria; for him, both were sure signs of a neurological syndrome, characterized by disinhibition and automatism. A hypnotic state was compared to hallucinations, dreams, and spiritual trances. These related mental states were characterized by a loss of will and regarded as either approaching mental illness or as virtually indistinguishable from it. Charcot considered hypnosis as a clinical experiment aimed at evoking typical symptoms of hysteria; he used it as a diagnostic technique in his famous demonstrations of patients. Bernheim and Liébeault, by contrast, considered hypnosis not as a neuropathological but as a normal phenomenon; everyone was hypnotizable to some degree. The Nancy school emphasized the more general therapeutic value of hypnosis. Concentrating on the role of suggestion and persuasion, they developed a form of practice that focused on talking with patients about the motivations for their actions and urging them to change their behavior in the future (Shorter 1992, 246). Already before Freud, psychological analysis as a new therapeutic ideal, relying on the analyst's attentive ear as a major tool, began to be practiced by other French psychiatrists as well, including Pierre Janet (1859–1947), Binet, and Théodule Ribot (1839–1916) (Schrenk 1973; Schmitt 1983; Schmiedebach 1986; Gauld 1992).

1. For the controversy on hypnosis between the Nancy and Salpêtrière schools, see Laurence and Perry 1988, 194–214; Gauld 1992, 306–56.

Under the influence of the Nancy school, therapeutic hypnosis began to spread among psychiatrists in other European countries, and in its wake psychological approaches increasingly competed with psychiatry's anatomical gaze. There was much resistance in central European medical and psychiatric circles against hypnosis, opposed as it was by people like Meynert and Kraepelin, but from the mid-1880s on various German, Austrian, and Hungarian physicians and psychologists—among them Forel, Dessoir, Breuer, Freud, Moll, Schrenck-Notzing, and Krafft-Ebing—began to follow the French examples. For a large part, hypnosis gained ground in mental medicine because of the particular interest in sexual pathology and psychology (cf. Gauld 1992, 298). Krafft-Ebing, always open to French influences, was one of the pioneers using hypnosis in psychiatry (Hauser 1989). Already in the 1870s he had published two articles on "states of dreaming and semiconsciousness" (1898b). Between 1886 and 1900, he published two books and twelve articles on hypnosis. Like Charcot, he used it as a diagnostic tool and in clinical experiments. Krafft-Ebing believed that hypnosis was a valuable method for investigating the psyche, its unconscious side in particular (1886; 1889c, 1186). But at the same time he borrowed ideas from the Nancy school by using hypnotic suggestion as a therapeutic technique in his treatment of hysterical patients and perverts, homosexual men and women in particular (1889/1890a; 1889/1890b; Ps 1903, 318–25). Furthermore, in 1896 he referred in a positive way to Freud's and Josef Breuer's hypnotic treatments of hysteric patients (1896c, 28).[2] Similarly, Krafft-Ebing discussed, albeit with caution, the possibilities of using hypnosis for the treatment of more or less mild psychoses and neuroses that were of a functional, nonorganic nature. Successful therapy, Krafft-Ebing emphasized, depended on the personality of the patients and the seriousness of their complaints. A certain level of self-consciousness and self-control was desirable; superficial and impulsive characters were unfit for hypnotic treatment (1891d, 11).

Krafft-Ebing's most remarkable work on this topic was his best-seller *Eine experimentelle Studie auf dem Gebiete des Hypnotismus* (1888), of which, in addition to three German editions, Swedish, Russian, English, and Italian translations appeared. It was in fact a very extensive case study of a woman, the twenty-nine-year-old Hungarian Ilma S, who Krafft-Ebing subjected to several, occasionally rather bizarre, hypnotic experiments. After having been arrested for petty theft, she was admitted to Krafft-Ebing's clinic in Graz because of her confused mental condition and her

2. When Breuer treated the hysteric Bertha Pappenheim (alias Anna O) in 1881, he consulted Krafft-Ebing. However, Krafft-Ebing's visit was not very effective: the patient got very upset by his presence (Hirschmüller 1989, 103–4).

claim that she was not aware of her offense. The first part of the case history deals with Ilma's eventful and troubled course of life. During her stay in the clinic, she wrote a comprehensive autobiography, while Krafft-Ebing obtained reports on former hospitalizations in Budapest. It appeared that she had suffered from hallucinations, had committed several thefts while being in a trancelike state, and that she had passed as a man for three years, taking female lovers. After being arrested by the police, she stayed in several hospitals in Budapest and was diagnosed with "hystero-epilepsy." Some of the doctors subjected her to a series of experiments with hypnosis, suggesting to her in some of the sessions that she was a dog, in others that she killed one of the doctors, or that the cold piece of metal that they pressed to her body was very hot (after she was admitted to Krafft-Ebing's clinic, he evidently found several scars on her skin). When she found out that accounts of the experiments were publicized in the local newspapers, she fled to Graz.

Although Ilma S claimed that the hypnotic experiments were the main reason that she had left the hospital in Budapest, Krafft-Ebing hypnotized her no less than ninety times during her seven-month stay in his clinic. During these sessions he tested a whole range of physiological and psychological reactions to posthypnotic suggestion, and he discovered that there were three separate layers in her consciousness while she was under hypnosis. He also applied hypnosis therapeutically to influence her sleeping pattern, and she was one of the first patients whose homosexual leanings he tried to cure by hypnotic suggestion. Krafft-Ebing included her case history in several editions of *Psychopathia sexualis,* and he also used her in demonstrations to large medical audiences in Graz, which resembled the variety shows of lay hypnotists and which, again, were widely publicized in the local press. Ilma, who was an intelligent and well-educated woman, showed considerable aversion to these experiments and after the sessions she suffered from fits, but Krafft-Ebing nonetheless continued to do sessions with her, asserting that hypnosis could do no harm as long as it was practiced by a qualified doctor. After seven months he claimed that her condition had improved, and he concluded that hypnotic suggestion was a valuable therapy to treat functional nervous disorders. After she was discharged from Krafft-Ebing's clinic, however, she was transferred to a mental asylum in Budapest, where her therapy would last another two years. Krafft-Ebing even made her travel from Graz to Budapest while in a hypnotic state.[3]

Krafft-Ebing's demonstrations with Ilma S were repeatedly criticized, and his experiments with hypnosis became even more controversial when

3. Postcard of Krafft-Ebing to Oberwärter Glasy (July 1, [1888]), Autograph 213/61–2, Österreichische Nationalbibliothek, Vienna.

he began to hypnotize at social gatherings to entertain the guests. Attending a séance where Krafft-Ebing gave a demonstration of hypnosis, the famous surgeon Theodor Billroth (1829–1894) even denounced Krafft-Ebing as a swindler, and Meynert equally attacked him by characterizing hypnosis as charlatanry (Szeps-Zuckerkandl 1939, 165–66; Johnston 1972, 234; Kraepelin 1983, 57). Kraepelin, who in 1888 witnessed Krafft-Ebing hypnotizing a patient, was not impressed, mainly because the patient—she may have been Ilma—lapsed into a hysterical fit (Kraepelin 1983, 58). More public attacks followed in 1893, when at a public meeting of the Verein für Psychiatrie und Neurologie in Vienna, Krafft-Ebing hypnotized a certain Clementine Piegl, a thirty-three-year-old Viennese woman who was not a patient but an enthusiastic volunteer. After having hypnotized her, he suggested that she was a girl of, respectively, seven, fifteen, and nineteen years old, whereupon Piegl indeed talked and behaved accordingly. Moritz Benedikt dismissed such sessions as "a stupid swindle" and "fantastic humbug" (1893a, 29). To counter such attacks, Krafft-Ebing repeated the experiments at the request of Piegl, not only to prove that earlier stages of the "Ego" could be reproduced and that this was a serious psychological phenomenon and not some occult or spiritist mystery, but also to demonstrate that healthy people could be hypnotized—which is why he insisted that Piegl was quite a healthy, ordinary, and all but hysterical woman.

Although hypnosis had meanwhile gained some scientific acceptability, it was still controversial because the patient was the passive instrument of whatever the hypnotist deemed appropriate. There were allegations that hypnosis could be used to abolish the willpower of those who submitted to it, to manipulate them and instigate them to commit crimes, and even to sexually seduce and rape women. In two articles, both dealing with the moral and legal aspects of hypnosis, Krafft-Ebing tried to set himself apart from lay stage-hypnotists. In the first one he advocated a legal ban on the use of hypnosis by nonmedical practitioners (1897c; cf. 1891e).[4] However, because he also felt that physicians should be given complete freedom to apply hypnosis as they wished, legal rules to prevent the abuse of patients were unnecessary in his view. In the second article, a forensic contribution, he argued that spiritistic circles run by lay hypnotists should be forbidden because such sessions constituted a danger to public health (1897d). The way Krafft-Ebing dealt with hypnosis aptly characterizes the inherent tensions and ambiguities of his professionalizing efforts in general. On the one

---

4. At the end of the nineteenth century in many European countries, legislation was adopted to restrict the use of hypnosis to the medical profession (Laurence and Perry 1988, 223).

hand, he used his publications, experiments, and demonstrations to publicize, popularize, and legitimize psychiatric knowledge, but, on the other hand, he made great play with psychiatric expertise in order to monopolize that kind of knowledge.

In addition to hypnosis, Krafft-Ebing advocated free and easy talking as a significant therapeutic device. Being able to listen carefully to the patient was of crucial importance for the psychiatrist: "Talking with the patient is the central point in the psychical diagnosis. . . . The object of the examination is not a chemical substance, but an ever-changing human consciousness, which is intensely influenced by the manner in which the examination is carried out" (1897e, 233). In his private practice as well as in his sanatorium Mariagrün, talking or the so-called psychical therapy was a prominent aspect of the treatment. Not only did the physicians quote statements of their patients like "trust has loosened my tongue, which gave me enormous relief," but they also theorized about the therapeutic value of verbal, cathartic communication (Gugl and Stichl 1892, 136). Accepting the authority of the doctor and trusting his abilities were central to this talking cure. Krafft-Ebing also used the term *psychotherapy*, which he described as "a purposeful methodological medical psychagogy, in which the patient, while being fully awake, was influenced by suggestions" (1896c, 27; cf. 1897e, 153). He saw hypnosis and "psychical therapy" or psychotherapy as general means to influence and strengthen the will of patients, and as means to encourage them to break with bad habits and obsessive behaviors in particular. In this process, the moral authority of the psychiatrist was essential, but the effectiveness of these psychological therapies depended in large part on the patient's sense of responsibility and willpower.

Krafft-Ebing's methods of hypnosis and talking cure were still quite different from modern forms of psychotherapy that are largely aimed at self-knowledge. His psychic therapy, which he once compared to confession, was rather authoritarian. However, it took shape in a relatively new psychiatric setting. Apart from private practices, the first forms of psychotherapy were generally developed in a neurological setting, rather than in psychiatry. A major role was played by private nerve clinics, which targeted middle- and upper-class neurotics and which, ironically, advertised physical therapies to avoid the stigma of mental illness (Shorter 1997, 137). The patients Krafft-Ebing treated with psychological therapies were not representative of the population in asylums and psychiatric wards of hospitals. It was especially in his private practice and his sanatorium, which catered to middle- and upper-class patients, that he stressed the usefulness of hypnosis, suggestion, and talking. The application of such an array of psychological therapies by psychiatrists was part of their effort to break out of the confines of the asylums and psychiatric clinics and broaden and diversify their territory, in an attempt to enhance their social prestige. During the days of Krafft-Ebing, the therapeutic domain of psychiatry was extended beyond the walls of the asylum and the clinic. The psychological approach enabled psychiatrists to make their field more attractive for individuals who showed relatively mild neurotic and mental disturbances and who in most cases did not need to be hospitalized. If diagnoses like monomania, moral insanity, and psychopathy had been at the heart of psychiatry's expansion in the middle of the nineteenth century, various forms of nervousness, especially neurasthenia, hysteria, and sexual perversion, played an analogous role for the psychiatric profession in the 1880s and 1890s (cf. Goldstein 1987, 321).

In the last decades of the nineteenth century, psychiatry began to appropriate clients who were more affluent and socially respectable than the inmates of public asylums. This new category consisted of individuals who basically counted as ordinary citizens, who generally did not disturb the public peace, and who commonly lived at home while making periodic visits to their psychiatric doctor. The demand for psychological services among members of the bourgeoisie grew stronger, in part because regular physicians, who increasingly had training in the natural sciences and were influenced by new bacteriological theories about contagious diseases, were no longer as willing to listen patiently to endless stories of their patients' troubles. To clinical psychiatrists like Krafft-Ebing, however, the subjective accounts about all kinds of mental complaints were often quite instructive and even crucial for a proper diagnosis. By meeting the needs of an economically more prosperous clientele, psychiatrists created the possibility of building up a private practice. Because of their interest in psychological symptoms and because of the fact that their patients tended to have the same social or intellectual background, in many cases a closer relationship between doctor and patient was established. Krafft-Ebing applied hypnosis and developed psychical therapy, in part because several of his patients more or less expected and sometimes asked to be so treated. The proto-psychotherapeutical approach rationalized close, concerned contact between doctor and patient. As we will see in part 3, it was especially in the field of sexual perversions that Krafft-Ebing appeared as the emotional confidant of many of his patients.

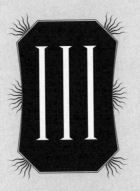

Articulate Sufferers

PERVERSION AND AUTOBIOGRAPHY

AS WE HAVE SEEN IN PART 2, CHANGES IN THE INSTITUTIONAL CONTEXT of psychiatry gradually generated a shift from the dominant somatic approach toward a more psychological viewpoint. From the beginning, Krafft-Ebing was a key figure in this development, particularly regarding issues involving abnormal sexuality. Although he continued to view degeneration and heredity as the underlying causes of perversion, he steered the medical discussion away from explaining sexuality as a series of interrelated physiological phenomena, and in his work a psychological understanding came to the fore. Perversion, he felt, was not so much rooted in physical as in functional disorders. In this new psychiatric style of reasoning, functional diseases were disorders of an instinct that could not be located in physiology, be it a specific organ or tissue. Like Freud, Krafft-Ebing viewed human sexuality as distinct from the instinctual sexuality of animals. The basic materials for developing his professional views and theories were provided by the stories of his patients. This explains why case histories and (auto)biographical accounts were so important in the development of his understanding of sexual pathology.

One of the leading clinically oriented psychiatrists of his time, Krafft-Ebing was even specifically known for his extensive case histories. He illustrated his work, that on sexual pathology in particular, with literally hundreds of observations. Initially, many of these observations were borrowed from colleagues, or he used cases of patients hospitalized in asylums and those of the moral offenders whom he examined as an expert witness. As his work progressed, though, more and more of the case histories used in Krafft-Ebing's writings were based on the stories of the patients hospitalized in the university clinics in Graz and Vienna where he was a medical superintendent. Furthermore, a growing number of individuals contacted Krafft-Ebing as private patients or corresponded with him because they had recognized themselves in one of his published case descriptions. Increasingly, he also relied on their narratives, which often took the form of rich and detailed (auto)biographical accounts. Some of the correspondents sent their life history to Krafft-Ebing, hoping to see it published in the next edition of *Psychopathia sexualis*, of which new and updated versions appeared continuously from 1886 on. While at first most case histories he used in his work were quite short and factual, they became more extensive from the 1880s on. By incorporating his patients' narratives into his own work and by also quoting from them at length, many of the case studies foreground subjective experience and thus do justice to the personal character of each individual's story.

Of a total of 627 case histories pertaining to sexual disorders and perversion that I have been able to collect, Krafft-Ebing borrowed 187 from existing legal-medical and psychiatric sources. Since these cases were first described by others, I excluded them from my analysis of Krafft-Ebing's empirical materials; my concern here is therefore with the 440 cases he himself collected. They deal with patients whom he treated or with whom he corresponded. One hundred seventy-six of these histories and autobiographies were published in one or more of the fourteen editions of *Psychopathia sexualis* that appeared between 1886 and 1903 (including two editions of *Neue Forschungen auf dem Gebiet der Psychopathia sexualis*), while 238 of them appeared in other monographs and articles. Twenty-six case histories that I found in Krafft-Ebing's estate were, as far as I have been able to determine, never published.

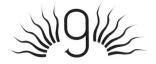

Sexual Disorder in the Asylum
and in Court

Although *Psychopathia sexualis* counts as a milestone in the development
of what later became sexology, Krafft-Ebing probably never intended to
establish a new medical discipline. His interest in the broader aspects of
sexual deviance grew out of his experience in asylum psychiatry, where he
was confronted with sexual disorders of patients in connection with already
established mental pathologies. Yet his particular concern for sexuality was
perhaps even more fostered by his involvement in forensic psychiatry.

In some of his early writings, published around 1870, Krafft-Ebing discussed abnormal sexual behaviors, like sexual precociousness, excessive
masturbation, and debauchery, not as diseases in themselves but as symptoms of hereditary madness, degeneration, or moral insanity (1868b, 200;
1869a, 454; 1871b; 1872a). Feeling that moral consciousness and social
attitudes depended on a healthy sexual development, he stressed the importance of the psychiatric diagnosis of sexual disorders. An intense, uncontrollable sex urge that manifested itself at a young age, often as excessive masturbation, and that could result in other sexual derangements at a
later stage in life was proof of a constitutional weakness of the nervous
system. In two articles Krafft-Ebing dwelled on the possible connections
between masturbation and insanity (1875b; 1878a). Although he believed
that masturbation was a symptom rather than a cause of mental disease,
he stressed its pathological nature: excessive masturbation caused nervous
exhaustion, and it was often accompanied by paranoia as well as hallucinations.[1] Not so much the loss of semen, as popular belief had it, but the waste

---

1. Krafft-Ebing especially pointed to olfactory hallucinations: according to him not only
masturbating men but also menstruating women often showed nasal disorders. For that reason
he assumed a special physiological link between the nose and the genitals (1878a, 136; *Ps*
1903, 27–29). In the 1890s, the Berlin ear, nose, and throat specialist Wilhelm Fliess (1858–
1928), at that time a close friend of Freud, would develop a theory on this link.

of nervous energy was detrimental to one's health. In these first articles on deviant sexuality, Krafft-Ebing presented eleven case histories, all of men. Ten of them, including two priests, were hospitalized in the Feldhof asylum, while the other one was treated in the university clinic in Graz. Again and again, Krafft-Ebing would point to masturbation as a crucial symptom of perversion in his later works on sexual perversion.

Krafft-Ebing's earliest published case histories in which sexuality played a major role were of two female patients hospitalized in the Illenau asylum (1869b; 1869c). The first involved the thirty-four-year-old Sara A, who was diagnosed with "hysteric neurosis," melancholia, paranoia, and "erotic madness." Although Krafft-Ebing referred to her unhappy marriage and the death of one of her children as triggers of her mental distress, he focused on the fact that she had developed full-blown "sexual insanity." She had obsessively fallen in love with a family friend and although he did not require her love, she imagined that he also loved her, but that others conspired to break up their relationship. In the asylum, one of the doctors became the object of her exalted protestations of love. Krafft-Ebing treated her with medication and hydrotherapy: she was put in a warm bath with a shower pointed at her head. Eventually Sara A returned to her family, where Krafft-Ebing visited her after a year and concluded that she had become a diligent and happy housewife. The syndrome from which she suffered and that Krafft-Ebing later relabeled as *erotic paranoia* would turn up frequently in his later casuistry. It involved men and women who constantly accused their partner erroneously of being unfaithful or who obstinately believed that their (unrequited) love for someone, often a higher-ranking person, was reciprocal and who in both cases tended to interpret everything as positive evidence of their view. The other female patient, a twenty-year-old farmer's daughter, was treated for excessive masturbation, which had started after her first menstruation at sixteen and which resulted in mental disturbances. After having treated the patient with "methods of coercion" and hydrotherapy to no avail, Krafft-Ebing discovered that she masturbated continually because she was vexed by maggots. After treating this problem, she quickly recovered and was released from the asylum.

Regarding women's sexuality, Krafft-Ebing concerned himself mainly with pregnancy and menstruation as common causes of mental and nervous disturbances. Both conditions intensified the irritability of the nervous system, he explained, and especially women with a hereditary taint were at risk (1868d; 1878b). An article on neuropathic and psychotic disorders during menstruation, published in 1878, was illustrated with nineteen case histories of, for the most part, lower-class women who were either hospitalized in the asylum or treated in the university clinic. Later in his career, Krafft-Ebing came back to what he called "menstrual insanity" or "menstrual psychosis," publishing an article and a monograph on the subject with altogether forty-seven observations, all of women who were hospitalized—with the exception of one or two private patients—or who had committed crimes under the influence of this disorder (1892a; 1902a). He often prescribed bromide to treat it; as an ultimate remedy he also suggested castration, which, according to him, was not dangerous given the advanced medical skills and antisepsis. Among his patients suffering from menstrual psychosis, however, there was only one whose ovaries were indeed surgically removed.

Apart from his treatment of mental and nervous disorders that were related to masturbation, pregnancy, menstruation, and "erotic paranoia," Krafft-Ebing's initial interest in sexual pathology was also intrinsically linked to forensic issues; Psychopathia sexualis was largely intended for lawyers and doctors discussing sexual crimes in court. He regularly acted as an expert witness of courts by writing forensic-psychiatric reports on the mental condition of moral offenders. His first published forensic report dealing with sexual pathology was on a thirty-eight-year-old worker who, ironically, appeared to lack any sexual desire (1875a). The man had been arrested because he tried to castrate a boy. He accounted for his deed by criticizing social injustice: the problem of widespread poverty could be solved by stopping people from propagating. Castrating children, thus the man reasoned, was the first step in getting rid of poverty. Krafft-Ebing concluded that the man, who had tried to castrate himself earlier, was mentally disturbed. His defective sexual urge, which according to Krafft-Ebing explained his antisocial behavior, pointed to degeneration. On his psychiatric advice, the court decided that the defendant should not be sent to prison but be hospitalized in an asylum.

Three years later Krafft-Ebing published a forensic examination of the psychological condition of a twenty-three-year-old female worker, Eufemia A (1878c). Apparently, she had been seduced by two young men into having sexual intercourse with them. Since she was known to be mentally disturbed, Krafft-Ebing was asked whether Eufemia A, at the time of the incident, was aware of what happened to her and disposed of free will. If not, according to Austrian law, the two men could be prosecuted for rape. He diagnosed her and found that she suffered from fits of temporary insanity, especially when she had her period. Her illness manifested itself as nymphomania and seriously affected her presence of mind. His conclusion was that she could not be held responsible for what had happened, but at the same time he doubted whether forced sexual intercourse had actually taken place: nymphomaniacs like Eufemia A often provoked men sexually and tended to confuse fantasy and reality.

Over the years, these forensic cases were followed by many others addressing rape, sexual violence (ranging from murders for lust to biting one's lover's nose), sexual harassment of the feebleminded or children under the age of consent (fourteen years old in Austria and Germany), homosexual intercourse, bestiality, public indecency by exhibitionists, and lesser crimes committed by fetishists and women suffering from menstrual insanity. Some of Krafft-Ebing's forensic reports were based on medical observations by other doctors, but in most cases the examination was carried out or supervised by himself on the request of courts, while the defendants were hospitalized.

A more or less typical forensic case—though never published—involved a twenty-nine-year-old tailor, named X, who had been arrested for homosexual behavior in a public toilet.[2] To verify his accountability, X was observed in the psychiatric clinic in Vienna in 1899. In the case report, written down by one of Krafft-Ebing's assistants, several interconnected elements led to the conclusion that he suffered from inborn contrary sexual feeling. The deceased mother of X, an alcohol and morphine addict, had suffered from nervousness and hysteria and had been hospitalized in mental institutions. Even in old age his grandfather, who had died from softening of the brain, had indulged in sexual extravagances. One brother of X had committed suicide on account of an unhappy love affair; the other one drank heavily and suffered from megalomania. Other relatives were nervous and lacked willpower. As a boy, X had a weak constitution and was disease-ridden, had trouble learning, was introverted and unsociable, and played with dolls until after the age of fourteen. Additionally, he was ill-tempered, ostentatious, readily upset, and hypochondriacal, had difficulty making decisions, and was guided by obsessional thoughts. He had erections already at the age of ten and masturbated almost on a daily basis since the age of thirteen. Since puberty he also engaged in homosexual contacts. An attempt at having sexual intercourse with a prostitute failed. He nevertheless married and proved capable of having sexual intercourse with his wife, but only if he fantasized about men during the act. A physical examination of X brought to light that his genitals were fairly small and that the implant of his pubic hair as well as his subcutaneous layers of fat looked like those of a woman. Taken together, all these data on X's relatives, past, character, fantasies, conduct, and bodily constitution could only lead to the conclusion that he suffered from an inborn perversion: his misbehavior was not immoral, but it had been dictated by an irresistible urge, for which he could not be held accountable. Although Krafft-Ebing—as psychiatrist and in his role of expert witness—was not expected to formulate a legal

2. Case history of X (February 6, 1899), Nachlass Krafft-Ebing.

judgment, the judges must have noticed that his diagnosis was aimed at exonerating X of further legal persecution.

While some of Krafft-Ebing's forensic reports were clearly in the interest of defendants, others suggest that his psychiatric judgment could also bolster arguments in favor of outright suppression of perversion. A thirty-four-year-old German lawyer who, as guardian of some boys, had spanked and felt up two of them and who defended himself with the argument that these were pedagogic measures was sentenced to a prison term of two and a half years. Krafft-Ebing criticized the sentence, but at the same time he argued that this did not mean that the man deserved clemency. On the contrary, he stressed that society should be protected against such perverts and that prolonged hospitalization in an asylum and forced psychiatric treatment served this purpose much better than a basic prison sentence (1900c, 555–56).

Somewhat peculiar is the forensic report Krafft-Ebing wrote in 1891 on behalf of a businessman and inventor from Cologne, Paul Gassen. This man was charged with distributing lecherous leaflets advertising one of his inventions, a device for men who had problems with upholding an erection. He had visited Krafft-Ebing earlier in order to demonstrate this so-called "erector" and thus obtain medical authorization. Since Krafft-Ebing came across impotency among nervous patients quite regularly and did not know of a cure, he took a serious interest in the device. "Mr. Gassen produced a double-winding spiral with bulges on either end . . . and since there was no test subject available, he decided to demonstrate the device on his own body" (1897a, 217). Apparently, the psychiatrist was impressed: he stated that the erector served its purpose and deserved the attention of doctors. After Gassen was prosecuted on immorality charges, Krafft-Ebing wrote a sympathetic report, stressing the usefulness of the device and exempting Gassen from the charges, upon which the man was acquitted. Much to Krafft-Ebing's surprise and indignation, though, the shrewd businessman immediately began to advertise the erector again in newspapers and leaflets, using the forensic report as an extra recommendation.[3]

In his first systematic, classificatory work on sexual pathology, an article published in the *Archiv für Psychiatrie und Nervenkrankheiten* in 1877, Krafft-Ebing focused on the lack and pathological increase of the sexual urge, murders for lust (including cannibalism and necrophilia), and contrary sexual feeling. The article was illustrated with seventeen observations, nine of his own patients and eight derived from medical literature.

3. Letter of Paul Gassen to Krafft-Ebing (November 24, 1896), Nachlass Krafft-Ebing.

Two of the three male patients suffering from a lack of sexual desire were hospitalized in the asylum, one after a suicide attempt and the other for hallucinations. The third, the forensic case of the man who had tried to castrate a boy, had been published by Krafft-Ebing two years earlier. In the category of a pathological increase of the sexual urge, later labeled as *hyperesthesia* or *satyriasis* (in men) and *nymphomania* (in women), there were four case studies. Two of them—a man and a woman—were examined by Krafft-Ebing himself, and the other two involved much older cases borrowed from the psychiatric literature. The male patient, a forty-five-year-old engineer whose sexual urge was so intense that, according to the report, "he made no distinction between humans and animals when it came to satisfying his lust," was prosecuted for rape (1877, 297; Ps 1999, 408). This was a typical forensic case. The second patient—a woman of forty-seven who told Krafft-Ebing that she suffered from "monomania for men"—had been hospitalized in the asylum with the diagnosis of melancholia and persecution delirium, caused by a severe concussion (1877, 298; Ps 1999, 405). Under the rubric of murders for lust, Krafft-Ebing presented two older cases that he had found in the medical literature. Although he listed necrophilia under the perversions, he did not illustrate it with a case history. Instead, he presented another borrowed observation that he apparently could not classify; it was about a medical student who derived sexual pleasure from polluting women by urinating on them.

The remaining case histories presented in this article addressed homosexual behavior. Significantly, in these accounts Krafft-Ebing used the term *contrary sexual feeling* for the first time. In earlier publications on moral offenses, he had referred casually to sodomites and pederasts, together with necrophiles and committers of incest, and also to "certain instinctive pederasts" in connection with moral insanity and degeneration (1868b, 200; 1872b, 33). Three of the seven cases on contrary sexual feeling were borrowed from the medical literature, while the other four, two men and two women, were about his own patients. Not homosexuality in itself, but other derangements—neurological complaints, melancholia, nervousness, persecution mania, megalomania, and *folie raisonnante*—were the main reason for their psychiatric treatment. These cases are different from later ones because sexual deviance was only revealed more or less by accident during hospitalization and because Krafft-Ebing viewed homosexuality as inborn in only one case, that of a twenty-five-year-old civil servant, while in the other three cases he saw it as a temporary deviation of the normal sex urge. However, some of the characteristic elements that would turn up again and again in his later casuistry of contrary sexual feeling were already present: parents, brothers, sisters, and other relatives who were not normal (suggesting degeneration); irritability, nervousness, eccentricity, and frequent masturbation from an early age on; dreams as well as fantasies with a same-sex purport; continuous absence of heterosexual desire; and, in men, the failure to have intercourse with women.

All the observations published in the 1877 article were brief and factual, many not longer than a page, most not even twenty lines. In the majority of the cases, the content was limited to a bare listing of medical facts. By and large, Krafft-Ebing's initial theory of sexual pathology was premised on a comparatively small number of generally severe cases of moral offenders, often derived from older medical literature and criminal proceedings, and of patients who were hospitalized in the asylum or in his clinic, not because of perversion but because of other mental disturbances. Abnormal sexual behaviors were as of yet hardly diagnosed as individual psychiatric syndromes, but as part of a much wider range of mental and behavioral derangements that were often connected to degeneration and moral insanity. In his *Lehrbuch der gerichtlichen Psychopathologie* (1875), sexual crimes were not treated as a separate category, and in his *Lehrbuch der Psychiatrie*, there was only a small four-page section on abnormal sexuality (1879–80, vol. I, 67–71). In the forensic textbook only 9 out of 167 observations dealt with sexual derangements, and in the psychiatric textbook only 11 out of the 159 case histories, while in both textbooks they were always discussed in the context of other mental disorders such as feeblemindedness, senility, dementia, moral insanity, melancholia, paranoia, hysteria, raving madness, and menstrual insanity.

The pattern that characterized Krafft-Ebing's discussion of abnormal sexuality in the 1870s can still be observed in the first edition of *Psychopathia sexualis*, published in 1886 and containing fifty-one case histories. In more than half of the cases he reviewed, the sexual derangements were part of other psychiatric and nervous disorders such as imbecility, feeblemindedness, epilepsy, hysteria, paranoia, persecution mania, and "transitory insanity." Most of the other observations had a forensic background because they involved violence, public indecency, or theft. They concerned murderers for lust, so-called *Mädchenstecher* (men who were sexually excited by wounding women), exhibitionists, a necrophile, and some men who were guilty of, as Krafft-Ebing described it, "paradoxical acts," meaning that they were sexually aroused by certain garments (like aprons and nightcaps), handkerchiefs, certain fabrics (especially fur), or ladies' footwear. Those belonging to the last group, who would later be categorized as fetishists, came to the attention of doctors because they had been arrested for theft of their desired objects or, in cases of so-called sadifetishism, for harassment of women in possession of them. Thus, numerous times the same fetishist with a penchant for ladies' handkerchiefs was arrested for stealing them and sentenced to prison terms, ranging from fourteen days up to four years

(1893b). The majority of the cases in the first edition of *Psychopathia sexualis* had been adopted from other publications: out of the fifty-one case histories, only five involved Krafft-Ebing's own patients. Moreover, there were only four cases of homosexuals, two of which had been published earlier. This is striking, not only because in later editions contrary sexual feeling would be the category illustrated with the most observations, but also because in the early 1880s Krafft-Ebing had already published a series of conspicuous case studies of urnings.

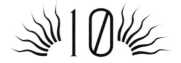

Plato Was Not a Filthy Swine

Krafft-Ebing's interest in contrary sexual feeling or uranism was stimulated by one of his patients, the lawyer Karl Heinrich Ulrichs, who consulted him in 1869 when Krafft-Ebing was in practice as a nerve doctor in Baden-Baden. Early in 1870 they met in Nice and together they did some sightseeing in Monaco (Krafft-Ebing 2000, 129, 133, 137). From 1866 on, Ulrichs had sent him his writings on uranism. Ulrichs had made himself publicly known as an urning; he considered it a normal biological phenomenon and strongly advocated its decriminalization. In 1879 Krafft-Ebing wrote to Ulrichs that his writings had been a major impetus to investigate "this highly important, interesting, and puzzling phenomenon" (Ulrichs 1898 [1879], 108). Ulrichs, for his part, frequently quoted Krafft-Ebing's works, especially to emphasize that contemporary psychiatry no longer viewed homosexuals as sinners or criminals and that Krafft-Ebing was promoting a "humanitarian" approach.[1] However, later he also identified Krafft-Ebing and other psychiatrists as his scientific adversaries, criticizing them for drawing their observations from lunatic asylums and prisons only (Ulrichs 1898 [1879], 122).

As far as Krafft-Ebing's observations in his first article on sexual perversion—published in 1877—were concerned, Ulrichs's criticism was to the point. However, it did not hold true for all of the twelve case histories on contrary sexual feeling that Krafft-Ebing published in the early 1880s in three prominent psychiatric journals and in the second edition of his *Lehrbuch der Psychiatrie* (1883). These histories, all but one of men, were based on his own work with patients or they were derived from the candid letters men wrote to him. The case descriptions differed from the ones published before in

---

1. Ulrichs 1898 (1864a), 34, 56–57; 1898 (1864b), 27; 1898 (1869a), 5, 59; 1898 (1869b), 39, 59.

three respects: with a length of at least two printed pages, they were much more extensive; the subjects primarily came from the upper and middle classes; and, most importantly, in these case histories Krafft-Ebing allowed for the voices of his subjects to be heard, both directly and indirectly.[2]

In the first article, which appeared in 1882 in the *Allgemeine Zeitschrift für Psychiatrie*, Krafft-Ebing stated that until then only fourteen concise case descriptions of contrary sexual feeling were known to the medical world. He suggested that the German and Austrian laws penalizing homosexual acts prevented those concerned from revealing their condition to doctors. Only by coincidence, Krafft-Ebing wrote, was he able to present three new cases. The first one dealt with the thirty-seven-year-old Count Z, who after studying law had embarked on a career in the army. As in the cases published in 1877, Count Z's homosexual leanings only became apparent after his institutionalization; he was treated for his "neurasthenia spinalis" and "masturbatory paranoia." In the asylum, he confessed that at the age of eleven he had been much aroused by a man and that from the age of thirteen men in general exerted an irresistible influence upon him. Z gave a detailed account of his youth, including his sexual experiences. It turned out that his father had been insane and that his mother had died after an apoplexy. Count Z remembered that as a child he was very emotional, worrisome, sensitive, and fanatical about art and literature, that he held "eccentric" opinions and preferred girls to boys as playmates, while his dreams were dominated by men. From the age of eleven he masturbated, and at twenty his effort to perform intercourse with a prostitute proved a miserable failure. He was entirely indifferent to women, but merely the handshake of a man, watching male acrobats perform in a circus, or even a statue of a man would arouse him sexually "from head to toe," as he told Krafft-Ebing (1882, 213).

The striking element in this case history was not only that Krafft-Ebing devoted attention to Count Z's subjective experience of his sexuality by suggesting, for instance, that his love for men really was not different from that of normal men for women, but also that he rendered his patient's viewpoint:

> It was at our first meeting that the patient could be induced to discuss the secret of his sexual life. The patient is neither unhappy about the inversion of his sexual feeling, nor capable of recognizing it as unhealthy.

2. This was not the first time that Krafft-Ebing verbally reproduced statements of his patients. In his 1875 article about masturbatory insanity, two priests who were hospitalized in the asylum were quoted extensively. Krafft-Ebing was not the first doctor to publish writings of homosexual men. In the 1850s and 1860s, the forensic expert Johann Ludwig Casper had published the diary of a certain Baron von Malzan, who had been arrested by the Berlin police, as well as an autobiography that an anonymous man had sent to him (Müller 1991, 182–88).

He is even less capable of doing so, since he feels morally dignified, happy, and relieved because of the contacts with men. How could it be unhealthy, that which makes a man happy and inspires in him beautiful and lofty things! His only misfortune is that social barriers and penal codes stand in the way of "naturally" expressing his urge. This is a great hardship. (1882, 213)

Krafft-Ebing did not argue with Z. On the contrary, he informed him of proposals aimed at the reform of criminal law that would doubtlessly be to his benefit, thus encouraging the man to provide even more detailed information about his sexual preferences and experiences.[3] Count Z told him that he despised pederasty (anal penetration) and that he found sexual gratification in embracing and mutual masturbation. He also gave a precise description of his sexual proclivity:

He feels himself completely effeminate vis-à-vis the male. It appears to him that he has a completely female character and that the form of his pelvis is entirely female. He believes that he is a kind of hermaphrodite and that in addition to male genitals he has a female ovary. According to him, his sexual disposition is as natural as that of others. In his relations with men, he feels sensuality and delight; with them, he feels free, happy, and gratified. (1882, 214)

The intelligent and talkative Count Z easily won over Krafft-Ebing's sympathy. The man was well-mannered and the poems he had written and that he showed to Krafft-Ebing left no doubts about his high-mindedness and his sensitive character. Notwithstanding his female inclination, the psychiatrist asserted, his outward appearance was masculine in all respects; there was nothing in his looks or behavior that betrayed his deviant sexual preference.

The second case description, that of Dr. Phil G, was even more striking. This fifty-year-old man, who made a living as a writer and private tutor, had been arrested in Graz on immorality charges while traveling from Italy to Vienna in the spring of 1880. A soldier who had sex with G for money reported him to the police. They apparently did not know how to handle G when he openly and in plain terms began to defend his inclination. It was reason for the police to call into question G's mental state, and so he ended up in Krafft-Ebing's clinic. G, having "a horny expression and a cyni-

3. Krafft-Ebing probably referred to the new criminal code, which the predominantly liberal Austrian government proposed to parliament in 1867 and which questioned the penalization of homosexuality. However, it failed to materialize beyond the stage of a proposal: "vice contrary to nature" would remain punishable by law in Austria until as recently as 1971 (1894a; cf. Brunner and Sulzenbacher 1998, 31–33).

cal coquettish manner," appeared not to be very impressed by his arrest. With "cynical frankness," according to Krafft-Ebing, he related that he had been in prison for two weeks a few years earlier owing to a similar affair. He also made it clear that he considered himself neither a sinner nor a patient. On the contrary, he was perfectly happy, especially because he often stayed in Italy, where, unlike in Austria and Germany, homosexual intercourse was not punishable. "With great delight and apparent cynicism," Krafft-Ebing wrote, G claimed to have an "inborn contrary sexual feeling" (1882, 214–15; cf. Ps 1999, 590–91).

At one point, G entered into an argument with Krafft-Ebing and his assistants. They posited that contrary sexual feeling was against nature and interfered with the survival of the human species, upon which G remonstrated that he considered his sexual behavior not a vice but a natural force that left him no choice. As long as G could remember, he was cursed with a "horror feminae"; from his early youth on, a "dark impulse" had pushed him toward members of his own sex. He told them that at the age of five he was already fascinated by the male sexual organ, that he masturbated long before the onset of puberty, that as a boy he liked to dress in women's clothes, and that his sexual dreams were all about men. Referring to famous predecessors like Frederick the Great and Plato—who, according to G, "was certainly no filthy swine" and who had already adequately explained same-sex love—he even stated that it was elevating. Like Z, he wrote poetry:

> G points, with a great feeling of self-satisfaction, to his poetic works, and puts forward that persons with attributes like his were poetically endowed. . . . His greatest pleasure is to have a sympathetic young man read his verses to him. . . . He says that the love of urnings is a passionate, inner fire. . . . He feels happy in his peculiar sexuality, which he certainly considers abnormal, but which he does not regard as unhealthy or unjustified. He thinks that nothing remains for him and his pals, except to raise what is unnatural in themselves to the supernatural. He looks upon the love of urnings as the higher, ideal, as the divine, abstract love. (1882, 215–16; cf. Ps 1999, 591–92)

Contrary to Count Z, G did not win much sympathy with Krafft-Ebing, though, perhaps because of his sweeping statements or the crude language in which, for example, he reported his visits to brothels to observe young men having sex: he characterized himself as "a rival of whores" (1882, 215). According to Krafft-Ebing, there was no doubt that G was crazy:

> This is proved by his cynicism; his incredible frivolity in applying his views to religion, in which direction we can not follow him without

overstepping the bounds set by scientific inquiry; his perverse philosophical ideas with reference to his sexual perversion; his perverse worldview; his ethical defect in all directions; his vagabondism; and his perverse character and appearance. G makes the impression of an original madman. (1882, 216; cf. Ps 1999, 592–93)

The third case history, dealing with the thirty-year-old Von H, most likely involved a forensic case, even though there was no legal persecution. Quite possibly his relatives had him placed under legal restraint because of his profligate lifestyle. In the case description, it is stated that the man could not handle money, had financial debts, and, moreover, had caused a scandal. Maybe his relatives wanted to have him institutionalized against his own will and Krafft-Ebing was the one asked to assess his mental state of health. During the examination, he discovered that the indolent Von H had had effeminate leanings from childhood on and that he spent his money on toiletries, fineries, odds and ends, and antiquarian and artistic objects with which he packed his "boudoir." For male activities like hunting and military science, this nobleman showed no interest at all. Except for female activities involving needlework, cooking, and other domestic practices, he was only interested in the creative arts, praising his own paintings and poems. The link between Von H's idiosyncrasies and his sexuality was soon established, even though he was less talkative than either Z or G and despite his saying that his feelings for men did not go any further than friendship; he could even imagine himself as a married man, as long as he did not have to fulfill the "marital duties."

Krafft-Ebing, however, had also acquired information from others about Von H's wheelings and dealings. Among other things, he learned that the man was rumored to have challenged young men sexually in an inn; when he confronted him with this information, his response was one of embarrassment. Moreover, his outward appearance left little to be guessed: his dress, the way he walked, his eye glance, hair, the white powder on his face, the high-pitched voice, the broad thighs, the sparse bodily hair, and the distribution of bodily fat clearly indicated that effeminacy in the case of Von H was not restricted, as with G and Z, to his character only. Although Krafft-Ebing established that Von H was mentally abnormal and incurable, he concluded that he could not be declared of unsound mind in a legal sense, as a result of which forced institutionalization was not at issue. Despite being placed under legal restraint, he would still be able to lead his life on his own, even though because of his inclination he would be in constant danger of getting into trouble and having to face criminal court; if so, the inborn and diseased dimension of his deviation should have to be put forward in mitigation.

On the basis of these three cases, Krafft-Ebing came up with a number of new insights. In comparison to the earlier cases published in 1877 in which three out of the four cases involved more or less temporary aberration, he now put emphasis on the inborn and unchangeable nature of contrary sexual feeling. Although he criticized Ulrichs, maintaining that uranism was a pathological phenomenon because it was usually accompanied by signs of degeneration and mental deviations, he could not deny that some of those involved did not consider themselves to be ill at all. The words of Count Z and Dr. G amply illustrated that they were not so much bothered by their sexual preference as by the social denunciation and penalization. Furthermore, the casuistry revealed that, in addition to the lascivious urnings, there were also those who were morally and aesthetically high-minded. "Contrary to nature" was not by definition the same as "immoral." Similarly, contrary sexual feeling should not be confused with pederasty (anal intercourse); even G, who entirely seemed to go his own way not bothered by anything or anyone, explained that he "looked on the behind with disgust, because it was a secreting organ," suggesting that he could not morally justify this particular sexual practice (1882, 216; Ps 1999, 592). He also considered masturbation as reprehensible: onanism was a miserable and also harmful surrogate for morally high-minded and vitalizing same-sex love. In addition, Krafft-Ebing suggested that evident feelings of love among urnings were comparable to those of normal people and that they experienced their desire as a natural one. In part on the basis of these new insights, he argued to restrict the penalization of homosexuality to pederasty. In doing so, he opposed a trend in German and Austrian jurisprudence that precisely sought to widen notions like "unnatural vice" (according to the German Paragraph 175) and "vice against nature" (according to the Austrian Paragraph 129) to include not only anal penetration but also so-called "coitus-like acts"; thus judges could mark several homosexual contacts as punishable.[4]

The fourth case history appeared in the second edition of Krafft-Ebing's *Lehrbuch der Psychiatrie*. The thirty-three-year-old married businessman from Hungary who sought professional advice because of insomnia and neurasthenia was a private patient, perhaps the first homosexual who consulted Krafft-Ebing on his own initiative. The psychiatric examination of the causes of his complaints resulted in the patient's confession that he was inflicted with an abnormal sexual urge, whereupon Krafft-Ebing incited him to tell "the tale of his life and woe" (1883a, 85). The man, who

---

4. Sievert 1984, 15; Müller 1991, 136–38; Brunner and Sulzenbacher 1998, 38, 57; Sommer 1998, 43–57.

stated that his inborn inclination toward men manifested itself already
when he was three years of age, deplored his marriage and attributed his
physical and nervous complaints to his abstention from homosexual intercourse.

In 1884, a year after publishing the case of the Hungarian businessman,
Krafft-Ebing introduced his second article on contrary sexual feeling,
which appeared in *Der Irrenfreund* with the statement that, for the sake of
social and legal justice, the task of science was to fight ignorance and prejudice, to differentiate pathological perversion from mere immorality and
crime, and thus to improve the social position of these unfortunate people.
The article presented six extensive case histories, five of men and one of a
woman. Strikingly, all of them, like the Hungarian businessman, were his
own private patients, and with one exception—a wealthy twenty-nine-
year-old Polish landowner sent by his family—they consulted Krafft-Ebing
on their own initiative, mostly because of nervous and neurasthenic complaints. None of them was institutionalized in an asylum; three patients
were hospitalized for a limited period in Krafft-Ebing's clinic, and the other
three he met in his consultation room.

The first of these case histories was in fact based on a letter from a thirty-
eight-year-old businessman. The man had read Krafft-Ebing's first article
on contrary sexual feeling with great interest and approval, and he offered
his life history to him in order to contribute to scientific research that, he
hoped, would result in a more enlightened public opinion on the matter.
The man expressed his deep gratitude for the article, suggesting that he and
thousands of others were rehabilitated "in the eyes of every sensible and
reasonable man. . . . You yourself know very well how men like me are de-
rided, despised, and persecuted" (1884c, 2; cf. 1888c, 566). The businessman had emigrated to the United States because of a conviction for "unnatural vice" and the ensuing prison sentence that had socially ruined him.
He felt that grievous wrong had been done to him and that in a moral sense
he was not guilty at all, although he regretted that his family had also suffered because of the scandal:

> And yet I had to say to myself "You have sinned, yes, grievously sinned
> against the common ideas of morality, but not against nature." A thou-
> sand times no! Part of the blame at least should fall upon the dated law
> which confounds the urning, forced by nature to satisfy his instinct, with
> the depraved criminal. (1884c, 4; cf. 1888c, 569)

A similar statement was made by a German count of thirty-four who
consulted Krafft-Ebing because of his neurasthenia and his, as he put it,
"baroque" sexual urge. The psychiatrist wrote in his report that the patient
did not feel unhappy "in his perverted sexual feeling, but that the highest

sexual enjoyment is denied to him for social reasons makes him often feel very sad, unhappy, and embittered, and increases his neurasthenic symptoms" (1884c, 7; cf. 1888c, 572). The count, who was married, felt attracted to young men, but he was not averse to women, although normal intercourse, "this 'crushing' into the 'cloaca' of a woman," as he phrased it, horrified him, while women's breasts were unappealing to him since they reminded him of cows' udders (1884c, 6). He did find sexual gratification, though, if a prostitute kicked him, gave him a flogging, or had her feet licked by him. According to the count, such forms of sexual contact—the term *masochism* was not current yet—were a surrogate for homosexual intercourse, which he did not dare to practice because of moral reservations and penalization.

The American businessman and the German count were not the only ones who attributed their problems to social restrictions rather than to their disposition. A thirty-six-year-old upper-class man who suffered from a nervous disorder had arrived at the conclusion that only in contacts with men could he find lasting happiness. He saw a close connection between his neurasthenia and the need to hide his leanings all the time and suppress his sexual desire. Krafft-Ebing wrote that the "sensitive and frank" man told him with tears in his eyes that he was "most unhappy,"

> partly because of his fatal sexual position and partly because of his nervous disorders and the resultant fear to become insane. The most painful feature of his situation is that he must repress his desires and thereby suffer deeply in mind and body, and that he cannot give expression to his feelings and desires and live up to them. This throws a shadow over his whole life, in particular because of the constant danger that his secret will be discovered and his social position thereby destroyed. (1884c, 9–10; cf. 1888c, 575)

From another case history, it was even more evident that nervous and mental troubles might be related to the forced suppression of contrary sexual feeling. The twenty-nine-year-old Polish landholder—sent to Krafft-Ebing by his relatives because he suffered from neurasthenia and hallucinations while also showing symptoms of hypochondria and paranoia—spent months in the psychiatric clinic in Graz. The man entrusted to Krafft-Ebing that he had felt attracted to men from the age of nine, that they aroused him sexually at the slightest provocation, that he did not consider his sexual preference a disease, and that homosexual interaction gave him a feeling of well-being. In the anamnesis, countless neuropathological disorders and inbreeding in the family of the patient were reported. At first sight, the man seemed a typical case of degeneration, but the next episode reported in the observation also allowed for other conclusions about the causes of his complaints (although Krafft-Ebing did not state this explicitly). After Krafft-Ebing treated the Polish man with electrotherapy, which according to the case description had a beneficial effect, the patient left for Venice, where he contacted fellow urnings and began a relationship with a young man. For some reason, he became the talk of the town, upon which he saw himself forced to leave Venice. On his way back to Poland, he visited Krafft-Ebing, who was surprised by his former patient's healthy physical and mental condition: all symptoms of neurasthenia had completely disappeared and his paranoia was only latently present. Back in Poland, however, where he had no opportunities for homosexual interaction, the former complaints resurfaced and finally the man was institutionalized.

In contrast to the men who distanced themselves from thinking about their condition in terms of disease, a married fifty-one-year-old Polish count did consider his leanings as pathological, even though he simultaneously admitted not to be unhappy at all. The count suffered from severe neurasthenia, which got worse after he was convicted to seven years detention for high treason and had been deported to Siberia. Possibly because the man indicated that his homosexual desire was in large part platonic and because until the age of twenty-five he had had sex with women, Krafft-Ebing decided to treat him not only for his neurasthenia but also his perverse inclination. Electrotherapy had the effect desired, according to Krafft-Ebing: after twenty treatments, the patient felt attracted to women once again.[5] He returned to Poland and wrote to Krafft-Ebing with pride that he was again capable of performing sexual intercourse with his wife and that this also fully gratified him.

Among these case histories on contrary sexual feeling, there was only one that involved a woman, and in some respects it differed from the others. The unmarried thirty-eight-year-old woman spent several months in Krafft-Ebing's clinic and suffered from a "neurasthenic-hysterical neurosis" that was accompanied by hallucinations, fits of cramps, and insomnia. In addition, she had become addicted to morphine. Treatment with electrotherapy had a positive effect on her neurosis, but from the moment the woman appeared in his consultation room, Krafft-Ebing had suspected that more was going on with her:

> Already at our first encounter the patient attracted attention by her clothing, features, and behavior. She wore a man's hat, short hair, spectacles, a gentlemen's cravat, a sort of coat of male cut covering her dress, and boots with high heels. She had coarse, fairly male features, a rough and rather deep voice, and, with the exception of the bosom and female

5. As in other case descriptions in which Krafft-Ebing mentioned electrotherapy, he did not go into the details of this treatment.

contour of the pelvis, she looked more like a man in woman's clothing than like a woman. (1884c, 13–14; cf. 1888c, 580)

Initially, however, his observations did not lead to more or other information; only with great difficulty did Krafft-Ebing and his assistants incite her to reveal that as a young girl she loved horses, that she preferred male activities, and that later on she cherished warm feelings for young ladies in particular. Her family confirmed some of the information, and Krafft-Ebing discovered that she maintained a platonic relationship with a young woman to whom she wrote intimate letters. Significantly, in contrast to the talkative male patients, this woman hardly showed any willingness to tell Krafft-Ebing about her love life.

Krafft-Ebing's third article on contrary sexual feeling appeared in 1885 in *Jahrbücher für Psychiatrie und forensische Psychologie* and included the elaborate autobiographies of, as he put it, two sincere and intellectually gifted urnings. He believed that their life histories, which displayed striking similarities, offered a faithful account of the homosexual condition. Both men reported extensively on the medical histories of relatives; on their own delicate physical constitution, character, childhood, and puberty; on their effeminate predilections, interest in the arts, dreams, sexual development and activities; and on their awareness of being different, their inner conflicts, and their special penchant for soldiers. As one of them suggested: "My sexual inclination is that of a woman to the core, my taste is about the same as that of a Bohemian cook" (1885a, 39). Both had read some of the writings of Ulrichs, and one of them was also familiar with Krafft-Ebing's work. Yet Ulrichs's work in particular had revolutionized their lives because it disclosed to them that they were not alone. As one of them claimed:

> I cannot describe how much I felt relieved when I heard that there are many other men with the same sexual disposition, and that my sexual feeling is not an aberration, but an inner, natural sexual inclination. I opened my eyes and soon found kindred natures. For the first time I enjoyed sexual satisfaction by touching a male body. No longer did I try to suppress my deeply rooted inclination in vain, and since giving free reign to my urning-nature, I am happier, healthier, and more productive! (1885a, 46)

The other man also showed great relief when he noticed that "the earlier inner turmoil about the wickedness and immorality of my inclination had disappeared; no longer did I consider myself as worse than any other young man in love" (1885a, 41). There was no ground to consider his inclination for men as pathological, he argued, if not for his being cursed with a peculiar and unfortunate passion that he experienced as quite painful: his sexual fantasies focused on young men being caned.

Krafft-Ebing's introduction to these two autobiographies clearly reveals that his insights were in part influenced by his homosexual patients and correspondents. Concerning the penalization of homosexual activity, it was advisable, he claimed, not only to consider the acts committed, but to look at the overall (neuropathic) personality. Although he felt that the prosecution of pederasts was justified, his casuistry also revealed that most urnings, whose desire for their own sex was innate, did not commit anal intercourse. They found sexual gratification in other ways, including mutual masturbation, feeling, hugging, and *frictio in corpore alii*; none of this was harmful, and hence there was no reason at all to punish urnings. The legal definition of punishable "unnatural vice" and "vice against nature" should be limited to anal penetration.

Furthermore, Krafft-Ebing believed that urnings were generally not so mentally disturbed that they could not be held responsible for their actions. What exonerated them, though, was their inescapable natural predilection, for which they could not be blamed. Their strong sexual drive was hard to control because of their neuropathical constitution; some entered a state of sexual arousal at the slightest provocation. The Polish landholder told how a hug, a kiss, and even another man's handshake could trigger an orgasm, while for the Polish count the mere look of handsome men or even statues of well-built men were enough for him to find sexual fulfillment. In many cases, forced abstention caused unhealthy onanism or worsened their neuropathic condition. Urnings deserved compassion rather than contempt, Krafft-Ebing maintained; if society, and legal authorities in particular, would take account of their situation, then fewer urnings would be prone to commit suicide or fall prey to blackmail. Strikingly, Krafft-Ebing mentioned three literary works in which same-sex love was treated in an intelligible way: Adolphe Belot's *Mademoiselle Giraud, ma femme* (1871), *Fridolins heimliche Ehe* (1875) by Adolf Wilbrandt (1837–1911), and *Schatten im Licht: Bric-à-brac* (1882) by Count Emerich von Stadion (1838–1901). Finally, he held a plea for more scientific research and a widening of the casuistry. At that point, the international casuistry published on homosexuality comprised only thirty-two cases on men and five on women. Therefore, he strongly appealed to those involved to come out and thus contribute to the advance of science.

It did not take long for responses to pour in. A year later, in the first edition of *Psychopathia sexualis*, Krafft-Ebing included an extensive autobiography of a married homosexual physician who in his youth was seduced by a family doctor. The forty-year-old man considered himself not so much a patient but an informant of Krafft-Ebing. He emphasized that he came from a perfectly healthy family and regretted that he was often unfaithful to his wife because of his inborn inclination. He claimed to have had sexual contact with at least six hundred urnings, many of them belonging to the social elite. Their sexual desire had manifested itself already at a young age, the physician reported, and their sexual drive tended to be strong. Only 10 percent of them would be inclined to enjoy female activities, but female bodily characteristics—like sparse bodily hair, a tender skin, a high-pitched voice, or the abnormal development of breasts—would occur a little more frequently.

In the introduction to the second edition of *Psychopathia sexualis* (1887), subtitled *Mit besonderer Berücksichtigung der konträren Sexualempfindung*, Krafft-Ebing stated that a number of lawsuits in which the accused homosexuals had been treated unjustly had given him occasion to draw special attention to these unhappy "stepchildren of nature." In the introductions to ensuing editions of *Psychopathia sexualis*, he encouraged them to contact him, and they responded by consulting him as private patients and sending him letters and their life histories. After 1887, therefore, the casuistry grew rapidly, and quite soon urnings comprised the category in *Psychopathia sexualis* with the largest number of case histories. The majority of these accounts consisted of autobiographical narratives and letters (or fragments thereof).

The subjects of Krafft-Ebing's observations in his publications on sexual pathology were drawn from different social groups. Whereas most of the cases discussed in the previous chapter involved lower-class people, the ones described in this chapter predominantly dealt with aristocrats and members of the upper middle class. Consequently, class is an important variable in understanding the individual differences among Krafft-Ebing's various case histories (see table 1). This was in part closely connected to his endeavor to broaden psychiatry's base by changing the institutional settings in which he worked and by actively selecting his patients, as we have seen in part 2. Whereas hospitalized patients and suspected moral offenders generally had no other choice than to conform to standard medical procedures and have their stories recorded by Krafft-Ebing and his assistants, many of his aristocratic and bourgeois patients, who more and more began to contact him on their own accord, were given ample opportunity to speak for themselves (see tables 2 and 3). Several masochists and fetishists would soon follow the example set by articulate homosexuals in the sense that they were eager to reveal their lives to the psychiatrist. They were the spirited sources of the life histories and self-observations that in ever larger numbers and with ever greater detail appeared in the expanded and updated versions of *Psychopathia sexualis*.

Table 1 Social Position of Krafft-Ebing's Patients and Correspondents

aristocracy	24
bourgeoisie	206
lower middle class	28
working class	82
unknown	100

Table 2 Patient Status of Krafft-Ebing's Patients and Correspondents

prosecuted for a sexual offense (forensic)	55
hospitalized in an asylum	50
hospitalized in a university clinic	44
hospitalized in an asylum or university clinic	34
hospitalized in a sanatorium	2
consulting Krafft-Ebing's private practice	172
consulting or informing Krafft-Ebing through correspondence	47
unknown	36

Table 3 Authorship of/Voices in Krafft-Ebing's Case Histories

psychiatrist	299
psychiatrist, patient/correspondent paraphrased	54
psychiatrist and patient/correspondent	38
patient/correspondent	49

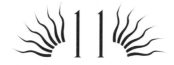

Superior Degenerates

Between 1886 and 1903, fourteen editions of *Psychopathia sexualis* appeared, two under the title *Neue Forschungen auf dem Gebiet der Psychopathia sexualis*. Krafft-Ebing continuously added new case histories; the last edition of *Psychopathia sexualis* edited by himself contained almost 250 numbered observations and another 50 unnumbered, scattered through the text. Many of these cases can be found in multiple editions, while some first appeared in one of the countless articles Krafft-Ebing published aside from his main work.[1] Some were borrowed from other authors, but as his career progressed, the number of cases derived from his own psychiatric practice increased, both proportionately and in absolute terms. After the first edition, the character of *Psychopathia sexualis* changed in no small degree. Whereas initially the majority of the cases were borrowed from other physicians and often involved forensic issues, from the second edition on, Krafft-Ebing's own patients and correspondents acquired a more prominent role with each new edition. He also introduced new categories of perversion, of which fetishism, masochism, and sadism were the most significant ones, but pedophilia, zoophilia erotica, and zooerasty were also identified as specific forms of perversion, whereas stercoracism and coprolagnia were discussed as variations of masochism. Like contrary sexual feeling and its subgroups, he considered most of them as forms of psychopathology in their own right, as existing independently of other psychiatric diseases, and in the subsequent editions they were illustrated and supported by a growing number of case histories. Exhibitionism, nymphomania, satyriasis, paranoia erotica, necrophilia, and incest were discussed under the broader label of sexual pathology as part of other neurological and mental disorders (epi-

1. Where I cite from these case histories, I refer to the publication of Krafft-Ebing in which they appeared for the first time.

Table 4   Diagnosis of Krafft-Ebing's Patients and Correspondents According to Sex and of Borrowed Case

DIAGNOSIS	MALE	FEMALE	BORROWED
anesthesia sexualis	9		9
attempted castration	1		
contrary sexual feeling	143	25	11
defilement with urine			1
epilepsy-perversion	2		1
exhibitionism	2		13
fetishism	35		31
frottage	1		3
hyperesthesia sex/satyriasis/nymphomania	9	2	5
hysteria-perversion			1
incest	2		
insanity after rape		2	
Mädchenstecher/Blutigstechen	1		4
masochism	47	3	16
masturbatory insanity	12	3	
moral insanity-perversion			3
murder for lust	2		16
necrophilia			2
neurasthenia sexualis	4	2	
nocturnal emission in women		1	
paradoxy	1		
pedophilia	9		1
pseudohermaphroditism	1		
psychosis menstrualis		65	16
public indecency			1
sadism	17		14
sexual abuse of feebleminded			1
sexual abuse of minors	9		13
sexual abuse of an unconscious person			1
sexual insanity		1	
sexual/erotic paranoia	24	14	2
sexual bondage		3	1
stercoracism/coprolagny (scatology)	5		3
transitory madness-perversion	1		5
zoophilia erotica/zooerastie/bestiality	3		8

lepsy, imbecility, dementia, paranoia, and transitory insanity) or they were considered in the forensic context (see table 4).

A great number of the perverts who contacted Krafft-Ebing after the first publication of Psychopathia sexualis called on him because they were unable to accept their own sexual inclination, as a result of which they were tormented by feelings of shame and guilt. Whether they were familiar with the medical-psychiatric world or not, many of these patients failed to conceive of their sexual feelings other than as unnatural and sickly. For example, one thirty-year-old man who experienced his homosexuality as highly painful and who therefore wanted to get rid of it told Krafft-Ebing that he considered himself as "a kind of moral insanity character" (1894e, 346). Others characterized themselves as an outcast, outlaw, or "in opposition to the whole world," as well as an "error of nature," a "moral monster, devoid of human feelings," or an "unnatural human being, beyond the laws of nature and society."[2] Many of those who contacted Krafft-Ebing had already fought a long but vain struggle against their sexual leanings, which they considered abnormal. For some, Krafft-Ebing represented their final hope. As one Hungarian homosexual with masochistic leanings wrote to him: "In depression and despair over a life that shuts me out from all that makes human happiness, I come to you with the last gleam of hope to be rescued from a condition that can only end tragically when it persists" (1891h, 12; Ps 1999, 530).

Some of Krafft-Ebing's patients were so desperate that they were on the verge of suicide, if they did not actually commit it. There is one case history on a twenty-four-year-old civil servant, diagnosed as masochistic and coprophileac, who called on Krafft-Ebing to be cured of his perversions. The psychiatrist wrote about him: "He told me that he always carries a pistol now (which he does indeed), but that he is too faint-hearted to shoot himself. . . . I am his final hope." The hypnosis applied by Krafft-Ebing brought no relief: "After the third session I have never seen him again and suspect that he at last has found the courage to put an end to his sad existence" (Ps 1903, 144). The minds of others, though, were eased by Krafft-Ebing: "Over and again his confession was interrupted by severe hysteric attacks," he wrote in a case history of a man who was deeply troubled by his homosexuality, but, as he added, "comforting words, the prospect of help calmed him down" (Ps 1890, 228). Some patients had consulted other physicians before ending up with Krafft-Ebing. Commonly, doctors did not quite know what to do with them; they played down their complaints or encouraged them to look for a diversion, to suppress their sexual fantasies, or to go to the countryside in search of quietude. The naivete displayed by some of Krafft-Ebing's colleagues is remarkable. One of his homosexual patients told him, for instance, that he had already been examined for his sexual problems by another physician: "When the doctor examined my genitals, I immediately had an erection. I lost all inhibition, fell upon his neck and ejaculated. The doctor laughed and said I lacked nothing but a woman" (Ps 1888, 92).

Many patients were not willing to simply accept their fate to be a "stepchild of nature" and were looking for a cure. When a thirty-three-year-old man who had earlier reconciled himself and lived up to his homosexual

2. Ps 1886, 66; Ps 1999, 560; 1891h, 13; 1891h, 102; 1899d, 150; Ps 1901, 263; 1901a, 34.

urges read *Psychopathia sexualis*, he was titillated by some of the passages. Yet he changed his mind:

> The farther I read in the book, however, the more I saw its moral earnestness, the more I felt disgust with my condition, and the more I saw that I must do everything possible to bring about a change in my condition. When I finished the book, I was determined to seek aid from its author. (1891h, 101; cf. *Ps* 1999, 604)

Another patient had been intimidated by reading Krafft-Ebing's study: "After reading *Psychopathia sexualis* he became afraid of himself and of coming in conflict with the law, and he avoided sexual relations with men" (*Ps* 1901, 273; cf. *Ps* 1999, 318). A thirty-five-year-old masochist wrote: "Since reading your book . . . , I have actually not reveled in my fantasy, though the masochistic tendencies have recurred at regular intervals" (1891j, 19; *Ps* 1999, 133). Many were hoping to be cured. Two homosexuals and a fetishist told him they were considering castration (1890e, 57; *Ps* 1898, 155; *Ps* 1901, 266). Two patients had themselves indeed castrated: a woman suffering from psychosis menstrualis and a seventeen-year-old student who believed that his severe neurasthenia was caused by his excessive sexual urge and masturbation. The student decided in favor of castration after hypnosis had failed to bring him relief. Krafft-Ebing advised against this drastic intervention, but the young man turned to a surgeon who was willing to operate on him. When the operation did not exactly have the desired result, he called on Krafft-Ebing once again, who this time successfully kept him from undergoing an even more radical operation he had set his mind on: the amputation of his penis (1899i, 191–92). In another case a female patient who suffered from neurasthenia sexualis was advised by her gynecologist to have a clitoridectomy to put an end to her sexual obsessions. Although at first she was reluctant to undergo such an operation, ultimately she agreed to have her clitoris removed (1892f, 372). It is the only case of clitoridectomy that I found in Krafft-Ebing's casuistry.

Krafft-Ebing did not believe that perversion could be cured by castration; it influenced the forcefulness of the drive but not the direction or object of sexual desire (1899i; 1901b, 133; *Ps* 1903, 324). During the 1880s he treated some homosexuals with electrotherapy, while sometimes he also recommended taking a rest cure or hydrotherapy as treatment for the nervosity and neurasthenia he frequently found in patients. Since the middle of the 1880s, he applied hypnosis in particular. After Krafft-Ebing publicized the successful therapeutic results that he achieved with suggestion under hypnosis, many homosexuals and some masochists and fetishists contacted him with the request to cure their perversion. One of the first cases in which he applied therapeutical hypnosis involved a homosexual academic who asked him in 1888 if he could be cured because he felt unhappy and wanted to marry. Although Krafft-Ebing clearly suggested that the "innate, fundamentally constitutional" contrary sexual feeling of the man was hard to remedy, he still tried to do so, both out of compassion and scientific curiosity, as he wrote. After having hypnotized the patient, he, as Krafft-Ebing noted, "in a drawling voice, repeated the following suggestion: 'I feel that, from this time, I am sexually indifferent to men, and that I am as sexually indifferent to a man as I am to a woman'" (1889/1890a, 10; Ps 1999, 615). This treatment with hypnosis was repeated on a daily basis for a week, after which the psychiatrist tentatively concluded that he had reason to assume that the patient was cured.

The treatment of another patient that same year convinced Krafft-Ebing even more of the therapeutic effect of hypnosis. Although the twenty-five-year-old wealthy landowner, sent by his relatives to be cured by Krafft-Ebing after a painful case of blackmail, did not see himself as ill and although he said that the famous hypnotist Hansen had tried to hypnotize him in vain, he gave his consent to the treatment. According to Krafft-Ebing, this would likely be useful because the young man also displayed some heterosexual inclinations—having told him of his successful visit to a brothel—and therefore he was not "a thorough and hopeless homosexual" (1889/1890b, 62; Ps 1999, 377). In combination with moral treatment and hydrotherapy, the repeated application of hypnosis turned out to have a positive result indeed: Krafft-Ebing reported that the patient became more sexually focused on women. When a year afterward he published this case history once more in a new edition of Psychopathia sexualis, he reported that the patient's cure had been permanent. Not only had the patient's father sent him a letter to let him know his son was doing well; Krafft-Ebing in fact met the young man in person on one of his trips, and there was no longer any trace of homosexuality in the man—he claimed to have had intercourse with a woman and was even considering marriage. Krafft-Ebing hypnotized him again and it turned out that the suggestions were still active: "an excellent example of the possible duration and power of post-hypnotic suggestion," according to the psychiatrist (Ps 1890, 234; Ps 1999, 379).

Case histories like these seemed to evince that it was relatively easy to cure perverse sexuality. In the early 1890s, many private patients came to Krafft-Ebing's clinic in search of treatment by means of hypnosis. Some even thought that they were capable of curing themselves by applying one aspect of the therapy, the suggestion, to themselves. One homosexual, for instance, claimed that he could control his drives through self-suggestion. A proud thirty-three-year-old man contacted Krafft-Ebing to tell him that after reading Psychopathia sexualis he had cured his own masochism and fetishism without outside help. He had bought a pair of elegant ladies' shoes after which he constantly told himself that it was nonsense to get aroused by merely a piece of cured leather. This act of self-suggestion is supposed to have been effective: "the erections disappeared, and finally the boot impressed him only as a boot." The only thing left to do for Krafft-Ebing was to congratulate the man (Ps 1898, 115; Ps 1999, 156).

Around 1890 Krafft-Ebing even gained public fame as an expert in the craft of therapeutical hypnosis. However, numerous case histories indicate that the results of this treatment were mixed at best, something he himself admitted as well. Success was never guaranteed, since not everyone could be hypnotized, and, moreover, as Krafft-Ebing hinted, the likelihood of a cure became proportionally smaller as the perversion was more deeply embedded in the individual's constitution (1891c; 1899a). As far as contrary sexual feeling was concerned, patients with acquired leanings and psychic hermaphroditism, who he assumed still possessed a rudimentary heterosexual desire, offered the best therapeutical opportunities. Many others had to reconcile themselves with the idea that their condition was incurable, that, as one of the patients posited, "nature could not be argued with" (Ps 1887, 85). The same held true for fetishists whose sexual preference came from a particular mental association that over the years had rooted itself firmly at a deep level of the personality. Many homosexuals, fetishists, and masochists had no other choice, according to Krafft-Ebing, than to accept that their natural leanings could not be altered. The way he concluded the consult of a fetishist, who was sexually attracted to crippled women only, is typical of the matter-of-fact attitude that Krafft-Ebing frequently displayed:

> I enlightened the patient on the subject, and told him that it was difficult, if not beyond medical capacity, to obliterate a fetishism so deeply rooted in old associations, but expressed the hope that if he made a limping maid happy in wedlock he himself would also find happiness. (Ps 1898, 155; cf. Ps 1999, 202)

Krafft-Ebing rejected the therapeutic nihilism of the Vienna medical school, but the effort to find a cure for perversions was still of marginal importance in psychiatry at that time. It is true that he experimented with hypnosis to cure perversion, but in general he seems to have applied this remedy only when patients asked for it. Moreover, in later publications he tended to qualify the effect of hypnosis. He warned against "the illusions about the true value of hypnotic therapy"; what was involved was not the veritable cure of patients but, as he claimed, a psychological maneuver, a "suggestive training" (1901b, 133; Ps 1903, 324; Ps 1999, 379–80). In this respect, it is important to note that in many cases psychiatric intervention was limited to treating symptoms: it involved attempts, occasionally with the help of bromide, to control sexual urges or to reduce the common nervousness and neurasthenia of patients. Some patients explicitly indicated that it was not so much their sexuality that they wanted to see treated. A twenty-three-year-old homosexual, for instance, was "completely pleased with his vita sexualis"; he did not pursue any changes on that level and consulted Krafft-Ebing "only because of neurasthenic symptoms" (1894e, 355).

The theory of hereditary degeneration found resonance with many of Krafft-Ebing's private patients and informants. The state of health of parents, brothers, sisters, and other relatives was a recurring theme in their life histories. Only one or two tried to locate the cause of their perversion in bad habits, sexual extravagances, or a failed upbringing. Most of them believed that their abnormal sexuality was inborn, and several stated that they did not want any children out of fear that their offspring would suffer the consequences. Quite a number of homosexuals believed that their parents were to blame for their leanings, some pushing this idea to extremes. One homosexual thought, for instance, that at the moment of his conception, his father had wished for a girl (Ps 1887, 93). Someone else reported that at the time of his birth, his father was said to be "sexually ill" and his mother "to have often gone out in male attire, worn short hair, smoked a long pipe, and in general to have been remarkable for her eccentric character" (Ps 1891, 97; Ps 1999, 599). Another urning claimed that his father at the climactic moment of the procreative act had been weaker than his mother, so that he had inherited more female than male qualities. Again others looked for a cause in the fact that the parents were both very sensitive and irritable persons, or that their mother was plagued by strong emotions during pregnancy (1891h, 123, 127). Cerebral abnormalities were also mentioned as cause. One patient believed that he was equipped with a female brain, while another claimed that something was missing in his brain, namely, "the site in the brain where the feeling for women might be located" (Ps 1890, 116). One of Krafft-Ebing's clients had worked out an elaborate and sophisticated explanation of contrary sexual feeling on the basis of the bisexual stages in the development of the embryo. Later in life this original bisexuality manifested itself physically as well as psychically in various forms and combinations of "latent hermaphroditism." This explanation was all but discarded by Krafft-Ebing, as it resembled the biogenetic theories of Kiernan, Lydston, and Chevalier, which he himself was to give ample consideration in his work (Ps 1893, 227–30; 1895c).

Although such explanations postulated that sexual organs could show signs of hermaphroditism, there were hardly any instances of it in Krafft-

Ebing's casuistry. The thirty-six-year-old lesbian who was convinced that something was wrong with her genitals was an exception (Ps 1901, 294). Various homosexual men indicated that nothing was lacking in that respect, and in most cases Krafft-Ebing, who regularly examined the genitals of patients, could only agree. Inasmuch as other physical defects were reported, they were generally minor, whereas many patients had none at all. Craniometry was frequently reported in the case histories, but only in three of them is direct reference made to an anatomical examination of the brain. Two of them involved homosexual women: one was hospitalized in the asylum because of her "manic-erotical" condition, and the other was admitted to the sanatorium for "hysterical-epileptic attacks," "spinal irritation," and a morphine addiction. Both died while being treated; the autopsy of their bodies disclosed no degenerative anatomical defects in the one patient and lesions in the kidneys, uterus, and an ovary in the other. The examination of the brain, however, did not reveal any particularities in either case (Ps 1886, 70; Ps 1903, 300). The other case involved a pianist who suffered from "sexual metamorphosis": he felt entirely as if he was a woman. After a residency of almost ten years in the Illenau asylum, he died there, upon which a postmortem anatomical examination was done with particular attention devoted to the genitals, but no irregularities were found (Ps 1888, 132).

To a certain extent, Krafft-Ebing's private patients and correspondents applied the biological concept of hereditary degeneration for their own purposes. Of those who considered their perversion a disease or hereditary defect, only a minority may have looked for a cure; many interpreted such qualifications even as rather comforting and soothing, as a counterbalance for the moral repudiation they encountered in the outside world. For example, one urning who was appalled by what he had read in Psychopathia sexualis also found consolation in the idea that he had to be ill (Ps 1890, 228). Someone else considered Krafft-Ebing's explanation of uranism as an innate phenomenon "depressing on the one hand and soothing on the other" (Ps 1888, 80). And a masochist who did not want to give up "the feelings that had become so dear to him" came to Krafft-Ebing with the rhetorical question "whether he was detestable like a vicious man, or an invalid who deserved pity" (1890e, 13–14; cf. Ps 1999, 136–37). The psychiatric concern for hereditary causes was used by patients to underline that their leanings, no matter how regrettable, were part of nature, and therefore unchangeable. Often they jumped at the label of pathology to excuse or justify their sexual conduct, like the forty-year-old factory owner Y who although he was desperate after having been blackmailed and having lost his social position, still did not regret that he had given way to his urges:

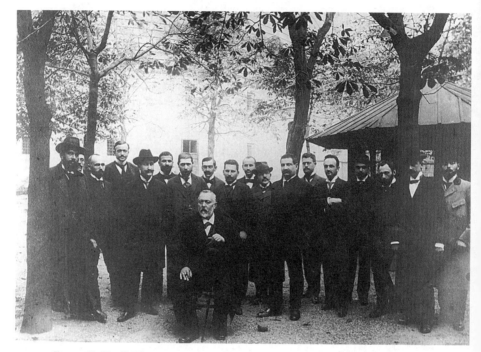

Figure 12. Krafft-Ebing among his colleagues and assistants. (Krafft-Ebing Family Archive, Graz, Austria)

Y recognized the pathological character of his sex life early in his life, but he considered his way of satisfying these abnormal needs to be in accordance with nature. He states that he set aside scruples against yielding to such instincts, although he is sensitive and adheres to strict morals. . . . [H]e felt forced by nature to seek satisfaction in his own manner. (Ps 1901, 263; cf. Ps 1999, 305)

"She recognizes the pathological nature of her sexual inclinations," Krafft-Ebing wrote about the famous Hungarian countess Sarolta V, who had passed as a man under the name of Count Sandor and married a woman, but she "has no desire to have them changed, inasmuch as she feels both well and happy in this perverse condition" (1890a, 453; cf. Ps 1999, 358). Sarolta V, who had been charged with deceit by her father-in-law, defended herself with the argument that God had created her with this disposition:

> Gentlemen, learned in the profession of law, psychologists and pathologists, do me justice! Love led me to take the steps I took; all my deeds were conditioned by it. God put it in my heart. If he created me so and

not otherwise, am I guilty or is it the eternal, incomprehensible way of fate? (1890a, 452; cf. Ps 1999, 357)

This argument met with some approval by Krafft-Ebing: in his forensic report on Sarolta V, he concluded that her behavior was rooted in an inborn disposition and that therefore she was not guilty in a legal sense. The court granted pardon and she continued to present herself as Count Sandor.

A few cases suggest that some clients or their lawyers asked Krafft-Ebing to support their defense in court. Thus the chemist Dr. S, aged thirty-seven, and his close friend, twenty-year-old G, who had both been convicted of "unnatural vice," had appealed an earlier verdict and tried to back up their case with medical and psychiatric reports. The two traveled from Germany to Graz to see Krafft-Ebing, who not only examined them in his consulting room, but, as he wrote in his report, also secretly observed them while they were having dinner in a restaurant together with the wife and brother of S. Krafft-Ebing concluded that the relationship between S and G was based on an intimate, emotional friendship, but that they were not pederasts. His report contributed to the reversal of the court's judgment and both men were cleared of all charges (Ps 1890, 287–88).

Another typical forensic homosexual case involved the upper-class Berlin landlord R, whose lawyer called in Krafft-Ebing's help. His client had been convicted for sexual abuse of several of his servants, but the lawyer tried to reverse the sentence by proving that R suffered from a pathological mental disturbance that had eliminated his free will. Since there is no forensic report by Krafft-Ebing left (in his estate I only found letters from the lawyer and copies of the court's verdict), we do not know the content of his expert testimony in this case. However, the request itself evinces that lawyers and accused homosexuals who were able to pay for it—Krafft-Ebing was promised "a proper fee"—tried to buy his psychiatric expertise to benefit their own cause.[3]

Many of Krafft-Ebing's patients indicated that their perverse desires were inextricably bound up with their personality. They generated memories from their early youth to make clear that their sexual condition had already manifested itself long before puberty. The urning who wrote that "as far as I can remember, I have always had this elementary longing for a male lover" was typical for many patients and correspondents (1891h, 123; Ps 1999, 577). Homosexual men frequently noted, for instance, that already as a small child they preferred playing with girls while feeling attracted to boys or men. A businessman recalled that as a three-year-old he

3. Letters of Dr. S to Krafft-Ebing (January 10 and 31, 1894), Nachlass Krafft-Ebing.

had looked into a fashion magazine and that only the depictions of men captured his attention: "I kissed the pictures of the most beautiful men until the paper was torn to tatters, but paid no attention to the female figures" (Ps 1887, 75; cf. Ps 1999, 562). A masochist claimed that at the age of six he reveled in masochistic fantasies: "As a precocious child I devised a code of discipline for an imaginary school for girls, which was full of corporal punishments" (1899d, 159). Other masochists could vividly remember how as a child they were punished; sadists claimed to know exactly when they had witnessed a punishment and how it had aroused them, while quite a few fetishists said that they had already become obsessed by their particular fetish before the age of ten. That children could have sexual feeling was a supposition that was shared by many of Krafft-Ebing's patients and correspondents. Some testified to have been sexually aroused and to have had sexual fantasies already as a preschooler. Such youthful memories underlined that their sexual preference was deeply rooted in their personality.

Arguing that their "illness" was inborn and part of nature, several patients and correspondents stressed that it was beyond their power to change their behavior. Some of them even indicated that they were not unhappy at all and that they experienced their sexual conduct as wholesome. Thus one of Krafft-Ebing's homosexual correspondents, Dr. XY, who had left Germany to escape legal prosecution and who lived in Italy where he "indulged in perverse love," wrote to the psychiatrist that he did not see the point of a medical examination "inasmuch as his impulse to his own sex had existed from his earliest childhood and was congenital" (Ps 1890, 171; Ps 1999, 310). Perverted sexual behavior often resulted in inward conflict and qualms of conscience, to be sure, but it is striking how many patients and correspondents told Krafft-Ebing that they had experienced their first sexual contact as liberating. A homosexual lawyer, aged twenty-seven, wrote how relieved he felt after his first sexual experience with a soldier: "I knew positively that my whole temperament would find happiness and satisfaction in this, and I resolved to find a human being whom I can love and from whom I would never separate again. I don't have any qualms about my way of acting" (Ps 1889, 150).

"Embracing a male invigorates him physically and morally," Krafft-Ebing noted in the case history of a businessman (Ps 1890, 116). Another businessman also pointed to the salutary effects of frequent sexual contacts:

> In this, I experience the greatest pleasure, the purest happiness, and I feel myself refreshed and invigorated. . . . I am absolutely unable to exist without male love; if I am compelled to forgo it, I become depressed, weary and miserable, and have pain and pressure in my head. (Ps 1887, 77; cf. Ps 1999, 565)

He was not the only one who put forward that homosexual behavior was not so much detrimental to one's health as abstinence was. "Sexual satisfaction was obtained by passionate embraces and kissing of a loved man, especially when he lay on top of him," read the case history of a high-placed thirty-six-year-old man:

> Then he would almost immediately have an ejaculation, producing extraordinary gratification. It seemed to pervade his whole body like a magnetic current and he felt stimulated and happy. Every ten or twelve days he would experience this need, and if he could not satisfy it, he became nervous, irritable, moody, and suffered from all sorts of nervous symptoms. (1884c, 9; cf. 1888c, 574–75)

Not only several urnings claimed that the realization of their sexual desires was wholesome; also masochists and fetishists confirmed that it was beneficial to their physical and mental health. "The adjustment of his vita sexualis strikingly stimulates him mentally as well as physically," Krafft-Ebing recorded in the case history of a nineteen-year-old masochist, "so that it was easier for him to study, he gained energy, got rid of his neurasthenic troubles, and enjoyed physical health" (1899d, 158).

Just as their consideration of heredity, the appreciation of their sexual behavior is an example of the way several patients and correspondents were able to apply medical thinking to their own purposes. The medical drive model indeed suggested that (male) sexuality was a forceful instinct that had to be released in some way; therefore, many of them argued that sexual gratification was inevitable and had to be condoned. Sexual interaction with prostitutes was a recurring topic in the life histories of the male patients and correspondents. For masochists and fetishists, prostitution offered opportunities for satisfying certain perverse desires. Several urnings reported that they frequented brothels in order to "cure" themselves of their homosexual leanings, in general only to find out that they were impotent with women. For them prostitution caused embarrassment in another way: in some circles, such as among students, a collective visit to a brothel was more or less a natural thing to do and without a valid reason it was hard to back out of it.

Among Krafft-Ebing's patients and correspondents, the often positive evaluation of sexual intercourse was sharply contrasted with the common view of masturbation—also the prevailing medical opinion—as harmful to one's physical and mental health. Although virtually all of his male patients resorted to it as soon as they entered puberty and although most of them did not believe that it caused their perversion, only a few did not bother with it at all. Many attributed their nervous disorders to excessive masturbation, and a few men even believed that it had resulted in sexual

perversion. Some referred to writings warning against the dangers of masturbation. There was wide agreement that it was a poor substitute for sexual
intercourse. Several men posited that homosexual interaction precisely
kept them from harmful masturbation. Its supposed harmfulness was even
used as an argument to extenuate one's sexual misbehavior. A pedophilic
private teacher who was sentenced to a prison term of one year on account
of unnatural acts with boys and who after his release came into contact
with Krafft-Ebing claimed that he had put his moral concerns aside "as he
presumed that youths do this anyway among each other and that mutual
masturbation was more healthy for them than solitary onanism" (1899c,
122). Another homosexual correspondent told Krafft-Ebing that as a youth
he had been seduced by a physician into mutual masturbation as well as
pederasty. The man, who also sodomized his own two sons, warned him
against solitary masturbation because it would be injurious to his health
(Ps 1886, 65).

Although many of Krafft-Ebing's patients had trouble accepting their
abnormal sexuality, there were as many who explicitly indicated that
they did not experience their sexual deviation as painful or immoral and
that they did not want to deny their leanings. "He would rather die than
give up male-to-male sexual contacts," Krafft-Ebing quoted one of them;
these were "invigorating and cheering" (Ps 1890, 153–54). Stressing that
his urge was inborn and natural, another urning strongly rejected treatment
with hypnosis:

> Although his contrary sexual feeling is the misfortune of his life, he is
> desperately attached to this kind of love which affords him with a little
> bit of happiness. He would rather not become another person nor lose
> his sweet memories. If he would be cured of loving men, he would be
> unhappy. He cannot and does not want to "swing around," for his whole
> ethics, etc. have developed around this peculiar sexuality. (1890e, 58)

Others expressed themselves in similar ways. "Suddenly I felt like a fish in
the water and I have never noticed any scruples about it," one homosexual
wrote to Krafft-Ebing after he had found contact with some of his peers
(1890e, 50). A musician who had met with many sexual partners while
traveling all over Europe indicated that he, like many others, did not feel
unhappy. "The inherent disadvantages (social intolerance, the endless lies,
and simulation) are amply compensated by the mysterious and magical
charm of the matter" (1890e, 60–61). Emphasizing that he had found most
of his sexual partners in perfect health and with nerves of steel, he hoped
that his confession would be encouraging to others.

Whereas Krafft-Ebing probably had expected perverts to be nervous and effeminate "degenerates," many of his private patients and correspondents indicated that they enjoyed perfect health and that they were physically indistinguishable from their fellow men. Many urnings, for example, stressed that their appearance and behavior was masculine and did not betray their leanings. Nor should they be considered as inferior in character, declared one of Krafft-Ebing's informants:

> It would be wrong to consider the urning as an inferior being. He can be the most perfect creature of nature. I know some, whose character is so noble as I have never observed in normal human beings. . . . He loves his fellow men and feels pity for their shortcomings and weaknesses, because he knows from his own sad experience how powerful the inborn instinct is in man, be it for good or evil. In him the tenderness of female feeling is joined with male strength and willpower, and if he also has— as is often the case—a beautiful appearance, than he really is the model creature of nature. (Ps 1890, 114)

Furthermore, it is striking that many homosexual men put forward that their feelings of love were not different in any respect from those of heterosexuals. One of the correspondents who had sent his life history to Krafft-Ebing told the story of how he had experienced his first love affair, because, as he wrote, he wanted to show that

> among our loathed and objectionable group, the soul, i.e., the complete inner being, is perhaps even more inclined to feelings of sympathy than among people with a normal disposition. . . . I don't think that a man who feels normal can love a woman more ardently and passionately than I did then. (1890e, 47–48)

Another urning, who rejected Ulrichs's proposal that urnings should be allowed to marry, nevertheless stated:

> Our love also bears the most beautiful and noble blooms, develops all noble drives and stimulates the spirit, as much as the love of a youth for his girl. One finds the same devotion, joy in sacrifice, . . . the same pain and sorrow, the same exultant mood and happiness as with real men. (1884c, 5; cf. 1888c, 570)

Among Krafft-Ebing's private patients and correspondents, many were doubtlessly seeking confirmation of their odd feelings. Several of the autobiographies and letters reveal a strong rhetorical effort toward self-justification. They often asserted that their sexual behavior could not be immoral or pathological because they experienced their desire as "natural." Few of them suffered from mental problems beyond fear of exposure and disgrace or beyond uneasiness about their position in society and the difficulty to find love and sexual gratification. An American artist "considered his sexual anomaly as inborn and yielded to it; he felt only unhappy in this situation as far as he had to hide his inclinations, suppress his drives, or did not find his love requited" (1890e, 59). "Most 'aunts,' like myself, do not regret their abnormality," said another urning, "but would regret if their condition were changed. Furthermore, we all are convinced that this inborn condition cannot be influenced. Therefore, all of our hope is pinned on a change of the relevant law" (Ps 1890, 175; cf. Ps 1999, 315).

Discussing the legal aspects of same-sex behavior in the second edition of Psychopathia sexualis, Krafft-Ebing included a long letter from a high-placed man from London who criticized him for holding on to the opinion that homosexuality was a disease:

You have no idea what a constant heavy struggle we all still must endure nowadays—particularly those of us who have the best minds and finest feelings—and how we suffer under the still prevailing false ideas about us and our so-called "immorality." Your opinion that the phenomenon under consideration is primarily due to an inborn "pathological" disposition will, perhaps, make it soon possible to overcome existing prejudices and awaken pity for us poor, "abnormal" men, instead of the present repugnance and contempt. Much as I believe that the viewpoint expressed by you is possibly beneficial to us, I am still not willing, in the interest of science, to accept unconditionally the word "pathological."

Psychological suffering and mental pathology were indeed widespread among urnings, the man continued, but experience had taught him that the cause was not so much their inborn disposition as the legal and social suppression with which they had to contend:

According to my firm belief, the greater number of cases, by far, of mental disturbance or unhealthy disposition observed in urnings are not to be attributed to the sexual anomaly. Instead, they are caused by the existing false notions about uranism, the current laws which are connected to these, and the dominant public opinion on this matter. Whoever has any idea of the mental and moral suffering, the anxieties and worries that the urning must endure; the constant hypocrisy and secrecy he must practice in order to conceal his inner drives; the endless difficulties which he meets in satisfying his natural desire—can only be surprised that more insanity and nervous disturbance does not occur among urnings. The greater part of these unhealthy conditions would not develop if the urning, like the dioning [heterosexual], could find a simple and easy way in which to satisfy his sexual desire; if he were not forever tormented by these fears! (*Ps* 1887, 139, 141–42; cf. *Ps* 1999, 480–81, 483–84)

This shift in the attention away from viewing homosexuality as a pathological condition toward a more concrete concern with the social restraints it involved was soon picked up by others as well. In the third edition of *Psychopathia sexualis*, Krafft-Ebing published the autobiography of a fifty-year-old urning from Belgium who explained that his nervousness was caused by the many obstacles that made it difficult for him to satisfy his sexual urges and by the fact that he continuously had to hide his nature and pretend.

> Neither can I acknowledge, even though I am an urning, that my nature is an "unhealthy" one, otherwise you would have to classify other categories of men who are usually considered normal as unhealthy as well. . . . I lack the desire for the female sex, as other people display a marked aversion to other things; since most men don't lack this desire and since those who also lack it, don't say so, we are labeled as "sick" for we appear to be the unnoticed minority. . . . We are considered sick for another reason, which, unfortunately, is a completely valid one, namely, that we have really become sick. But people have confused cause and effect. . . . We certainly become sick, just as animals are stricken by rabies if they are prevented from engaging in the sexual act appropriate to their nature. (*Ps* 1888, 82)

Although this statement contradicted Krafft-Ebing's medical opinion, he did not censor such criticism. On the contrary, in the following editions of *Psychopathia sexualis*, more and more letters and autobiographies were included in which urnings posited that medical theory was one-sided and that they were not seeking a cure since it was not their disposition that made them unhappy but the social condemnation. A thirty-one-year-old employee wrote: "Although I suffer greatly because of my anomaly, I am not unhappy because I love young men, but because the satisfaction of such love is considered improper, and therefore I cannot gratify it without restraint" (1891h, 108; cf. *Ps* 1999, 554–55). In his elaborate autobiography, a cosmopolitan man of thirty-six insisted:

> I cannot believe in the least that my condition might appear unnatural, for as far back as I can think I have always felt the same way. . . . Morally I endured a lot, quite a lot, however, not because I considered my instinct as unhealthy, but because of the general contempt we encounter all around us. (1890e, 55)

To consider contrary sexual feeling a disease, a German engineer contended, was a serious fallacy.

> For in every disease there is a means of cure or amelioration, but no
> power in the world can take from an urning his perverse natural constitu-
> tion. Even suggestion, which has been used with so much apparent suc-
> cess, cannot induce any enduring change in the mental life of an urning.
> In us, effect is mistaken for cause. We are considered diseased because
> eventually the majority of us actually become ill. I am almost convinced
> that two-thirds of us in later life—if we live so long—have a mental
> defect of one kind or another and that is only too easily explained. Con-
> sider what strength of will and nerves is required for one to constantly
> dissimulate, lie, and feign all of his life! How often in the society of nor-
> mal men, when the conversation turns to contrary sexual feeling, must
> one agree with words of abuse and contempt, while every one of them
> hurts the heart. On the other hand, there are always the tiresome and
> indecent jokes and talk about women that are so popular today in so-
> called "good society"—and one must feign interest and give attention to
> them! To daily and hourly see so many handsome men and not be able
> to reveal oneself; to be compelled to go out without a friend, the com-
> panionship we desire so much; to say nothing of the constant and fearful
> anxiety of betraying oneself before the eyes of the world, only to stand
> covered with ignominy and shame! . . . [W]e need all our strength of will
> and all our power of endurance for the struggle with our fate. How injuri-
> ous it is to our nerves to constantly be compelled to hide all such
> thoughts and feelings in our hearts. (1891h, 131; cf. Ps 1999, 585)

A thirty-one-year-old employee, who wrote that he "no longer [had] any
moral scruples" because of his "anomalous inclination," also criticized contemporary thinking on homosexuality, especially the argument that it was
immoral because of its sterility. As he pointed out, ubiquitous prostitution
and the use of contraceptives showed that it was far from simple to pass
moral judgment on sexual behavior on the basis of the norm of procreation.

> It seems questionable to me that only sexual gratification having this
> purpose is moral. Certainly, sexual satisfaction not directed to procre-
> ation is contrary to nature, but it may have other purposes which are
> unknown to us; it is not clear, and, even if it were purposeless, it would
> not necessarily be despicable (since it is not certain that the measure of
> a moral act is its functionalism). (1891h, 109; cf. Ps 1999, 555)

Other correspondents not only criticized Krafft-Ebing and other doctors for
surrounding uranism with the stigma of pathology; they also fiercely rejected current legal thinking on homosexuality. Thus a businessman wrote

to Krafft-Ebing that he suffered from nervousness, which, according to him, was "first acquired as a result of the cursed contempt from which we suffer."

> How can the view of society be changed as long as there is a law that strengthens it in its false morality? The law must correspond with public opinion, to be true, but it should not be in harmony with the erroneous public opinion. It should, instead, accord with the ideas of the thinking and scientific circles among the people, and not with the obscure wishes and prejudices of the populace. Truly thinking minds cannot much longer be satisfied with old ideas. (Ps 1890, 164; cf. Ps 1999, 570)

A letter from another businessman who had read one of Krafft-Ebing's articles on contrary sexual feeling was equally unambiguous in this regard:

> Your work "Die conträre Sexualempfindung vor dem Forum," which I just put down, greatly aroused my interest. It is, to be true, but a poor attempt at making the abnormal phenomenon—which occurs more often than you assume—clear to wider circles and at proving that the expressions of the natural drive, even if different from the conventional form, cannot be punishable. If truly wise men would create laws, they should say to themselves that one cannot punish people for inclinations which nature has planted in them. (Ps 1890, 113)

Whatever two persons voluntarily do with each other in private and without harming others should never be part of the criminal code, one thirty-four-year-old musician claimed:

> In our in other respects so enlightened and prudent age, the time should be ripe to do justice to these millions of individuals, on whom nature has played a dirty trick and who are indeed completely innocent. After all, improper behavior is forbidden in public, but what two individuals do in private with mutual consent without harming a third person should not be forbidden by human laws. (1890e, 61)

Even two pedophilic teachers, who were prosecuted because of their sexual abuse of some of their pupils, criticized the criminalization of their behavior. One acknowledged that he had misbehaved as a teacher, but as a human being, he argued, he could not accept that his leanings, which were natural to him, were punishable (1899c, 121). Neither did the second one, a priest who was observed in Krafft-Ebing's clinic, admit that he had committed a crime. The man stated that he was pitiful rather than guilty and appealed to a statement of the apostle Paul: "I acknowledge the law, but another one prevails in my limbs" (1900b, 266). Another pedophile, a twenty-year-old gymnasium student, equally suggested that his leanings were unchangeable and had to be accepted: he wrote that being exiled to a land where "such things are permitted" would be his only rescue (1899c, 124). Compared to perversions like homosexuality, pedophiles generally considered their leanings not as particularly serious.

By publishing the sometimes lengthy, assertive arguments of urnings without adding any medical or moral judgment, Krafft-Ebing gave a clear signal to his readers. Repeatedly, in fact, he pointed out that these accounts powerfully illustrated the feelings and sufferings of their authors. Moreover, in *Psychopathia sexualis* as well as in several articles on contrary sexual feeling, he came back again and again to its legal aspects. At first he did not attack the German and Austrian laws criminalizing homosexual intercourse, but merely stressed the need to distinguish crime from disease and to punish pederasty only. Whereas in 1882 he still concluded that one of his patients, Dr. G, who criticized German and Austrian legislation, showed "incredible cynicism" and was mentally deranged, a few years later, after having published several life histories that showed the harmful effects of penalization, he himself began to favor judicial reform. In the early 1890s Krafft-Ebing put his name to pleas for the abolition of Paragraph 175, and in *Psychopathia sexualis* he added that the book should contribute toward changing the law, thus making an end to "the errors and hardships of many centuries."[4] He deplored that politicians and lawyers showed so little interest in the latest medical opinion on the matter and that innocent people were stuck with the consequences.

In 1891 and 1892 Krafft-Ebing published the letters of a high-level German civil servant and a lawyer who both had formulated elaborate well-founded pleas against the criminalization of homosexual intercourse (1891f; 1892c; 1892i). In the epilogue that Krafft-Ebing wrote to the article of the "renowned" lawyer, who wanted to keep his anonymity, he stressed that he fully agreed with his arguments in favor of the abolition of Paragraph 175. Uranism was not immoral and most urnings experienced their strong sexual urge as natural. There was no rational justification for Paragraph 175: the interests of third parties were not infringed upon. Moreover, the definition of "unnatural vice" was vague and open to question, and consequently verdicts were often arbitrary. This legal provision only benefited blackmailers, while everybody who was prosecuted under it suffered from social ostracism.

In his introduction to the autobiography and the legal argument of the

---

4. Surprisingly, Krafft-Ebing aimed his arrows at the German Paragraph 175 in particular, while showing much more reserve regarding the Austrian Paragraph 129. He had become an Austrian citizen and probably, because of his position as *Hofrath* and the most prominent professor of psychiatry in the Habsburg Empire, he held back in order not to antagonize government officials and colleagues.

civil servant, Krafft-Ebing stressed that his correspondent's views deserved serious attention, even if they came from a layperson. Referring extensively to juridical literature, the man critically discussed Paragraph 175 and concluded that this law was based on prejudice and ignorance: the legal prosecution of homosexuals was the modern equivalent of the witch trials of the past. In the same way, medical science did not escape the harsh criticism of this correspondent, who stressed that his own health left nothing to be desired and that he did not suffer from any hereditary defect. It was wrong to equate the abnormal with the pathological, he contended, and what had been instilled by nature could not be immoral: "Thus not nature is guilty of our misfortune because we feel well in our special way of being . . . , but our human judges and persecutors who don't know what they are doing are guilty" (1892i, 8). Medical scientists had the duty to enlighten the general public rather than to cure homosexuals. He concluded his apologetic with a straight appeal to Krafft-Ebing:

> But what keeps a scholar invested with the highest authority in his field from presenting the case to the public in a proper way, excluding all unpleasant details, and instruct them: that nature has planted the love for one's own sex in many of our fellow beings, including noble, highly valued men; that a natural drive is not a vice and crime; . . . that society, under the spell of a delusion, is committing a grievous sin by daily sacrificing thousands of fellow men. The doctor should devote himself to this task. To cure the perverted instinct is to little avail, even if he succeeds in a few cases; for the born urnings all remedies are at least precarious anyway, and hypnosis is no exception to this. Just consider a hardly less valid experiment: to hypnotize a normalsexual and burden him with contrary sexual feeling. However, if the physician would be concerned to free the world of its misguided view, thus he would bring about a mass cure of the ignorant as well as of their victims, which would provide him with the gratitude of thousands of sufferers. (1892i, 43)

Soon afterward, in his *Der Conträrsexuale vor dem Strafrichter* (1894), Krafft-Ebing began to echo some of these arguments against the penalization of homosexuality, which, he pointed out, was inspired by prejudices. In Germany penalization was justified on the basis of popular opinion alone, and the persecution of witches in the past had proven that this was a poor justification indeed. He tried to disprove three widely held misconceptions in particular: that homosexuality was a crime instead of a disease, that it was the same as pederasty, and that urnings lusted for young boys. His casuistry illustrated that the moral standards of the average homosexual were as high as those of the average heterosexual person. Those who were convicted by public opinion and jurisdiction were often not inferior beings, he stressed: many of them were gifted *dégénérés supérieures*. Homosexual love was not even incompatible with national greatness, Krafft-Ebing asserted, "for during the flowering of Hellas, pederasty was widespread" (1894a, 11). He further argued that criminal law was not the appropriate tool for protecting the state against moral decay. Ultimately, he claimed to favor legislation that was modeled on the French system, in which homosexual activity was only punishable if it was accompanied by the violation of public decency, the seduction of minors, or the use of force or violence. He did advocate a legal minimum age of eighteen with regard to homosexual activity as well as regulations against male prostitution.

Krafft-Ebing sent *Der Conträrsexuale vor dem Strafrichter* to Ulrichs. Although Ulrichs regretted that Krafft-Ebing did not acknowledge his pioneering work in this respect, he praised him for advocating the decriminalization of homosexual behavior. A year before his death in 1895, Ulrichs wrote: "I sowed the seeds; all fell on gravel or thorny bushes. Only one fell on a human heart. . . . The ice is broken" (cited by Kennedy 1988, 224). When, at the end of the nineteenth century, other homosexuals began to organize themselves, they referred to Krafft-Ebing as a scientific authority who was on their side, and he indeed supported the homosexual rights movement that was founded in Berlin by Hirschfeld in 1897. In his *Die Enterbten des Liebesglücks* (1893), Otto de Joux (pen name of Otto Rudolf Podjukl) from Vienna mentioned a petition of a group of urnings in Germany in which Krafft-Ebing was praised and thanked because he stood up for their rights (De Joux 1893, 15, 72–73). The Berlin-based Comité für Befreiung der Homosexualen vom Strafgesetz, which in 1899 published a pamphlet—"Aufruf an alle gebildeten und edelgesinnten Menschen!"— apparently also viewed Krafft-Ebing as an ally, because they sent him a copy of it (Nachlass Krafft-Ebing). In a letter to Hirschfeld written early in 1902, he praised Hirschfeld's *Jahrbuch für sexuelle Zwischenstufen* and expressed his willingness to contribute to the "good cause."[5] Hirschfeld would continue to claim Krafft-Ebing as an ally of the homosexual rights movement until long after Krafft-Ebing's death. After Krafft-Ebing had signed Hirschfeld's petition advocating the abolition of Paragraph 175, he admitted in his last article on contrary sexual feeling, published in *Jahrbuch für sexuelle Zwischenstufen*, that its medical conception had been one-sided and that there was truth in the point of view of many of his homosexual correspondents. Having earlier referred to the decline of Greece and Rome as cautionary tales from the past, he now believed that contrary sexual feeling in itself should not be viewed as psychic degeneracy or even as a disease; it was not incompatible with mental health or even with intellectual superi-

---

5. *Jahrbuch für sexuelle Zwischenstufen* 5 (1903), first unnumbered page.

ority, as was proved by many writers, poets, artists, generals, and statesmen of all nations (1901a, 6). It was not so much a disease as a biological and psychological condition that had to be accepted as a more or less deplorable but natural fate. Emphasizing homosexuality as a psychological condition, rather than as a specific kind of sexual activity, Krafft-Ebing—unlike most of his contemporaries—attributed equal moral value to same-sex love and heterosexual love.

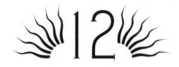

Orgies of Fantasy

The letters and personal narratives of Krafft-Ebing's patients and correspondents reveal that perverts, in their interaction with the psychiatrist,
did not play a passive role by definition. Their writings betray a considerable degree of suffering because of their sexual leanings as such, but also
because of the social condemnation, the repressive legal situation, the need
to disguise their real nature, the apprehension of being blackmailed, and
the crippling fears of losing their social status. In the words of medical historian Roy Porter, they were "articulate sufferers" and their sincere stories
certainly touched a nerve in Krafft-Ebing (Porter 1985, 176). The confessional writings that were specifically addressed to him caused him to adopt
a more sympathetic attitude toward their authors. Over the years, he gradually introduced new and more subtle differentiations within the field of
sexual pathology on the basis of these writings and his evaluation of their
contents. Some perverts were indeed mad, violent, dangerous, immoral,
and unscrupulous, he found, but others were pathetic rather than horrific,
while many appeared to be just harmless, good-natured, sensitive, and even
civilized, respectable, and socially integrated. Krafft-Ebing's sustained
study of his subjects' self-analyses and commentaries prompted a shift from
his predominantly forensic and biomedical focus toward a considerably
broader concern for the psychology of human sexuality in general. Seeking
to understand all aspects of perversion, the psychiatrist and his patients
not only fixed their attention on heredity, degeneration, and physical and
mental health, but they looked more closely into personality formation as
the defining factor of sexual identity as well.

Krafft-Ebing's views were shaped by his interactions with urnings, but
some masochists also left their mark on his way of thinking. In fact, masochism as a label was suggested to him by an anonymous correspondent

from Berlin who referred to the novels of Sacher-Masoch. But also for his psychological explanations of masochism, the psychiatrist depended heavily on the ideas of this same "well-educated man," as Krafft-Ebing characterized him. The man counted as one of his main informants on masochism, and Krafft-Ebing consulted him when he became engaged in a dispute with a Russian lawyer about the discovery of masochism.[1] Emphasizing that he did not consider his sexual leanings in any way as painful or pathological, notwithstanding his neuroses and obsessional thoughts, the man sent Krafft-Ebing an extensive life history, including meticulous self-analysis and elaborate depictions of his sexual fantasies. In a cover letter, he also reported his observations of prostitutes who were experienced in dealing with masochistic clients. The man, who was widely read and who recognized himself in Rousseau's *Confessions* and Sacher-Masoch's novels, had thoroughly reflected on his perversion.

The crucial thing, the Berlin man suggested, was the role of fantasy: the essence of masochism was "a process of inner consciousness" (1890e, 25; *Ps* 1999, 528). As a youngster he spent hours indulging in fantasies about prison scenes in which he was kicked, beaten, and tortured in other ways by a woman. He imagined himself to be in chains and kneeling down in front of an ideal mistress, exposed to humiliations and agonies designed to amuse her. He reveled in these "orgies of fantasy," as he phrased it, and indicated that he felt more at home in the world of the imagination than in that of reality. To nourish his fantasy, he devised, wrote down, and drew erotic scenes that excited him. Explaining that he was swayed by a peculiar obsession, he unwittingly mirrored a typical hang-up of contemporary psychiatry: the craving for elaborate classifications of mental diseases.

> My most peculiar obsession may be the urge to design systematic divisions without any reason or purpose. Then I make every effort to classify a series of things I love according to clear principles and a symmetric structure of the categories. Even my sexual imagination and fantasies have become the object of this passion; for weeks I have made strenuous efforts to list all maltreatments and humiliations which a woman can inflict on a man, and to classify them in clearly delimited categories and subcategories, which I indicated with Roman and Arabic numbers. (1890e, 21)

1. In 1891 Krafft-Ebing was informed by the Russian lawyer Dimitri Stefanowski that he had discussed this sexual aberration already three years earlier in a lecture for the Moscow society of lawyers, labeling it "passivism." In an article about the differentiation between what he called "sexual bondage" (of women) and masochism, Krafft-Ebing tried to make plausible that passivism was equivalent to the former and not the same as the latter. He argued that sexual bondage, though abnormal, was not a perversion (1892b, 210).

When, however, after many years of solitary fantasies, the Berlin man acted upon them by paying and instructing a prostitute, the experience proved to be an outright disappointment to him. The tragedy of masochists was that their attempts at realizing their fantasies frequently resulted in frustration and even revulsion. "What was done to me I felt to be rough, repugnant, revolting, and silly at the same time" was how he described his experience of being flogged (1890e, 19; cf. *Ps* 1999, 527). He posited that masochism was not about physical pain; maltreatments such as floggings were only symbolic acts of the psychological need of the masochist to be dominated by a woman. The masochist could only be fully satisfied if the staging of his "elaborate comedies" dovetailed with his fantasies. Yet the problem was that women generally were not inclined to dominance and not capable of instilling in the masochist man the feeling of truly being subjected; even prostitutes who specialized in playing the sadist's role, the man claimed, only tended to offer a poor substitute for the masochist's fantasies at best.

This Berlin man's intricate self-analysis and explanation of masochism was supplemented by numerous autobiographical reflections of other men who stressed the essential psychological nature of this perversion. "As for the essential element in masochism, I am of the opinion that the impression—i.e., the mental element—is the end and the aim," a thirty-five-year-old correspondent wrote to Krafft-Ebing.

> Everything which follows from the impression, be it onanism, coitus, or realization of the ideas, is in my view only an effect, but not the purpose. If coitus or other ways of getting satisfaction would be the purpose, then it would be difficult to understand why one keeps putting off as long as possible the satisfaction. This is because one knows very well that gratification all at once puts an end to the joy of indulging in fantasy. If the realization of the masochistic ideas (i.e., passive flagellation, etc.) is the desired goal, then it is in opposition to the fact that the majority of masochists never attempt realization, and if they indeed attempt it, they feel a great disillusionment; at any rate they do not obtain the desired satisfaction. (1891h, 17; cf. *Ps* 1999, 132)

What mattered was not so much the physical pain but the feeling of subjection and humiliation. A German civil servant of thirty-five, who only knew Krafft-Ebing's works on masochism from hearsay, stressed "that the point was not so much the suffering of physical pain as 'that the others made him feel their superiority in speech and behavior'" (1899d, 149). A twenty-nine-year-old engineer reported an analogous experience:

He twice visited brothels to have himself flogged by prostitutes. For this purpose he chose the prettiest girl he could find, but he was disappointed and did not even have an erection, to say nothing of ejaculation. He recognized that the flagellation was subsidiary, and that the idea of subjugation to the woman's will was the main thing. The first time he did not succeed, but the second time he realized this. When he had the "idea of subjugation," he was perfectly successful. (Ps 1892, 97–98; cf. Ps 1999, 121–22)

Not everybody succeeded in finding or creating a situation that corresponded to their fantasies. Again and again, masochists pointed out that the relation between imagination and reality was problematic. Many of them confessed that efforts to realize their desires were painful and not satisfying. Some of them, labeled "ideal masochists" by Krafft-Ebing, did not even try to act out their fantasies, not only because shame prevented them from doing so or because they failed to find the appropriate opportunity or suitable partner, but also because they knew beforehand that the actual experience would only result in deception. Thus one of them wrote:

I have never attempted to realize my very definite and characteristic impressions—i.e., to connect them with the world outside of me—but I have contended myself with reveling in my thoughts, because I was convinced that my "ideal" would not allow even an approach to realization. The thought of a comedy with paid prostitutes always seemed so silly and purposeless, for a person hired by me could never take the place of my imagined "cruel mistress." I doubt whether there are sadistically constituted women like Sacher-Masoch's heroines. (1891h, 16; cf. Ps 1999, 131)

For most masochists it was indeed not easy to find sexual satisfaction. A few of them stressed that a "proper staging" was important for achieving sexual gratification. The homosexual nobleman Z, for example, indicated how difficult it was to gratify his desires:

Only one among many, a young man, whose photograph Z carries with him, was able to play such comedies so skillfully that the illusion and its effect were realized. Z complains excitedly that this is rarely possible, for fantasy is the essence of his masochistic passions and this is not as easy to satisfy as his contrary sexual feeling in itself. If his "friend" does not perform his role well or if he beats too hard, Z does not satisfy his masochistic passions. (1899d, 153)

Another masochist, however, highlighted the advantages of this perversion:

> So the indulging in fantasy is the main thing, and this offers indeed an
> extraordinary pleasure, which causes one to forget all troubles and worries. The most beautiful thing is that fantasy knows no limits and that
> one can stage all the fitting conditions—such as location, personalities,
> their outward and inner characteristics—as one wishes and deems necessary. Such an effect cannot be realized in real life; every attempt to do
> this must therefore be considered as a failure in advance. A great advantage of this pure psychic side of masochism is therefore also that one does
> not come into conflict with the outside world, the state, and moral rules.
> One has no need for other men, children, animals or the like. Only a
> willing prostitute will suffice—voilà tout! (1891h, 17–18)

Krafft-Ebing backed up his theory of the inborn nature of this perversion
with detailed information of his informants. They put forward that their
aberration could not be rooted in mental association. One of them, for
instance, failed to remember whether he was ever physically punished during childhood, while he was certain of having had masochistic fantasies
way before puberty: "At that time the impressions were sexless. I remember
that when I was a boy it affected (not to say excited) me when an older
boy addressed me by my first name while I spoke to him in the third person"
(1891h, 20; Ps 1999, 134).

Two cases of female masochists were quite remarkable because the medical world itself was implicated in their fantasies and sexual gratification.
The twenty-one-year-old Miss X fantasized about being hospitalized in a
lunatic asylum:

> I fell upon this idea while reading the story about a director of an asylum
> beating a lady with a cane and a riding crop after he had pulled her by
> the hair from her bed. I longed to be treated in the same way in such an
> institute. . . . I prefer to imagine brutal, uneducated female warders beating me mercilessly. (Ps 1894, 139; cf. Ps 1999, 171)

The other case was communicated to Krafft-Ebing by one of his colleagues
of Vienna's General Hospital. It involved a prostitute who used to call on
doctors to give her a gynecological examination, instructing them to proceed even if she resisted. The doctor who had granted her request told
Krafft-Ebing that this was a clear case of masochism since "it was apparent
that orgasm was not induced by mere palpation of the genitals, but that it
was the effect of the act of violence which was intended, in the sense that
rape had the same effect as coitus" (Ps 1903, 150; cf. Ps 1999, 173).

To a large extent, Krafft-Ebing's psychiatric conception and interpretation of masochism relied on the self-observations of some of his most articulate patients and correspondents. Masochism should not be confused with flagellantism, he contended, even though it was true that many masochists loved to be whipped. He also rejected the term *algolagnia* (lust for pain)—which was used by the German psychiatrists Albert von Schrenck-Notzing and Albert Eulenburg (1901b, 143). Lust was derived not so much from the actual physical pain as from the indirect, symbolic implications involved in the experience of power and subjection; thus it was primarily a psychological pursuit. The same basically applied to sadism, which Krafft-Ebing believed to be different from the rapes and the murders for lust that he had described earlier on in his career. For many sadists, cruelty and physical punishments were just a means toward a goal, namely that of achieving a feeling of hegemony and superiority. Krafft-Ebing diagnosed some of them as "ideal" sadists: they were perfectly happy with their sadistic imagination alone while not having any eagerness to act on their violent fantasies. "The urge to punish others was never very strong," Krafft-Ebing noted in one of his case histories, adding that fortunately the patient found "more satisfaction by indulging in fantasies about flagellation scenes" (Ps 1891, 71). About another "ideal" sadist who complained of impotence, he remarked: "Strikingly this man has not hit the idea to use his latent sadism as a cure of his impotence, and as a doctor I did not see any reason to call his attention to this" (1899e, 164).

The case histories and narratives of both urnings and masochists display not only a concern for self-justification, but also efforts toward self-understanding. Many perverts were eager to confess the true nature of their inner self and seemed delighted to find their words represented in a scientific context. "I will say everything here, since I wish only to write the truth and nothing but the truth," guaranteed one of the homosexual autobiographers who disclosed to nourish the same passion as the one evoked by Sacher-Masoch in his *Venus im Pelz* (Ps 1890, 162; cf. Ps 1999, 568). A thirty-one-year-old urning assured Krafft-Ebing that he would seriously try to give a faithful account of his condition, his sexual impulses and feelings in particular: "I have brooded so much on my oddity that I believe that I can faithfully depict my feelings" (1891h, 124). Responding to Krafft-Ebing's call to urnings to contribute to his casuistry, a forty-eight-year-old academic introduced his life history with the following words: "In the interest of science I won't make a fuss about giving you an autobiography that is as detailed as possible and in which I will attempt to give all data as objectively as possible" (1885a, 42–43). A businessman, aged thirty-four, also made clear that in his autobiography, in which he presented many details about his sexual life, he strove for absolute truth, no matter how shocking it might come across:

> I will strive for the most severe objectivity in my communications, and, above all, I note concerning my drastic, often even cynical style, that I want to be true. Thus, I will not avoid strong expressions because they characterize the matter I am discussing most strikingly. . . . I could not choose my expressions, because my object here has been to furnish material for the study of an urning's existence, and therefore absolute truth was essential. (*Ps* 1888, 88, 91; cf. *Ps* 1999, 586, 589–90)

Another homosexual, a physician, excused himself to Krafft-Ebing for his explicit language, but, as he stated, such details were essential for a complete and true picture of his case: "I hope that the following statements will not awaken your repugnance. At first I intended to omit them; I am including them only for the completeness of this communication, for they serve to enrich the clinical material" (*Ps* 1890, 173; cf. *Ps* 1999, 312).

Not just Krafft-Ebing took great satisfaction in scrupulous analysis and the invention of new categories and subcategories of sexual aberration: several of his patients and correspondents displayed sheer diagnostic and explanatory zeal as well. The thirty-eight-year-old factory owner, in whose case history Krafft-Ebing noted that already at an early age he had started "to ponder on his peculiar sexual condition," was exemplary in this respect (1894e, 348). On the one hand, the life histories tend to be personal and at times very emotional, but, on the other hand, they testify to a certain intellectual detachment vis-à-vis their own feelings, thus making it easier to analyze and interpret them. In writing up the account of their life, some, like Von R quoted in the introduction, strictly adhered to the conventions, rhetoric, and schemes of the psychiatric case history genre, and they divided their self-analysis into neat categories like family roots, childhood, first experiences with sex, physical condition, mental condition, character, favorite activities, moods, sexual desire and behavior, fantasies and dreams (*Ps* 1887, 86–88). The way a thirty-year-old physician described himself shows how far the identification with the medical case history genre could go. There is nothing in this man's self-presentation that sets it apart from objectified medical diagnostic narrative:

> Medium height, gracefully formed. Skull dolichocephalic, with prominence in the occipital region; circumference, 59 centimeters; frontal prominence marked; glance somewhat neuropathic; pupils medium, teeth very defective; musculature strong and tense; abundant hair, blond. Varicocele on the left side of the scrotum; frenulum too short, hindering

me in coitus. I severed it myself three years ago. Since then ejaculation is retarded, and pleasurable feeling much diminished. Temperament choleric. Quick at comprehension; good at drawing conclusions; energetic; very persevering for one hereditarily predisposed. I learn languages easily, and have a good ear for music, but otherwise I have no talent for the arts. I am always ambitious to do my duty, but I am constantly troubled with *taedium vitae*, and only kept from attempts at suicide by my religion and the thought of my mother. Otherwise I am a typical candidate for suicide. I am ambitious, jealous, have a fear of paralysis, left-handed. I am filled with socialist ideas. I like adventures, and I am courageous. I have decided to never marry. (*Ps* 1892, 240; cf. *Ps* 1999, 543–44)

Few of Krafft-Ebing's correspondents proceeded this systematically and with such self-criticism and disregard for personalized narrative style. Yet by listing all the peculiarities of their own sexual condition, many nevertheless demonstrated their familiarity with the psychiatric approach and understanding of perversion. Several made no effort at all to put on a beautiful front; thus a thirty-four-year-old businessman wrote that he was irresolute, fickle, and manipulable:

Like a woman, I am moody and nervous, often irritated without reason, and sometimes mean. I am arrogant, unjust, and often shamefully insulting toward persons who do not please me. In all my conduct I am superficial, often frivolous, and have no deep moral feeling.

And he added:

I do not smoke or drink, and can neither whistle, ride, perform gymnastics, fence, nor shoot. I have absolutely no interest in horses or dogs, and have never had a gun or sword in my hand. My inner feeling and sexual desire is completely that of a woman. (*Ps* 1888, 88; *Ps* 1999, 586–87)

It is striking that among Krafft-Ebing's patients and correspondents, there are many doctors and medical students. Not only were many of them familiar with the medical literature on perversion; some of them also implicated their medical knowledge and practice in the fulfilling of their sexual desires. The physician cited above, who objectified his self-description, wrote that, as a boy, he was excited by stories about "injuries or operations that had to be endured by beautiful girls and ladies" and he "applied himself to the study of medicine with a real expectation of gaining an opportunity to satisfy or cure my desires. I cured them, thank God. After undertaking my first dissection of the lower extremity of a female, this unfortunate desire was removed from me" (Ps 1892, 238–39; Ps 1999, 541–42).[2] Another physician told the story of how, as a boy, he had been seduced by his father's friend, who was a doctor: "He practiced mutual masturbation with me and showed me our spermatozoa under the microscope. He also showed me pornographic works and pictures. . . . He dilated my anus with instruments upon which he practiced pederasty on me . . ." (Ps 1886, 65; cf. Ps 1999, 558).

Surely, Krafft-Ebing was not the only one who indulged in meticulous classification of sexual deviancies. One medical student with an irresistible urge to dress in women's clothes had exerted himself to get to the bottom of his anomaly. He had discovered, as he confided to Krafft-Ebing, that his case was complicated by fetishist as well as masochist traits. However, having absorbed himself in the study of psychopathology, he had not found a fitting category for himself in Krafft-Ebing's work. In order to get a full picture of his case and perhaps carve out a niche of his own in Krafft-Ebing's gallery of sexual anomalies, the student sent him a detailed self-description:

> Since I have not come to a full understanding as far as the diagnosis of my sexual life is concerned, not even after much reflection and the studying of your work on psychiatry & psychopathia sexualis, I have decided not to beat about the bush. If I take too much of your time, I apologize. I would not like to be too brief, because as a medical man I know that important diagnostic conclusions can be drawn precisely from apparent trivial statements. Giving much information, I hope at the same time to offer you something interesting from a scientific point of view.[3]

Others also turned to Krafft-Ebing after having searched his work for specific sexual aberrations in vain. "Recently I had your valuable book on 'Psychopathia Sexualis' delivered to me in order to find counsel on a peculiar case," a man from Glasgow wrote. "Unfortunately I did not find any case in it which resembles the one occupying me for weeks now."[4] The man was very worried about his brother who was engaged to a widow. The woman acknowledged that she had a sexual relationship with a younger man, but that she wanted to end it. It soon turned out, however, that she was unable to do so and that she was fully under the young man's spell, apparently against her own wishes. Most likely, Krafft-Ebing responded to the letter writer from Glasgow that this was a typical case of what he called sexual

---

2. The French psychiatrist Émile Laurent used the term *sadisme chirurgical* to describe this sexual perversion, which, according to him, could be found among physicians (Verplaetse 1999, 45).

3. Letter of K to Krafft-Ebing (June 2, 1898), Nachlass Krafft-Ebing.

4. Letter of BE to Krafft-Ebing (June 15, 1897), Nachlass Krafft-Ebing.

bondage, a form of sexual subjection that he distinguished from masochism and that was seen among women in particular.

A few correspondents who failed to discover their own sexual peculiarity in Krafft-Ebing's work wrote their life history in order to enrich his casuistry. A physician, aged forty-eight, who felt that he had gradually changed from a man into a woman—both in a physical and psychological sense—sent in the most extensive self-analysis ever published by Krafft-Ebing.

> It seemed a duty of gratitude to tell you the results of my recollection and observation, since I did not find an analogous case description by you; and, finally, I also thought it might perhaps interest you to learn, from the pen of a physician, how such an invalid human or masculine being thinks and feels under the weight of the obsession of being a woman. (1890e, 79; cf. Ps 1999, 267)

Some informants proposed new labels and categories as well as explanations to Krafft-Ebing. Thus a twenty-year-old technical engineer suggested introducing the term *pagism*—as a counterpart of masochism—to indicate the desire to act as a beautiful young woman's page:

> His conception was perfectly chaste, but piquant: his relation to her that of a slave, but absolutely pure—a mere platonic submission. This reveling in the idea of serving as a page to such a "beautiful creature" was colored by a pleasurable feeling, but this was in no way sexual. In it, he experienced an exquisite feeling of moral satisfaction, in contrast with sensually colored masochism, and therefore he could regard his "pagism" as something of a different nature. (Ps 1892, 98; cf. Ps 1999, 123)

Others entered in a debate with Krafft-Ebing about the possible explanations of their perversion. In the wake of Binet's association theory, which Krafft-Ebing largely adopted, many fetishists looked for the cause of their sexual obsession in a particular occasion that had triggered their sexual anxiety for the first time. However, in his own case, one fur and silk fetishist considered such mental association a fairly unlikely explanation because he did not remember an event that would have caused his predilection. At the same time, he discussed an explanation of fur and silk fetishism in terms of atavism, about which he had read. He also rejected this theory, however, especially because it suggested that the penchant for fur and silk was primitive and that it was related to cretinism and feeblemindedness.

> I distance myself from considering that the widespread fur fetishism can be viewed as an atavistic setback into the taste of the pelt-clad primordial man. That cretin just instinctively and shamelessly enjoyed his tactile sense, without necessarily involving a sexual-sensual dimension. In

the same way, many normal people like to caress cats and the like, even touch silk and fur, without being sexually aroused. (*Ps* 1892, 186)

Krafft-Ebing's Berlin informant gave a cultural and historical explanation for the dissemination of masochism among men. He believed it was closely linked to the rise of courtly love, which had put women on a pedestal, thus leaving men endlessly craving for their love. Another correspondent rejected Krafft-Ebing's idea that the masochist inclination of a man pointed to effeminacy by suggesting that both mentally and physically he was oriented toward masculinity. He felt that the relationship of master and slave should not be seen as a reflection of the sexual relation between man and woman; the relation between master and slave was more accurately compared to the way in which a man treated his dog or horse: "It is precisely this unlimited power over life and death, as exercised over slaves and domestic animals, that is the aim and end of all masochistic imagination" (1891h, 21; cf. *Ps* 1999, 134).

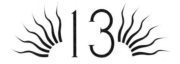

The Comfort of Togetherness

Both the productive involvement of several of the subjects of Krafft-Ebing's case studies in the genesis of his sexual pathology and his own encouragement of such an active stance substantially contributed to the dialogical nature of his work. This shared concern not only enabled medical treatment and other forms of restraint, but it also opened up the possibility for the individuals involved to speak out, to find a voice, and to be acknowledged. *Psychopathia sexualis,* though intended for professional physicians and lawyers, was read by perverts who recognized themselves in the case descriptions and by others interested in gratifying their curiosity about sexuality. It was a best-seller and in the history of medicine belongs to those books that had a pervasive influence on the lay public (Bullough and Bullough 1977, 62).[1] Although Krafft-Ebing's work has been regarded as a cultural defense against the corruption of morals and "decadence" of fin de siècle society, at the same time the study helped to make sexual variance imaginable and it enlarged the cultural space allotted to idiosyncratic desires. For many perverts, the book was the impetus to self-awareness and self-expression.

Some of the reactions to *Psychopathia sexualis* seemed to reveal a fear for its possible liberating effects. Mouthpieces of the German Purity League, for example, criticized the book as a serious undermining of the moral order. For them it was clear that Krafft-Ebing disseminated a materialist worldview and did not really believe in moral values. Since he declared that moral offenders were sick, rather than criminal, and that they lacked

1. The number of copies printed of each new edition of *Psychopathia sexualis* grew from 1,250 in 1886 to 2,500 in 1898 and subsequent editions. The book must have provided Krafft-Ebing with a considerable extra income; for the tenth edition he received a fee of 3,000 German marks, whereas his publisher paid him no more than 100 marks for other works (Verlagsverträge, Archiv Ferdinand Enke Verlag).

free will, perverts, they believed, could indulge in vice under the cover of nervousness and neuropathy. He was also attacked for favoring decriminalization of homosexuality for mere pragmatic reasons, for publishing "immoral" case histories, and for referring some of his patients to prostitutes. His work was considered dangerous in particular because it was widely read outside scientific circles: "From experience we can indeed report that, despite many Latin phrases, the book is eagerly read, even devoured, by numerous unauthorized persons, including workers" (Roemer 1892, 15).

Krafft-Ebing aroused antagonism in medical and government circles as well, not only because he challenged current moral and legal viewpoints, but even more, it seems, because of *Psychopathia sexualis*'s popularity (Benedikt 1906, 163; cf. Fuchs 1902, 263). They reproached him, saying that he catered to the general public's lust for sensation and that he had not prevented the book from being sold indiscriminately. Moreover, some of his colleagues suspected him of too much sympathy toward sexual deviants and of letting himself be misled by dishonest patients. By quoting so many urnings, he was disseminating "homosexual propaganda," and many believed that his pleas for decriminalization went way too far (Müller 1991, 140, 142). Moritz Benedikt, one of his colleagues in the medical faculty in Vienna, and Julius Wagner-Jauregg, Krafft-Ebing's successor as a professor of psychiatry in Vienna, felt that he explained away the immorality of homosexuality by wrongly stressing its inborn character and that he, as a forensic expert, gave the concept of criminal irresponsibility too wide a meaning (Benedikt 1906, 371–72, 391–92; Wagner-Jauregg 1950). Benedikt, who voiced widely shared views on this issue, saw three options for homosexuals: absolute abstinence from sexuality, imprisonment, or castration.

It appears that the stumbling block for many of Krafft-Ebing's critics was the popularity of *Psychopathia sexualis*, even more than its contents. Whether a work on sexuality was regarded as obscene largely depended on its availability and the size of its audience. This view, which bears witness to class prejudices and social fear, equally applies to pornography in the late nineteenth century. Earlier, pornography was mainly a literary genre for a sophisticated elite and thus was not considered a threat to public morality. But when the production and consumption of pornography began to flourish by the 1860s, fears about the sensuality of the masses grew accordingly. The late 1890s in Germany saw an upsurge in convictions for distributing obscene material. A new law that passed in 1900, the so-called *Lex Heinze*, made it no longer only illegal to distribute or display obscene works, but also to compose, manufacture, store, advertise, or publicly extol any obscene works or to give these to any person under sixteen years of age. Although persecutions rose dramatically, courts and legal scholars consistently made an exception for "true" works of art and scholarship, claiming

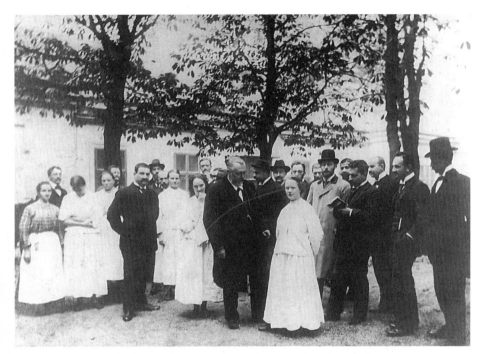

Figure 13. Krafft-Ebing with patients and students near his clinic in Vienna. (Krafft-Ebing Family Archive, Graz, Austria)

that these were never obscene per se (Keilson-Lauritz and Pfäfflin 1999; Stark 1981). Thus Krafft-Ebing's *Psychopathia sexualis*—though blurring the dividing line between science, scientific vulgarization, and pornography in the eyes of many—was safeguarded from legal bans. It was distributed beyond scientific circles, to be sure, but even critics could not deny that its author was a prominent man of science. Moreover, the book was published by the highly respectable medical publisher Ferdinand Enke. Krafft-Ebing persistently stressed that his book was intended for doctors and lawyers and that passages that might be considered offensive were translated into Latin. The importance of such precautionary measures can be illustrated by the fate of the German translation of an Italian study about sexuality by Paolo Mantegazza. Whereas a limited, expensive edition of this book was not persecuted, a low-priced popular edition of the same work with erotic drawings on the cover, issued by another publishing house, was banned.

In order to meet some of the objections after the first editions of *Psychopathia sexualis*, Krafft-Ebing translated into Latin an increasing number of explicit descriptions of sexual acts, which some might consider shocking

(*Ps* 1898, vi). As the following fragment on a man afflicted with masochism and coprolagnia shows, readers not schooled in this language missed out on some of the explicit language:

> What oppressed him was the unnatural desire, recurring every four weeks, for mictio mulieris in os suum. Asked how this perversion developed, he gave the following facts, interesting because of their genetic importance. At six years of age he accidentally put cum manu sub podicem of a girl who sat next to him in school. This caused him pleasure, and he did it repeatedly. The memory of these pleasant situations strongly aroused his imagination. Puerum decem annos agens serva educatrix libidine mota ad corpus suum appressit et digitum ei in vaginam introduxit. Quum postea fortuitu digito nasum tetigit, odore ejus valde delectatus fuit. This immoral act developed into a lustful fantasy that made him believe he was lying bound inter femora mulieris cumbere, coactus ut dormiat sub ejus podice et ut bibat ejus urinam. (*Ps* 1894, 134; cf. *Ps* 1999, 165)

However, most of Krafft-Ebing's educated readers will have had no difficulty reading such a passage.

The inclusion of Latin translations of some of the explicit language was Krafft-Ebing's only concession to scientific respectability. There is no indication that he ever instructed his publisher to have the sale of *Psychopathia sexualis* restricted to a professional audience. On the contrary, he proposed that the publisher increase the number of copies printed and was perfectly aware that his work was popular with a lay audience.[2] "Its unexpected commercial success is the best proof," he wrote in the foreword of the eighth edition, "that large numbers of unfortunate people look for and find in the book enlightenment and comfort with respect to enigmatic manifestations of their vita sexualis."[3] According to his former colleague and friend Heinrich Schüle, he was very attached to the book; each new edition was announced by the author with great satisfaction (Schüle 1902, 320). Apparently, Krafft-Ebing was self-conscious about opening up new psychiatric territory and proud of being a scientific pioneer in this field. Although he nourished strict personal moral views, at the same time he was liberalminded and convinced of his duty to contribute to a reduction in suffering. He believed that it was one of the tasks of medical science to enlighten the public (1891c). In the preface to the first edition of *Psychopathia sexualis*, he claimed that regarding sexual deviancy "the most erroneous ideas" and

---

2. Letter of Krafft-Ebing to Ferdinand Enke (February 16, 1894), Archiv Ferdinand Enke Verlag.

3. *Ps* 1893, vi; cf. *Ps* 1999, preface to the twelfth German edition.

"unjust decisions" prevailed and that medical science had to put itself in the service of truth (Ps 1886, v). He took the position that silence or ignorance about sexuality was more dangerous than having an understanding of what was involved; knowledge was necessary to prevent the spreading of sexual deviancy, and awareness of its pathological nature might deter people from engaging in such behavior (Ps 1903, 317).

However, Krafft-Ebing cannot have worried too much about the book's opposite effect. It evidently owed its success not only to its scientific merits, but also to its pornographic qualities. In addition to scientific expositions, Psychopathia sexualis contained extensive and detailed descriptions of a variety of sexual experiences and fantasies; accounts of the erotic temptations and amusements of big cities; examples from history, ethnography, and the Bible; fragments from literary and semi-pornographic writings; candid advertisements; letters from masochists to their mistresses; and journalistic descriptions of the underworld of prostitution and events like the Misogynists Ball for urnings in Berlin. "Last winter I bought your work about Psychiatry and Psychopathia sexualis," wrote a medical student ridden with a fetish for women's clothes, "and a new, completely unknown world was revealed to me."[4] Some correspondents confessed that certain passages in the book aroused them. One of them, who read the first edition of Krafft-Ebing's Neue Forschungen auf dem Gebiet der Psychopathia sexualis, in which masochism was introduced as a sexual perversion, confided to the author that the case history about a man with the desire to be ridden as a horse by a woman provided him with physical proof that he himself was also a masochist: "Reading the 'neuen Forschungen' impressed me tremendously, and how much I am a masochist myself became clear to me when reading the horse dreams caused me to have erections" (1891h, 19). Referring to the chapter in which Krafft-Ebing described transvestite behavior and pederastic relations among American Indians, a director of an estate, aged thirty-three, informed Krafft-Ebing:

Two or three weeks ago "Psychopathia sexualis" fell into my hands. This work has made an unexpectedly deep impression on me. At first I read the work with an interest that was undoubtedly lascivious. I was very excited by, for example, the description of the cultivation of mujerados. The thought of a young, powerful man being emasculated in this manner so that later he could be used for pederasty by a whole tribe of wild, powerful, and sensual Indians excited me to the point that I masturbated five times during the next two days, fantasizing myself as a presumptive mujerado. (1891h, 101; cf. Ps 1999, 603–4)

4. Letter of K to Krafft-Ebing (June 2, 1898), Nachlass Krafft-Ebing.

Another urning not only found sexual titillation but also consolation in Krafft-Ebing's book: "I find only pleasure in dreaming about my past happiness and in reading novels about urnings as well as the autobiographies in the 'Psychopathia sexualis'" (Ps 1890, 160). Although the book also excited a Dutch man with a penchant for ladies' gloves, the man expressed being somewhat disappointed because there were so few cases of this type of fetishism in the book. In a letter he asked Krafft-Ebing whether he was familiar with other literature on his idiosyncrasy and requested him to send some titles.[5] Another fetishist confessed that the very act of writing about his sexual feelings caused him to have intense erections.[6]

For some readers, the case histories could be an eye-opener, especially because several patients and correspondents made it perfectly clear that they knew just where to go to satisfy the perversions catalogued by Krafft-Ebing. Specialized forms of prostitution and meeting places had developed in response to masochistic and homosexual desires. His Berlin correspondent gathered a lot of information about masochistic practices and techniques among prostitutes in Berlin and Vienna as well as about the "comedies" they enacted to satisfy the sexual needs of some of their clients:

> It is always the same story: humble submission by the man, kicks, orders, faked lectures full of threatening and abusive language by the prostitute, followed by flagellation, beatings of different body parts and every possible maltreatment. The scene often ends with coitus, more often just with ejaculation without intercourse. Such prostitutes have shown me heavy iron chains with handcuffs, which their clients put on or which they have put on, and also the dried peas on which they kneel, etc. (1890e, 25)

Apparently there were bordellos with sadomasochistic facilities; one of Krafft-Ebing's patients, a sixty-six-year-old man, told him that as a young man he had visited a prostitute who had suggested a "masochistic scene" to him (Ps 1903, 118). Furthermore, he conveyed that masochism was particularly found in England and that masseuses frequently catered to masochistic desires. In Parisian bordellos some customers were referred to as "slave," Krafft-Ebing himself added. Other men stressed that masochism was widespread and that in big cities it was easy to find prostitutes who commonly treated men with whips, rods, and canes. These were used, as one informer explained, for normal as well as masochistic men. Prostitutes had told him

5. Letter of X (undated [1901/1902]), Nachlass Krafft-Ebing.
6. Letter of X (undated, 1899), Nachlass Krafft-Ebing.

that there are men who have themselves whipped simply to increase their sexual pleasure. These men, in contrast with masochists, regard flagellation as a means to an end. On the other hand, almost all prostitutes agree that there are many men who like to play "slave"—i.e., like to be so called, and have themselves scolded and trod upon and also beaten. (1891h, 19; cf. Ps 1999, 133)

Masochists also used newspaper ads as a way to contact women who were willing to meet their needs. In *Psychopathia sexualis*, Krafft-Ebing cited one from the *Hannover'schen Tageblatt*: "Sacher-Masoch. 109404. Ladies interested in and thrilled with the work of this author, and who embody its female characters, are requested to send their address, under no R. 537, to the offices of this paper. Strictest discretion" (Ps 1903, 126; cf. Ps 1999, 661). He found a similar ad in a 1895 issue of the *Vossische Zeitung*: "Ladies who like the works of Sacher-Masoch are requested to answer this advertisement. Letters under J. F. are forwarded by Rudolf Mosse. Berlin SW" (1899d, 132).

A need for group identification can be discerned among Krafft-Ebing's masochists, even though it was more difficult for them to find like-minded men than for homosexuals. Yet some masochists mentioned that they knew many men like themselves. The Berlin man ended his autobiography with a clear message to his "fellow sufferers," expressing the hope that it would be a reassurance to each one of them that "his abnormality is not unique" (1890e, 28). Krafft-Ebing also referred to a masochist who recognized himself in Sacher-Masoch's work and who had met numerous men who felt the same way as he did: "He only regrets that one can only rarely find a woman who fulfills the ideal of a masochist. . . . In a letter to another masochist this odd rainbow chaser proposed to look for like-minded men and sadistic women in order to establish a private society . . ." (1899d, 140). Similarly, a nineteen-year-old young man, who considered his "inborn" and "incurable" masochistic nature an inherent part of his identity, revealed that he "would consider it as the ultimate bliss to get to know other masochists" intimately because he wanted to share his experiences with them, "to hear their life history, to learn about their condition, and, if necessary, to advise and help them as much I can. The fact that many masochists feel unhappy hurts me deeply" (1899d, 160). The Dutch ladies' gloves fetishist also regretted that he did not know anyone who shared his fate and with whom he could exchange his experiences: "Unfortunately I don't know any man or woman with the same desire. . . . [H]ow much I would like to exchange with them ideas and . . . gloves! Yet I suspect that this group is more numerous than one knows."[7]

7. Letter of X (undated [1901/1902]), Nachlass Krafft-Ebing.

For urnings, in general, it was not so difficult to find like-minded men. A German physician who had been acquainted with Ulrichs and who had written a novel about the life of urnings was, like many others, familiar with the homosexual underground in Vienna and in several German and Italian cities:

> Since becoming conscious of my abnormal instinct, I have met thousands of individuals with a similar inclination. Almost every large city has some meeting place, as well as a so-called cruising promenade. . . . In my own town of 30,000 inhabitants, I personally know around 120 "aunts." Most of them, and I, especially, possess the capability of immediately determining whether another is like us or not. In the language of "aunts," such a person is called "reasonable" or "unreasonable." (*Ps* 1890, 174–75; cf. *Ps* 1999, 314)

On his travels across Europe, a thirty-four-year-old musician reported, he had found willing sexual partners everywhere. His recital is reminiscent of Leporello's famous aria "Madamina, il catalogo è questo" in Mozart's opera *Don Giovanni*:

> My lovers were: French counts and dukes, German soldiers, Swedish peasants, stable hands, elegant officers, English lords, Spanish marquises, Hungarian barons, artists, scholars, famous men (whose name may be known to all), but also the most vulgar chaps. . . . I had whoever I happened to meet. (1890e, 60)

Neither was another widely traveled urning short of sexual contacts. As Krafft-Ebing commented: "Wherever he goes, he has his connections. The number of male-loving men is so large, that they form a kind of secret union in all countries" (1890e, 57).

Not everybody was charmed by the loose sexual mores of the homosexual subculture though. When one of Krafft-Ebing's correspondents, a thirty-one-year-old entrepreneur, was taken by some other urnings to a bathhouse in Vienna, which proved to be a homosexual meeting place, the man was shocked. The spot well deserved the name of a male brothel, he believed: "I know that I am not one jot better than the customers of that bathhouse, but I had never encountered such disgusting lewdness and such a meeting of like-minded" (1890e, 41). Others, however, were relieved and delighted when they discovered the existence of such a homosexual underworld, especially because it fostered a sense of community. Thus a Hungarian civil servant, aged thirty-nine, related how a sexual encounter in a Viennese pissoir turned his life around: "This moment was decisive for the rest of my life." At that very moment he first realized "that I am not alone, and I only had one thing in my mind: getting to know the mysteries of my sex which had been hidden from me until then." Within a short time he got to know many companions in Vienna, Budapest, and Graz, and he entered a new world:

> Euphorically, I threw myself into the pleasures which, until that moment, had been unknown to me. It did not take long to be more or less acquainted and friendly with my companions in my hometown. Since then four years have passed; I have lost count of the number of men with whom I have enjoyed immense pleasure. . . . (1890e, 44–45)

A businessman of thirty-eight who had had his first sexual experience at a homosexual meeting place ten years earlier wrote to Krafft-Ebing that he had found such spots in many cities and that their existence had greatly relieved him, especially because they had solved his social isolation: "Thus you will understand that with this knowledge, I also felt consoled, because of the comfort of belonging together and not being alone anymore. The depressive feeling that I did not really belong to human society had been taken away" (1884c, 4). Another man, who once wrote a letter to an actor who was rumored to be an urning, described how his introduction to the subculture made him forget his sufferings. The actor took him to a large café,

> where also some other, older and younger, gentlemen were present; some of them were with their lovers and among them were several military officers. I found myself as if I was in fairyland. How unhappy I had felt before. . . . And now all this cheerfulness, this elated mood, and carefree enjoyment of life. Friendly eyes looked at me understandingly and that very evening I met someone who made me forget, at least for some time, all the suffering I had endured. (Ps 1887, 83–84)

Many of the psychiatrist's homosexual clients and correspondents reported that large urban centers offered plenty of opportunities for sexual encounters, not only because of the public meeting places, but also because of the male prostitutes and soldiers who offered their bodies for money: "Young men who can be talked into fulfilling our desires are around everywhere," one of them wrote (Ps 1887, 85). A thirty-three-year-old man who felt attracted to soldiers, sailors, and workers told Krafft-Ebing: "I have learned how easy it is to find men who, partly for money, partly from desire, yield to our inclinations" (1891h, 100; cf. Ps 1999, 602). Neither did a thirty-four-year-old businessman with a penchant for "real men" in close-fitting uniforms have any difficulty finding what he needed:

> My taste is by no means difficult to please—it is similar to that of a servant girl who finds her ideal in a dragoon guard. . . . Circumstances have

allowed me, during these years, to make about a dozen male acquaintances who, for a fee of a gulden or two per visit, serve my purpose. . . . Improbable as it sounds, I have always been able to find some coarse fellows who, in exchange for some extra earnings, will allow themselves to be used for this purpose. They learn these things while in military service, for urnings know that in such circumstances men are most cooperative in exchange for money. Once the guys are trained, in spite of their passion for the female sex, circumstances often compel them to continue the practice. (*Ps* 1888, 89–90; cf. *Ps* 1999, 587–88)

For some it was even possible to live together with a lover, "as if in marriage," as one of them wrote (1890e, 51). Dr. G, the man who shocked Krafft-Ebing with his direct statements, told him that in Naples and Paris there were districts where effeminate men, so-called *Effeminelli* and *Grisettes*, lived together with their male lovers, just like normal couples (1882, 215). Effeminate urnings might also find opportunities to indulge in travesty in public. Thus one of them, a twenty-two-year-old military officer of noble birth, told Krafft-Ebing that he had appeared as a ballet girl at a fancy dress ball. Proudly he presented the psychiatrist with a photograph of himself in his ballet skirt. "Dress and posture," Krafft-Ebing reported, "are impeccable, the pink dress charmingly adorned with flowers" (*Ps* 1887, 78).

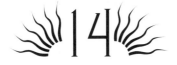

For Science and Humanity

By publishing his patients' letters and autobiographies and by quoting their statements verbatim, Krafft-Ebing enabled voices to be heard that were usually silenced. His case histories revealed to individuals with "odd feelings" that they were not unique in their experience. In doing justice to the subjective experience of patients in his writings, Krafft-Ebing represented a small minority within the medical world of his day. According to Müller (1991) and Hansen (1992), physicians were rather quick to generalize from a small number of cases and theorize without retelling individual life histories. As a last resort, physicians might even tamper with individual cases so as to construct a uniform set of evidence that perfectly fitted the established medical categories (cf. Klabundt 1994, 126). However, my investigation of Krafft-Ebing's case histories offers no support for such attitudes or practices. His unpublished case histories are in no way different from the published ones. In his writings, individual meanings did not automatically follow medical theories. Instead, contemporary readers could find subjective experience, dialogue, multivocality, divergent meanings, and contradictory sets of values in *Psychopathia sexualis*.

Those readers who recognized themselves in Krafft-Ebing's cases were left enough room to interpret their sexual feelings and experiences in their own way. The psychiatrist quoted the words of perverts not solely as evidence in support of his medical diagnosis; and, conversely, if their words challenged psychiatric doctrine, they were not censored. Some of the autobiographers took the opportunity to vent their criticism of current social norms. A twenty-year-old man was of the opinion that society did not have the right to ban homosexual contact:

Together with the majority of urnings, I claim that our sexual anomaly does not affect our mental condition or only slightly at best. Our desire may be abnormal, but it is as intense as the normal urge and not unnatural. Therefore, legislators do not have the right to deny to us cooperative boys and men, just as they have no right to deprive paralytics of their crutches. (*Ps* 1890, 161)

A thirty-six-year-old man who had lived a homosexual life in Paris, London, Rio de Janeiro, and in the United States stated that legal reforms were not enough to improve the social position of urnings:

> I myself don't foster any hope to witness a change for the better. That will be something of the future. Even if we will be treated by the courts in a more lenient way, there is still a question to be answered. . . . [W]ho will remove the prejudice against us, which from time immemorial has pervaded society? As long as that continues to exist, our moral suffering will not come to an end. (1890e, 55)

Even more militant was a medical student, aged twenty-three, who made it clear that he did not want a cure for his homosexual leanings. In his autobiography he stated:

> I intentionally and consciously curse contemporary moral standards, which force sexually abnormal people to offend against arbitrary laws. I think that sexual contact between two people of the same sex is at their individual discretion, without legislators having any right to interfere. . . . I only yearn for a time, when I can pursue my desires more easily and with less danger of being discovered, and thus enjoy a delight that will not harm anyone. (1890e, 63, 66; cf. *Ps* 1999, 571, 574)

Another urning wrote to Krafft-Ebing that his self-respect had been restored after he had read Plato's *Symposium* and a work by Gustav Jäger, but that his self-acceptance went hand in hand with a loathing of a social order that prevented him from organizing his life as he wished.[1] "From that moment, however, . . . a certain pent-up anger and an intense hate of modern social relationships took hold of me" (*Ps* 1887, 88). A technical engineer, too, was often, as he wrote,

> seized with bitterness and a deep hatred for the modern ideas that treat us poor urnings with such terrible harshness. For what is our fate? In most cases we are not understood, and we are derided and despised. Even when all goes well, and we are understood, we are still pitied like invalids

---

1. Krafft-Ebing's correspondent probably referred to the second edition of *Entdeckung der Seele* (1880), in which the zoologist and anthropologist Jäger, influenced by Karl Maria Kertbeny, differentiated different types of homosexuals. Some of them, Jäger argued, were not effeminate but masculine, even hypervirile.

or the insane—and pity has always been sickening to me. (1891h, 128; Ps 1999, 582)

The autobiography of a physician, which covered more than thirteen pages in small print and was published in several editions of Psychopathia sexualis, was also remarkable, because of its criticism of the medical profession. By recounting his life's story in a novelistic style, this man explained that he had changed into a woman. In a letter accompanying his autobiography, he advocated that women should be allowed to study medicine because they had a more intuitive understanding of the body than men:

> Finally, I wanted to present you with the results of my recollection and reflection to prove that one who thinks and feels like a woman can still be a doctor. I consider it a great injustice to bar women from medicine. A woman discovers the traces of many ailments through her intuition, while a man gropes in the dark, despite all his diagnostic skills, especially as far as women's and children's diseases are concerned. If I could have my way, every physician would have to live the life of a woman for three months. He then would have a better understanding and more consideration in matters affecting the half of mankind from which he himself is born. He then would respect woman's spiritual greatness, and at the same time also the harshness of their fate. (1890e, 79; cf. Ps 1999, 268)

Other correspondents criticized their fellow sufferers because they did not demonstrate any critical awareness of their condition. Thus a Hungarian civil servant asserted that most urnings were generally kind-hearted but also superficial and addicted to backbiting (1890e, 45). A technical engineer reported that among the fifty-five urnings he knew, he had found the same character traits and habits:

> Almost all of them are more or less idealists: they smoke little or not at all; they are bigoted, vain, desirous of admiration, and superstitious; and, unfortunately, I must confess that they embody more of the defects and reverse sides of both sexes than the good qualities. (1891h, 130; cf. Ps 1999, 584)

The impact of Krafft-Ebing's medical work was multifaceted: it not only served as a guide for professionals and experts, but also as a forum for the individuals concerned. The book opened up a space in which they could begin to speak for themselves and look for models with which to identify. Despite the medical bias, many case histories served as go-betweens, linking individual introspection—the self-conscious and frequently painful recognition that one was a deviant kind of person—and social identification, the comforting sense of belonging to a community of like-minded individuals. Because Krafft-Ebing distinguished himself as an expert who took a stand against traditional moral-religious and legal denunciations of sexual deviance, individuals approached him to find understanding, acceptance, and support, as one letter of a Belgian urning clearly illustrates:

> You will be able to empathize with what it means to lock forever within myself that which touches me deepest by far, and to not be able to confide in anybody, while I myself have often been the confidant in matters of great joy and grave suffering. You are the first to whom I open my heart. Use this letter in any way you please; maybe one day it will help lighten the fate of future men to whom nature will give the same feelings. (*Ps* 1888, 87)

Another urning, who regretted that he had not read *Psychopathia sexualis* earlier in his life because this would have prevented a lot of misery, confided to its author: "Nobody knows my true nature—only you, a stranger, you alone know me now, indeed better than father and mother, friend, wife, and lover. It is a real comfort to me to reveal, this one time, the heavy secret of my own nature" (*Ps* 1889, 138). Krafft-Ebing's humanitarian rhetoric did not ring hollow and had some real effect. In fact, many clients did not need medical treatment, because pouring out one's heart to someone was already something of a cure in itself: "Tout comprendre c'est tout guérir [To understand all is to cure all]," a thirty-five-year-old masochist wrote (1891h, 19; *Ps* 1999, 133). The psychiatrist's dealing with these men might be characterized as a form of "proto-psychotherapy." Several case histories create the impression that he showed an active interest in them, while simultaneously speaking reassuringly to them, thus making them feel at ease. A homosexual waiter, aged forty-two, was "pleased to obtain at last a professional explanation of the abnormal state that he had always considered a disease" (*Ps* 1887, 92; *Ps* 1999, 318). Being given a chance to tell their story in a leisurely, unhurried way and to explain themselves to the psychiatrist was frequently the first step toward self-acceptance. Writing their life history, giving coherence and intelligibility to their torn self, could result in a "catharsis" of comprehension: "I am very ashamed of myself because again I write down my confession, and yet it gives me great satisfaction to throw light on my condition," wrote the Dutch glove fetishist who had informed the psychiatrist earlier about his case.[2] Many suggested that his work had brought them relief: "I am very unhappy with my condition and have often considered suicide, but I was somewhat reassured after reading

---

2. Letter of X (undated [1901/1902]), Nachlass Krafft-Ebing.

the Psychopathia sexualis," a thirty-eight-year-old urning told Krafft-Ebing.[3] Another one wrote:

Your work "Psychopathia sexualis" gave me much comfort. It contains passages that I might have written myself; they seem to be unconsciously taken from my own life. My heart has been considerably lightened since I learned from your book of your benevolent interest in our disreputable class. It was the first time that I met someone who showed me that we are not entirely as bad as we are usually portrayed. . . . Anyway, I feel a great burden has been lifted from me. (1890e, 55)

To most private patients and correspondents, Krafft-Ebing was not simply a doctor treating diseases, but someone who answered their need to have themselves explained to themselves, an emotional confidant, and even an ally.[4] His German colleague Albert Moll, who corresponded with him on a regular basis, remembers in his autobiography that Krafft-Ebing was rather exceptional because his concern for his patients often went beyond mere professional commitment: he even answered letters of anonymous correspondents who were too ashamed to give their name (Moll 1936, 145). Displaying a humanitarian commitment to patients, Krafft-Ebing gained a reputation for trust and tolerance. For many he must have embodied the ideal of science as a means to improve their lot. "Your work 'Psychopathia sexualis' came to my attention a short time ago," a businessman informed Krafft-Ebing.

I saw in the book that you were working and studying without prejudice in the interest of science and humanity. If I cannot tell you much that is new, I will still speak of a few things that I trust you will receive as one more brick for the construction of your work: in your hands, I am confident, this will aid in improving our social condition. (Ps 1890, 161; cf. Ps 1999, 566)

"This is my general confession. I never would have suspected that I would ever speak out to a man who is not one of us," another urning confided to the psychiatrist.

3. Case history of K (October 20–29, 1892), Nachlass Krafft-Ebing.
4. Not only perverts consulted Krafft-Ebing to find an emotional confidant. A married Russian woman, for example, who was hospitalized in Krafft-Ebing's sanatorium confessed that her mental distress was caused by the fact that she did not love her husband and that she had a lover, but that her husband did not agree to a divorce because he feared a scandal. "I write to you because . . . I know for sure that you keep this between us. . . . I am infinitely grateful to you for your help, but, unfortunately, not everybody can be helped in this world" (Letter IB to Krafft-Ebing [January 24, 1901], Nachlass Krafft-Ebing).

Yet I have now opened my heart. Reading your work has warmed my heart; after all, contempt hurts, especially when one deserves only pity instead. Because of this low sexual drive, we are punished anyway. . . . I wish that public opinion on us unfortunate people would be alleviated. . . . A drowning person grasps at a straw. I hope to find something to hold on to, which protects me from sinking into the depths of misery and contempt. (1890e, 43)

Some of Krafft-Ebing's homosexual correspondents in particular believed that he was in a position to influence public opinion and to evoke more understanding for urnings in society. They appealed to him, not only to relieve their personal sufferings, but also with a call to mitigate the social ostracism of urnings in general. "Please, help to alleviate the painful pressure that burdens so many unfortunate men and carries them to despair," one addressed himself to Krafft-Ebing (Ps 1888, 93). What was especially depressing about his contrary sexual feeling, another autobiographer explained, was the fear that it might be revealed in public. He concluded his life history with an unequivocal appeal to science to enlighten the public: "Whoever will start to commit himself to the matter without prejudice, also before the general public? Science should discard its reservation and teach people about its insights" (1885a, 42). A thirty-three-year-old businessman declared that he was not the only one who was plagued with feelings of guilt and who had regularly considered committing suicide:

Thousands are in this terrible situation. Should not every effort be made to liberate these thousands from the depressed feeling of having to hide a secret, which, if revealed, puts them below the criminal. This secret freezes any intellectual and spiritual impulse and causes great talents to be numbed, if it does not lead to insanity and suicide. If it is in your power to protect these unfortunates from public opinion, then please do so: you will save many noble people from ruin, men of genius among them. (Ps 1890, 115)

Far from resembling "a cluttered Victorian mansion," as Krafft-Ebing's mind was once characterized, within the limits of the moral climate of his time, he managed to be open-minded and pragmatic (Robinson 1976, 26). As a promoter of psychiatry at the university, he was guided by the positivist model of natural science, but at the same time his treatment of patients was rooted in a humanitarian tradition of asylum psychiatry and an anthropological approach in clinical psychiatry. He impressed upon his students that kindness and trust were often more helpful to patients than medication.[5] In his private practice, categories were not simply abstractions;

5. Dornblüth 1902; Neues Wiener Journal (undated [1902]), Nachlass Krafft-Ebing.

"problems" were embodied in persons who often more or less stood on an equal footing with him. The letters of his upper- and middle-class patients suggest that he had a good relationship with many of them. With most of his private patients and informants, he shared a common bourgeois background, an attachment to individual achievement and independence, and a propensity toward a regular, well-ordered lifestyle. More than half of his patients and correspondents were members of the bourgeoisie or aristocracy, and the majority among them were private patients. Besides rich landowners, scholars, writers, artists, medical students, physicians, and engineers, there were also many common civil servants, businessmen, and employees. Apart from the unusual sexual life of some of them, most wanted to be respectable citizens. "After reading your work I hope that, if I fulfill my duties as a physician, citizen, father, and husband, I may still count myself among human beings who do not merely deserve to be despised," wrote one of Krafft-Ebing's correspondents (1890e, 79; *Ps* 1999, 268). A medical student who addressed himself to Krafft-Ebing because of his fetishism hoped "to become a useful employee, serving my country and science, in whatever position."[6] "I have a responsible occupation, and I think I can give the assurance," wrote a homosexual, "that my abnormal inclination has never, not even by a hair's breadth, caused me to deviate from the duty imposed on me" (1891h, 125; *Ps* 1999, 578–79). A high-level German civil servant who had sent Krafft-Ebing an extensive argument against the criminalization of homosexuality even reproached him for not being respectable enough, because *Psychopathia sexualis*, which might have contributed significantly to the improvement of the social position of urnings, contained so many "obscene details" (1892i, 43).

To many of Krafft-Ebing's patients and correspondents, however, bourgeois respectability with all its sexual and moral constraints also posed a problem, which in part explains why some preferably looked for their sexual contacts among the lower classes in particular. As a possible escape from the restraints of bourgeois respectability, the looseness of lower-class sexuality, though generally considered dangerous, still seemed enticing, especially for homosexuals and masochists. In fact, many middle- and upper-class urnings indicated that they preferred sex with lower-class men; some of them stated that they were not sexually aroused by men of their own class or that they were even impotent with them. One of them explained that his attraction to men of his own social standing was merely platonic and that his sexual desire focused on lower-class "masculine characters":

coarse, powerful men . . . who are mentally and socially beneath me. The reason for this strange phenomenon may be that my pronounced feeling

6. Letter of K (June 2, 1898), Nachlass Krafft-Ebing.

of shame and innate apprehensiveness, when combined with my cautious disposition, produces an inhibitory effect with men of my own social position, so that with them I can only rarely and with difficulty induce sexual excitement in myself. (1891h, 129; Ps 1999, 583)

Apparently, some social distance made it easier for these men to discard any psychological inhibitions they might have—in this respect their attitude did not differ from heterosexual men having sex with lower-class prostitutes.

For homosexual men there was another reason to prefer lower-class sexual partners. Many refrained from having sex with other urnings because they were after "real men." According to Dr. G, two urnings were easily put off by each other, just as "two whores" would be, simply for reasons of competition (1882, 215). Rough lower-class men who did not consider themselves urnings but still engaged in same-sex contacts were viewed as hypermasculine; soldiers were especially sought after as well. "Generally, I seek my lovers among cavalrymen and sailors, and, eventually, among workmen, especially butchers and smiths," an estate agent wrote, adding that he especially favored "robust forms, with healthy facial complexions" (1891h, 100; Ps 1999, 603). "I loathe sexual contact with urnings," another correspondent reported. "I prefer lower-class men, servants, stable hands, soldiers, for example, if they are powerfully built."[7]

A special fascination for crossing boundaries of class manifested itself in some of the case histories of masochists. Being dominated by someone of an inferior social position seemed extra humiliating. Thus a high-ranking civil servant of thirty-two, homosexual as well as masochistic, was fascinated by "sturdy, dirty working-class figures" (1894e, 351). An aristocratic military officer, aged twenty-eight, was aroused by lower-class men in shining boots who incited

> sensually colored ideas, such as being his servant's servant and pulling off his boots; the idea of being stepped on by him or shining his boots was extremely pleasing. . . . It was only servants' boots that aroused him; the same kind of boots on persons of a similar social position did not affect him. (Ps 1888, 120; cf. Ps 1999, 296–97)

Another aristocrat believed that his masochism was inborn, "for already when he was still a boy he had longed to wear ragged clothes and to get in touch with proletarians." Krafft-Ebing reported that this aristocrat's sexual urge was very strong and that he was solely attracted to "sailors, coachmen, servants, journeymen with big, callous worker's hands."

7. Case history of K (October 20–29, 1892), Nachlass Krafft-Ebing.

In order to experience such pleasure, it was necessary that he approached such men by changing his clothes, visiting cheap joints, etc. In his erotic dreams, which are all about masochist desires and sexual rape, only coarse masculine figures from the dregs of the nation play a role. (1899d, 151–52)

It is hard to think of a sharper contrast between this degraded milieu and the bourgeois and aristocratic worlds of many of Krafft-Ebing's private patients and correspondents as evoked in their stories and writings. Sent in by educated and often cosmopolitan men, several of these letters and personal narratives were filled with literary references, sophisticated self-analyses, and philosophical and medical speculations. Science was valued in particular. A thirty-four-year-old businessman declared:

Convinced that the enigma of our existence can be solved, or, at least, illuminated only by the unprejudiced thought of scientific men, my only aim in portraying my life is, as far as is possible, to throw some light on this cruel error of nature, and to be useful to my companions in misfortune among generations to come, for as long as men are born, there will be urnings. It is a fact that they have existed in every age. With the progress of science in our age, one will view me and those like me not as objects of hatred, but as objects of pity, who deserve the warm compassion rather than the scorn of their more fortunate fellow men. (Ps 1888, 87–88; cf. Ps 1999, 586)

Remarkably, perhaps, religious references are found only sporadically in the case histories and personal narratives.[8] With reference to Darwin, some pointed out that their religious conviction was undermined by modern scientific insights. It seems that many of them were quite active in tracing scientific and literary writings that could throw light on their condition, and frequently they knew Krafft-Ebing's publications or other popular and scientific works on sexuality. "Even though I have not consorted with other urnings, I am, nevertheless, fully informed about my condition," wrote a

8. Krafft-Ebing's own remarks on Christianity tended to be ambivalent. On the one hand, he praised this religious tradition for its contribution to the control of sexual urges and the institutionalization of marriage in which, as a rule, husband and wife were equal partners. On the other hand, notably in *Psychopathia sexualis*, he pointed to the darker sides of religious ecstasy, which, he believed, quickly degenerated into mysticism and zealotry. Sexuality and religion were both marked by transcendence of the self by means of love, surrender, and self-renunciation. The boundaries between various forms of Christian devotion and aspects of madness or sexual perversion, sadomasochism in particular, were fluid (1897e, 141). Although religiously inspired flagellants strove to move beyond the body by whipping themselves, the opposite was often the result, according to Krafft-Ebing (Ps 1903, 30; cf. 1879–80, 68). He also criticized celibacy: priests missed out on what he called "the ennobling influence exercised by love and marital life upon the character" (Ps 1903, 14; cf. Ps 1999, 16).

homosexual businessman, "for I have succeeded in consulting almost all the literature on the subject" (*Ps* 1890, 161; cf. *Ps* 1999, 566). Others referred to classical culture to justify their homosexuality. Although he was ashamed of himself, a twenty-six-year-old patient had accepted his leanings. As Krafft-Ebing noted: "If he thinks of the magnificent classical masterworks of art, then he cannot imagine that it would be wrong to love a living embodiment of them" (1894e, 357). Above all it was the shared access to art and literature, or, in short, *Bildung*, the broad neo-humanistic and cultural education that defined the habitus of the upper echelons of the central European bourgeoisie, and that provided the intellectual basis for Krafft-Ebing, his private patients, and his correspondents to communicate with one another as equals. The aim of *Bildung* as a cultural ideal was not only intellectual education, but also the development of character: the self and its formation were cultivated as objects of observation and concern—as objects of self-reflection.

Next to class and education, gender is a crucial variable in Krafft-Ebing's casuistry. In the nineteenth century, women were generally considered to be more susceptible to mental disorders than men, and they often outnumbered men in asylums; but as far as sexual perversions were concerned, men were overrepresented (cf. Showalter 1987). Most of Krafft-Ebing's patients and correspondents discussed here, 322 out of 440, were male. Moreover, in more than half of the 118 case histories involving women, the issue was not so much sexual perversion per se, but mental disorders related to menstruation. Among the sadists, fetishists, exhibitionists, pedophiles, and zooerastes or zoophiles in Krafft-Ebing's casuistry, no women at all were represented. And they constituted only a minority among the masochists and homosexuals: out of 50 masochists 3 were female, and out of 168 homosexuals only 25.

This underrepresentation of women was no coincidence, since medical definitions of sexuality in general and perversion in particular were gender-specific and closely connected to norms about normal sexual behavior of men and women. Men were supposed to be active and aggressive, women passive and docile. It was assumed, for example, that mainly men were exhibitionists. Women were hardly considered as perverts if they showed their bodies to men, because they were supposed to be sexually passive and make themselves accessible to the male gaze. Conversely, if a woman observed the naked body of a man, she was not so much seen as a voyeur as he was considered to be an exhibitionist. Exhibitionism by a man was seen as a perversion inasmuch as the man was making himself into a passive object for the female gaze (McLaren 1997, 205).

The reason for the rarity of masochism among women is, paradoxically, that subjection and dependence were considered by Krafft-Ebing and other physicians as part of women's normal condition. In addition to the three female patients discussed under the category of masochism, another three women were diagnosed by Krafft-Ebing with so-called sexual bondage, a one-sided, extreme emotional dependency of women on their sexual partner. Sexual bondage, though considered an abnormality, was not a perversion because it did not interfere with normal intercourse. Mainly in men, who were supposed to be sexually dominant, was subjection considered a perversion. Moreover, since masochistic men, by adopting the passive female role, did not follow the supposedly normal biological order, this behavior was related to inversion. Like male exhibitionists, masochists undermined active heterosexual masculinity.

All sadists observed by Krafft-Ebing were men. Sadism was indeed defined as a problem of men: as he pointed out, sexual aggressiveness was part of the normal masculine psyche, but it sometimes transgressed the limits of the normal. As such it was an "anachronism" in modern civilization:

> From cultural history and anthropology we know that there were times and that there are still tribes in which cruel violence, plundering, and even the knocking out of women by blows with a club took and take the place of courtship. Nowadays, among civilized people, we still see such anachronisms in the form of rape. (1890e, 1)

The medical definition of this perversion reflected changing norms about masculinity and it also was differentiated according to class. Before Krafft-Ebing gave it a psychiatric label, the term *sadism* was first used by literary critics who in the 1850s commented on the decadent themes found in the writings of Gustave Flaubert (1821–1880) and Charles Baudelaire (1821–1867), and it began to be widely employed in the 1880s when the Marquis de Sade's work was rediscovered. The literary notion of sadism referred to a cultivated libertinism and decadence, and it included an elitist disdain for conventional bourgeois society. However, the men whom psychiatrists first labeled as sadists were for the most part lower-class sexual delinquents. Their crude and violent sexual behavior was considered compulsive, and it clearly transgressed the boundaries of normal masculine sexual aggressiveness. New notions of civilized and restrained masculinity placed restrictions on male aggression (McLaren 1997, 169–70, 205). Bourgeois masculinity was not only defined by aggressiveness but also by self-control, reason, and willpower, qualities that lower-class compulsive sadists failed to possess. Yet, some bourgeois men who were diagnosed with "ideal" sadism by Krafft-Ebing seemed quite capable of controlling their violent urges: these men were cruel only in their own imagination.

All fetishists who appear in Krafft-Ebing's work were men. Although he listed fetishistic tendencies in women regarding abstract qualities in men involving traits and talents like courage, chivalry, self-confidence, and other nonphysical aspects, he stated that cases of perverse fetishism in women were unknown to him. Typically, fetishists, obsessed with female body parts or female clothes and ornaments, were presented as actively desiring subjects while women played the role of passive object (Matlock 1993). Women, however, were seen as actors in another context: especially in France in the 1880s and 1890s, psychiatrists were confronted with middle- and upper-class women shoplifting in department stores, not out of poverty, but because they were obsessed by the objects of female fashion and supposedly suffered from excessive vanity. Psychiatrists diagnosed these women as kleptomaniacs, and they might well have been considered as the female equivalents of male fetishists (O'Brien 1983). Kleptomania was viewed as a typical female mental disorder. Like other derangements in women, psychiatrists often connected it to the female reproductive system, and they also noticed that women derived sexual pleasure from shoplifting. However, kleptomania was not seen as a sexual perversion. In *Psychopathia sexualis* there is no reference to it, though Krafft-Ebing must have been familiar with the many case histories of kleptomania published by French psychiatrists. He probably saw no immediate ground to link this disorder to fetishism as French psychiatrists did, but, from the prevailing psychiatric perspective of his day, he might have done so with good reason (Rosario 1997, 113–14, 123–26).

In contrast to male homosexuality, female homosexuality largely remained a muted discourse in Krafft-Ebing's work, and his discussion of it was contradictory. On the one hand, he emphasized that lesbianism was comparable to male homosexuality and seemed as common as contrary sexual feeling in men:

> Careful observation of the ladies of large cities soon reveals that uranism is by no means a rarity. Females who wear their hair short, who dress in the fashion of men, who pursue the sports and pastimes of their male acquaintances, as well as opera singers and actresses who appear on the stage in male attire by preference may be suspected of it. (*Ps* 1903, 282; cf. *Ps* 1999, 328)

At the same time, however, he suggested that uranism was not as frequent among women as among men. Moreover, he contended that in the majority of cases, homosexuality in women was cultivated rather than inborn. Women were not only underrepresented in the casuistry, but they hardly spoke for themselves as well. In various case histories involving private female patients, who more often than men were sent by their partner or by relatives, Krafft-Ebing hinted at the fact that it was harder to elicit statements on their sexuality than from the men who consulted him (*Ps* 1887, 95; 1888e, 7). He seemed to have suspected that this might have been related to his own gender. "Details on the vita sexualis of women," he wrote as an aside in *Psychopathia sexualis*, "will come to our knowledge only when medical women enter into the study of this subject" (*Ps* 1903, 21; cf. *Ps* 1999, 22). He also suggested that, in comparison to men, women experienced their homosexuality as less of a problem. After all, female homosexuality was not punishable in Germany while it was hardly persecuted in Austria. Moreover, lesbian women were supposed to have fewer problems with heterosexual intercourse than urnings, which is why many were married and invisible to the outside world.

To Krafft-Ebing, especially the appearance of women—more often than that of men who were more eager to tell their life stories—suggested their homosexuality, and in his therapeutical interactions with them, it was thus a factor in his trying to raise this issue. The few case histories on women also reveal that they, if already displaying a self-conscious attitude, were taken less seriously than men. It seems understandable, therefore, that his female patients could identify themselves much less with the medical-psychiatric discourse on sexuality of those days. Moreover, around 1900 a distinct sense of lesbian identity was still hardly developed in central European societies. For women, there were no public meeting places or an established sexual underground, while most also lacked economic independence and freedom of movement. In Germany and Austria, a self-defined lesbian identity and subculture did not emerge until the 1920s (Hacker and Lang 1986, 13–17; Hacker 1987; cf. Vicinus 1989).

This is not to deny, however, that some women may well have recognized themselves in Krafft-Ebing's case histories and that his work may have reinforced their sense of identity, even though there are only slight and indirect indications for this. The novel *Sind es Frauen? Roman über das dritte Geschlecht* (1901), by Aimée Duc, the penname of the Austrian author Minna Wettstein-Adelt, is one of the first literary works picturing the life and viewpoints of self-confident lesbian women, among them Minotschka Fernandoff, the leading character, and her lover Berta Cohn. While some of the women are out for an evening in Geneva, they are joined at their table by two men, who, referring to Lombroso, argue that emancipation and intellectual pursuits cause nervous disorders and hysteria in women. Biting back, Minotschka mentions Krafft-Ebing. Upon hearing the psychiatrist's name, one of the men intervenes:

"Apropos: Krafft-Ebing! Is he not the one who stands up for perverse people?" Proudly he looked around the table. "Indeed," Minotschka said, "he is the same, the author of 'Psychopathia sexualis,' the book onto which many outsiders and uninitiated readers throw themselves eagerly and lustfully!"

Embarrassed, the men quickly leave the table:

"We have chased them away!" cheered Berta Cohn. "What a pity," replied Minotschka, "I would have liked to teach them a little more! I wanted to tell them that we also belong to these 'Krafft-Ebing people'! I think that they would have fainted!" (Duc 1976, 53–54)

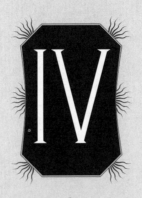

Psychiatry
and Sexual Identity
in Fin de Siècle
Culture

PSYCHIATRY, PRESENTING INDIVIDUAL SEXUAL EXPERIENCES AS TYPICAL
"cases," has played an important role in the making of sexual categories and identities—in what I have characterized as the modernization of sexuality. According to Michel Foucault, Jeremy Bentham's panopticum was the paradigm of the case history method in the medical and human sciences, while the case history itself was the prototype of modern identity. To Foucault, the psychiatric description is simply a modern version of the religious confession in which women and men not only reveal sinful transgressions, but also the often shameful truth of their inner being (Foucault 1975 & 1976; cf. Hahn 1982; Hacking 1995, 219). Since religious and medical authority determine what can and cannot be said, the confession and the case study are forms of representation that manipulate information so as to exercise power over individuals. In this line of argument, Krafft-Ebing's work, in which case histories were central, functions as an important stage in the development of what Foucault calls "a confessional science" that, in his view, not only imposed an identity upon individuals, but also controlled and disciplined them.

In the previous chapters, I have tried to demonstrate that the modernization of sexuality cannot be reduced to such a uniform model of medical stigmatization and control, even though physicians may certainly have purposefully heightened the problem of sexuality as a matter of health and disease in order to enhance their professional status. But nineteenth-century psychiatrists should not be viewed exclusively in terms of their theories or ambitions. Nor should psychiatry's concrete actors and elements—physicians, patients, institutions, therapies—be considered monolithically, as if there was little or no internal diversity or disagreement among them. Krafft-Ebing's sexual pathology was not shaped systematically by the logic of medical science, nor was it simply a means of controlling or disciplining deviants. Many of the case histories and autobiographical accounts from patients and correspondents that he used in his work suggest that they were not merely passive victims of the new psychiatric labeling. Moreover, they equally demonstrate that new ways of understanding sexuality emerged out of a confrontation and intertwining of professional medical thinking and patients' self-definition. The theory of degeneration and an emphatic understanding of individual predicaments existed side by side. Krafft-Ebing's work fluctuated between the stigmatization of perversions as mental diseases and the recognition of the individual's particular and unique desires. The medical model was employed by many of his private patients and correspondents to mitigate feelings of guilt and to maintain some sense of integrity and self-confidence. Medicine could be used to give perversion the stamp of naturalness and to part with the charge of immorality and illegality. Several perverts went to the psychiatrist, not so much seeking a cure, but to develop a dialogue about their nature and social situation. Sexual identities could not be formed in isolation; they had to be recognized, confirmed, and legitimized by others.

Sexual categories and identities were not only scientific inventions and imposed from above by the power of organized medical opinion. The medicalization of sexuality has to be viewed as a process in which new meanings were attached to existing behaviors and feelings. These new meanings were developed with the collaboration of some of the people concerned as they furnished psychiatrists with the life stories and self-observations on which medical interpretations were grounded. What is remarkable in Krafft-Ebing's dealing with the life histories of his patients and correspondents is that he did not manipulate their information for professional purposes, although he put them in a medical context. Even if they distanced themselves from medical thinking, he still published their letters and autobiographies uncensored, and he also acknowledged that some of them had influenced him. Medical theories would unlikely have evolved without the particular impetus of the personal confessions of sexual perverts themselves (cf. Silverstolpe 1987; Müller 1991; Hansen 1992). The construction of modern sexual identities was realized in a process of social interaction between individuals, who contemplated on themselves, and physicians, who shaped psychiatry and delineated perversion as a medical field. In the second half of the nineteenth century, well-educated, urban, and often cosmopolitan middle- and upper-class men increasingly began to fashion sexual identities self-consciously. Medical understanding of sexuality could only be successful because it was embedded in society and because psychiatrists like Krafft-Ebing and his patients shared the same cultural background and the same bourgeois values. Evidently, the case history method in psychiatry and the changing ways in which individuals understood themselves were not only closely associated with the expansion of a medical specialty, but they invoked a much wider cultural climate as well, involving transformations in the field of individualism, self-reflection, and personal identity as well as changes in the social structures of sexuality. The next three chapters will elaborate these broader nineteenth-century concerns and developments, while the fourth will focus on the culture of fin de siècle Vienna in particular.

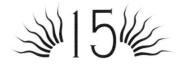

Autobiography and Sexual Identity

Krafft-Ebing's psychiatric explanations and the (auto)biographical case studies he used as empirical material reflected as well as shaped sexual experiences. He did not consider sexuality to be just a biological instinct; he presented it as something that was inextricably bound up with individual life histories, mediated by experience, and vested with personal meaning. Since sexuality played a core part in the narratives of self and perverse desire was linked to the individual mental makeup, it was burdened with significance. The autobiographical case histories were especially directed toward the discovery of one's authentic personal being. The experience of the self, as narrated by many patients and correspondents, was crucial in the development of Krafft-Ebing's sexual pathology. They were not just acting out a role on the basis of patterned behaviors, but they had internalized the idea that they were a special kind of person and many were aware that they shared this sense of self with others. A self-conscious sexual identity not only presupposes that one feels different but also that one belongs to a group.

The rise of sexual pathology in psychiatry did not so much cause this need for self-comprehension as channel it and magnify its effects. Krafft-Ebing's *Psychopathia sexualis* indicated, rather than provoked, a growing preoccupation not only with sexuality, but also with a vulnerable self. Medical explanations of sexuality took shape at the same time as sexuality became a subject for introspection and obsessive self-analysis in bourgeois milieus. The scientific "will to know" in psychiatry moved forward at the same pace as the concern for the authentic and voluble self and the searching scrutiny of the inner life (Perrot 1990, 453–547; Gay 1995). However, neither psychiatric case histories as reported by Krafft-Ebing nor autobiographies written down by his patients should be considered as unmediated voices of perverts or as direct reflections of internal psychological realities.

The way individuals experienced sexuality and gave meaning to it was determined not so much by inevitable facts of nature or a unique psychological essence, but by cultural codes and symbols as they circulated in social life. Sexual identities crystallized as patterned narratives and as such their content and form were of a social and historical origin, rather than of an individual and psychological nature.

Krafft-Ebing's case histories can be viewed as a specific version of the modern (auto)biographical genre as it originated in the eighteenth century and came to full development in the nineteenth century (Fleishman 1983; Buckley 1984; Peterson 1986). Personal narrative, to be sure, has older roots in accounts of exemplary heroic deeds or records of the events of inner religious experience. Since the Reformation (sinful) acts were not viewed apart and judged separately anymore, but evaluated in the context of an individual's whole life. The Christian—mainly Protestant—mode of spiritual introspection was characterized by a specific method of biblical hermeneutics called typology. Typological interpretation was the attempt to discover parallels between the actions of a biblical character and those of the autobiographer in order to find divine purpose and order in life. By applying types from the Bible to one's own life, the meaning and design of individual existence could be discovered. These spiritual autobiographies are narratives of conversion and deliverance (Hahn 1982, 418–25; Buckley 1984, 52–53). Modern autobiography, however, no longer highlights the presentation of a type or example to be followed, but ever more insistently explores the complex authentic individual ("like no one else in the world") by focusing on the protagonist's inner development. The term *autobiography* first appeared around 1775 and was not well established until the early Victorian period. Giambattista Vico (1668–1744), Johann Wolfgang von Goethe (1749–1832), and, above all, Jean-Jacques Rousseau (1712–1778) set a precedent for modern autobiography by moving away from the depiction of general human nature and its exemplary models to the portrayal of a distinctive, individual personality. In modern autobiography, the outward events matter far less than their effect upon the inner self and the depth of subjective experience.

The discovery of the "real" self and the attempt of being true to it constitute the hallmarks of modern autobiography. With his *Confessions* (1782, 1789), Rousseau was one of the first to claim that he gave a complete and sincere account of the most intimate experiences of his life, not concealing unsavory incidents and dark desires. In his autobiography he confessed, for instance, that he had abandoned all his children to an orphanage, while his sexual experiences involving masturbation, masochism, exhibitionism, and homosexuality were not suppressed. He broke new ground by emphasizing childhood and adolescence, the formative years of his character and the ideal of personal growth and authentic being, which could only be realized by safeguarding the autonomy of his consciousness vis-à-vis the outside world. The belief that there was a wide gap between artificial social roles and the real self was the crucial impetus for Rousseau's scrupulous self-inspection. Whereas the public world of social relations was generally considered of far more significance than the personal domain of inner experience, he replaced the fixed and average public self with the fluid and unique individual self, distinct from all others (Sennett 1974). Rousseau claimed to be completely sincere, to have thrown off all the dissimulation and pretense that he considered so characteristic of conventional social life. His revealing confessions of his unconventional sexual desires and fantasies proved that he strove for nothing less than the naked truth. (For nineteenth-century psychiatrists, Rousseau's autobiography would be a rewarding source for diagnosing him with several perversions.) His sustained self-examination served the purpose of impressing upon his readers the conclusion that he could not in any respect be false to any man because he had been true to himself.

Although it is questionable whether Rousseau really did live up to the requirements of his ideal of sincerity and authenticity, his example set the fashion for the autobiographical genre in the nineteenth century. Modern autobiographers are not expected to provide a mere chronicle of the events in their lives, but rather to reveal the cast of their mind, the style of their personality, and their voyage of self-discovery that is the more fascinating, the more it is interrupted by frequent misdirections and confused by inward struggles. Modern autobiographers are expected to be authentic and sincere, to tell the truth about one's own (private) existence, especially to be open about traits of character or actions that normally one would rather conceal (Trilling 1971). Calculated self-portrayal is never absent in modern autobiography of course, but at the same time the genre owes its existence and popularity to a deep-felt need for self-disclosure. Although baring one's inner life—which is inevitable for autobiographers who want to present themselves as interesting and unique personalities—might be risky in nineteenth-century bourgeois society because conventions were easily broken, autobiography was the preeminent literary genre to create space for the articulation of individual difference (Gay 1995, 113–14, 178, 343–45; Peterson 1986, 19). Rousseau had shown the way: he opened his *Confessions* with the statement that being different and unique was the source and measure of individual worth. Self-restraint and conventionality were characteristic of the bourgeois ethos, but at the same time a commitment evolved to unfolding the idiosyncratic self. Autobiographical self-understanding was crucial to the expression of subjectivity among the nineteenth-century bourgeoisie (Gay 1995; Baumeister 1986; Kaschuba 1993, 393). To be sure, introspection and self-revelation were not invented in the nineteenth century, but with the rise of a better-educated middle class, these practices found a broader social base. The inwardness launched by the Romantics was democratized, and the self became a major source of literary material. The growing number and circulation not only of autobiographies, but also of memoirs, diaries, and novels exploring inner consciousness indicate there was an audience that was preoccupied with the self.

Sustained self-reflection only became possible on a large scale with the eighteenth-century "invention of the self," which suggested the emergence of a new conception of personal identity, as well as with the separation of public and private spheres (Lyons 1978; Perrot 1990). Several historical developments affected self-definition and changed the way personal identity was defined and organized. Foremost is the process of individualization, the growing valuation of the unique and special characteristics of the person, which entailed a shift away from one's social role and position, community membership, or family descent as the determinant of identity. In premodern society, identity tended to be assigned: individuals did not have much choice because their identity was largely determined by fixed social structures and hierarchies. The breakup of restricted traditional communities and their stable and explicit codes offered individuals more freedom to choose their lifestyles and it also encouraged self-reflection. As assigned social identities lost some of their former significance, individuals were burdened with the task of defining themselves, even more so as consensual belief in the objective truth of a common set of values, morals, or religious articles was eroding. Nineteenth-century society developed in the direction of pluralism, and more and more the individual was thrown upon his or her own resources to decide what to believe in and what values and ideals to espouse. From the eighteenth century on, Western society has witnessed a shift in emphasis from the social, institutional components of identity to identity as a set of inner motives and impulses, personal desires and needs. Increasingly, individuals began generating self-definitions internally: personal identity was equated with the "real" or "true" inner self that could only be discovered in the private sphere. Closely connected to modern individualism is an awareness of internal space, the concept of the person having an inner self that is not directly shown in public life and that has a separate existence independent of one's position and role in society (Turner 1976; Baumeister 1986; Taylor 1994, 285–390).

Whereas in the eighteenth century the basic Enlightenment assumption was that the ideal, rational organization of society would be beneficial to individuals who supposedly shared a basic, constant rational human nature, the Romantics espoused the belief that society is oppressive to the individual and that human fulfillment has to be sought in the cultivation of one's unique sensibility and inner self. The Romantic notion of a deep-seated interior special to the individual person was seen as the foundation enabling all thought, passion, creativity, and morality. The self-contained personality offered the means to differentiate oneself from others and to achieve uniqueness. The preoccupation of the Romantics with the true self and their obsession with the deeper reaches of feelings left an irrevocable imprint on bourgeois culture. The cultivation of individual uniqueness and the view of the self as being in conflict with society depended largely on the social separation of the public and private domains of life. In the nineteenth century, more and more bourgeois sought individual happiness and fulfillment outside of public social relations, thus upgrading private life and essentially turning it into a refuge from society.

Individual authenticity became a preeminent value and a framework for introspection, self-contemplation, and self-expression. A public ready to believe that the interplay of emotions was necessary to one's full humanity and ready to tolerate and even welcome autobiographical confessions that rejected restrictive social conventions came into being. Self-disclosure was a means to show that to be honest to oneself could enrich inner life. Although solipsistic self-absorption might be viewed as more or less morbid in itself and detrimental to self-confidence, Freud was not the first and only one who believed that pursuing the self to its most secret hiding places was essential to a healthy and authentic life. The ideal of personal authenticity accorded some moral justification to the disclosure of much of what official bourgeois culture condemned and sought to exclude or ignore: loss of self-control, disorder, self-doubt, unreason, full play of emotions, and sexual desire (Trilling 1972, 11). Autobiographical disclosure accorded well with the intellectual trend in late-nineteenth-century culture that sought to unmask outward appearances and uncover their underlying, sometimes not all too pleasant, reality. Already before Freud, the inner self came to be understood as so vast and so well hidden that special methods of study would be necessary to achieve self-knowledge. Nor was he unique in asserting that the individual past remains active and continues to shape adult life. With the emergence of child psychology in the 1880s, the personal past began to be perceived in a new light and its effects on adult behavior highlighted. As the Christian soul became secularized, as it were, individual memory increasingly became the scientific key to define and study the self. In the 1870s and 1880s, psychiatrists and psychologists, developing new theories about remembering and forgetting, focused on memory as essential to self-understanding, moral consciousness, and personal identity (Hacking 1995).

In several ways, the wider reflective dimensions of modern self-identity are problematical, those of autobiographical analysis ambivalent. The effort of the self to achieve individuality and authenticity in writing has generated its own conventions and commonplaces. Autobiographers try to be sincere to themselves, because that is what they want their audience to believe they are and that is what the readers expect from them. However, to what extent do autobiographers just act at being themselves? Do they really offer insights into their inner life or are they just posing? Is writing autobiography just one mode of self-fashioning as part of a more general existential pursuit? Is a story about the self, directed to a public audience, simply a report about what is plainly already there, only to be discovered by introspection, or is telling a story about one's (inner) life an act of *creating* a coherent and presentable self? Modern autobiography is not only caught in the duality of efforts to reaffirm uniqueness in convention: it is also suspended between self-revelation and self-creation.

Writing one's life history in order to be read by an audience can never be entirely a private matter; in order to be understandable for that audience, autobiography has to be geared to the repertoire of socially available narratives. The paradox of modern autobiography is that a fully individual life can only be recounted within existing, established, and more or less authoritative frameworks and metaphors. Like any other genre, the autobiographical genre has its own rules, prescriptive forms, and prefigured narrative patterns. Conventions shape the ways of thinking about the self: information is borrowed from (or imposed upon people by) diverse cultural and social sources such as religion, literature, human sciences like psychiatry and psychology, psychotherapy, self-help groups and manuals, friends, social movements, the media, or movies. Thus individual self-understanding is embedded in culturally conditioned discourses. Narrative patterns that are common in autobiography refer to stability, regression, or progression, and they are borrowed from genres like tragedy (a progressive or stable phase in the life course is suddenly interrupted by a rapid regression), melodrama (a regressive phase is followed by a restoration of stability or progression), and the romantic saga (a series of progressive-regressive episodes) (Gergen and Gergen 1997, 165–68). Metaphors suggesting a lost paradise, a journey, a conversion, or a confession bestow on individual life stories something of the already familiar (Egan 1984; cf. Peterson 1986, 20; Kaschuba 1993, 394, 410).

Current theories of (auto)biography emphasize that it is a form of narrative, and that personal identity takes shape in the stories people tell about themselves (Hinchman and Hinchman 1997; cf. Porter 1997). Narrative is a form of discourse that arranges selected events in a sequential order, thus linking them up in a meaningful way, so that they can be understood by an audience as parts of a whole. The many memorized facts have to be selected and organized in one way or another. Authors can only make clear what sort of person they are if they indicate which particular events have special significance or which experiences were formative and if they arrange these events and experiences in such a way that unity, development, and purpose are established in their lived experience, as well as in the text. Autobiographers often relate the story of their life as a continuous process with an inner logic leading up to the present situation. Interpreting past events from a present point of view and anticipating the future course of their lives, they narrate their lives in terms of a basic plot formula. It is common to present one's life essentially as a *Bildung* process, the discovery of a vocation or destiny, or the fulfillment of (or failure to realize) one's desires, ambitions, or moral purpose.[1] In this way, personal narratives are not mere chronicles and do not merely describe, but also explore and explain: autobiography is a narrative embodiment of analysis and interpretation (Novitz 1997, 147–54). Autobiographical disclosure moves up and down between a continual self-dissection and efforts at reaching a narratively integrated and coherent self. On the basis of fixed patterns, individuals integrate the past, present, and future, thereby constituting more or less stable, coherent identities on both a personal and communal level.

Of course, autobiography is not simply lived life. Like all storytellers, autobiographers inevitably select and (re)arrange events from "real" life, while also remaining silent—intentionally or not—about particular events. The order of the facts in a life history depends on the narrative patterns and silences available in a culture. But does this suggest that autobiographers just impose an artificial form upon the bewildering variety of lived experience, which in itself is just a jumble of unrelated sensations and events? Are personal narratives and the identities to which they give rise just imaginative constructs that people adopt more or less arbitrarily? Many proponents of the social constructionist variant of narrativist theory argue that individual identities are not discovered through some sort of inner observation, but that they are constructed once individuals establish coherent connections among the events and experiences of their lives in the form of stories and shape them as systematically related and having a pur-

1. It has been argued that such coherent, pointed plot lines of autobiographical narratives are typically masculine and that life stories of women, organized around personal relationships, are less goal-oriented and more digressive and complex (Rosenwald and Ochberg 1992, 12).

pose. The self is viewed as a product of language rather than as expressing itself through language. Going one step further is the contention that personal identity is merely a narrative fiction, a free-floating work of art, necessarily distorting life as it "really" is lived (Fleishman 1983, 22; Kerby 1997, 114; Carr 1997, 11; Novitz 1997).

Not all narrativists, however, share the belief that the unity and coherence that autobiography confers upon the self is a mere illusive, artificial construct. According to the philosopher Alasdair MacIntyre, "man is in his actions and practice, as well as in his fictions, essentially a story-telling animal," and "stories are lived before being told" (1997, 254, 249). Like MacIntyre, supporters of a more realist version of narrativism contend that there is a continuity between human reality (as distinct from mere physical reality) and narrative, that real life shares with the stories about it many of the formal properties of narratives. Although life stories are not simply objective reflections of the course of events in real lives, the way they are told is deeply intermingled with the way individuals practically experience and organize their lives. The tales they tell are not only about their lives, but also part of it. Admitting that a purposeful life does not precede narrative but is constituted by it, advocates of a more realist perspective on autobiographical reflection emphasize that human consciousness is discursive: individuals in everyday life continuously reinforce their sense of self by linking their present states, plans, choices, and actions to both the past and the (imagined) future (Hinchman and Hinchman 1997, xviii).

Significantly, stories give direction to real lives. We cannot have a stable, continuous sense of self without remembering our past and anticipating our future. Without some narrative order, life would have no direction and be meaningless. Meaningful events are experienced, not as discrete instances, but as parts of a whole, ongoing life. Narrativity is anchored in the human, ephemeral experience of the world. Basically, autobiographical reflection—though most people do not spell out their life story at length—is a precondition for a sense of unity, orientation, and directedness amidst the confusing versatility and complexity of daily life. Not only can most people tell more or less coherent stories about their lives; they also experience their lives as narrative structures. The greater part of ordinary human action is purposefully oriented toward the future, toward projected ends, and as such it is always possible to tell a logical story about it. To a large extent, life narratives, be it on a primitive and fragmentary level, guide and regulate human behavior. Human action is continuously subjected to autobiographical reflection, especially when intentions and moral choices are involved. People need stories to know how to behave in a purposive and moral way: human action and narrative both have a teleological character (MacIntyre 1997, 245, 253, 254; cf. Carr 1997, 15–17).

In Krafft-Ebing's work, the genre of the medical case history and that of the autobiography seamlessly merged into each other: whereas in modern autobiography authors analyze the course of their life to arrive at self-knowledge, in psychiatric case histories a diagnosis was made by reconstructing the past life of the patient. In both types of discourse, all kinds of events and experiences were woven together to form the fabric of an individual condition or identity. It will be clear that the case histories and autobiographical accounts of Krafft-Ebing's patients and correspondents are not "true" pictures in the sense that their stories simply correspond to or mirror actual events of their lives. These stories should not be seen merely as (true or false) representations of lived lives. As examples of a specific discursive form, they can be studied in their own right. In this book, I have mainly analyzed the case histories and autobiographical accounts as sources of information about the way their subjects and authors gave meaning to their lives and (re)shaped their selves. These narratives say more about the inner life at the moment of composition than about the "real" facts of their past lives. What they presented as an intricate process of self-discovery involved to a large degree a specific interpretation of the events and experiences of the past in order to serve certain needs in the present. In these autobiographical narratives, present preoccupations and memory became so intimately connected that it is difficult to distinguish between the two.

In recounting the facts of their life history at a certain, often critical, moment in their lives, Krafft-Ebing's patients and correspondents selected, rearranged, and gave a specific color to their lived experiences. They endowed specific episodes with a symbolic meaning, turning them into fundamental transformations that explained and justified their present experience of their selves. Recurring plot elements included the first arousal of sexual feeling, the awareness of being different, fantasies, the first sexual contacts, and becoming acquainted with information about perversion and with like-minded individuals. Their autobiographies were not just straightforward accounts of their experiences, but contained specific elaborations of the "why" of the development of their selves as well. The emphasis on childhood experiences, for example, served the purpose of demonstrating that their sexual preference was not an arbitrary and fleeting impulse, but that they had been different from an early age on. And they came up with elaborate self-analyses to make clear that deviant sexuality was part and parcel of their personality. "Masochism is a crucial part of my thinking and feeling," concluded one of the correspondents (1899d, 160). Sexual identi-

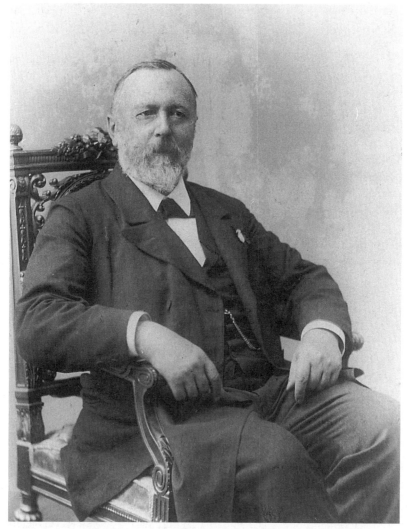

Figure 14. Krafft-Ebing in 1897. (Krafft-Ebing Family Archive, Graz, Austria)

ties, as expressed in Krafft-Ebing's work, presumed reflexive awareness and "autobiographical thinking," the ability to interrogate the past from the perspective of the present and to tell a coherent story about one's life history in light of what might be anticipated or desired for the future. As such, these autobiographical case histories may have had as much prospective as retrospective significance. Many of the more self-conscious and self-confident autobiographers not only recounted and justified their past lives, but also incorporated their past into a new perspective of their future life.

"Now I cannot keep silent any longer," a twenty-six-year-old fetishist introduced his autobiographical account: "I feel that a turning point is inevitable; all is either hopeful or lost."[2]

Self-clarification and self-justification are key functions of these sexual
autobiographies. They are typically "modernist tales" in that they are characterized by a sense of linear progression and the conviction that a truth is
being revealed. The autobiographers relied on detail and minute observation as signs of an underlying truth about their self, for example, that the
essential line in their life was a fixed, natural difference that had always
been there but was hidden and had to be traced. As we have seen in part
3, in some autobiographies there is a shift away from the biomedical vision
of a pathological, individual disposition toward a more socially reflexive
analysis, which focuses on the harmful effects of the suppression of sexual
impulses by the demands of society. As some autobiographers relate, this
critical awareness caused them to experience the gap between the true self
and the social environment more strongly as a problem than their sexual
impulses per se. Many of Krafft-Ebing's patients and correspondents had
fully developed a sense of themselves as objects of introspection, the more
so because they were obliged to keep up appearances in a society in which
they felt ill at ease, and because they suffered from their inability to communicate with others about their inner nature. They often appealed to ideals of authenticity and sincerity to bestow moral value on their sexual nature, and several of them complained that they continuously had to hide
their real self. "It is terrible to have to constantly act a farce," one of Krafft-
Ebing's patients, a thirty-one-year-old chemist, told him (Ps 1892, 343; Ps
1999, 609). "While crying, the patient pictures his endless moral suffering,"
one can read in the case observation of a highly-placed urning; "although
by nature he is a frank man, he is forced to dissemble continuously" (1890e,
58). "How sad to be afflicted with a condition, which one has to hide anxiously," another urning wrote; "this very concealment is the greatest threat
to one's inner peace" (Ps 1888, 96). A homosexual woman experienced it
as highly painful "that, to the outside world, she, like an actress, constantly
had to play a role that is foreign to her nature, namely that of a woman"
(Ps 1894, 224; Ps 1999, 271). Others expressed themselves in a like manner: "This is a sordid situation: time and again I am forced to act against
my nature, to throw dust in the eyes of other people" (1884c, 3). According
to a fetishist, he suffered most severely from the need to pretend:

> In only one way my perversion was a moral source of concern to me,
> namely that it could have a damaging effect on my character. I have a
> frank character and from my father I learned that lying is the most seri-

ous offense. And yet, how often I have had to resort to white lies because of my urge to dress in women's clothes.[3]

"I can no longer do without male love; without it I would always be out of harmony with myself," another man asserted.

Because this love is regarded as criminal, I am not in harmony with the outside world, although I am in harmony with myself in gratifying it. Therefore, I must necessarily be somewhat depressed, all the more because I have a frank character that hates a lie. The pain of always having to hide everything within me has induced me to confess my anomaly to a few friends, whose silence and appreciation I trust. Although my situation often seems sad, because of the difficulty of gratification and the general abhorrence of male love, I often feel a trace of pride that I have such anomalous feelings. (1891h, 107, 108–9; cf. *Ps* 1999, 553–55)

Since the need for an explicit, coherent story about the self is perhaps strongest in situations of crisis—when "authentic" feelings conflict with the demands and expectations of the social environment, when feelings and experiences are forbidden or not understandable, when a sense of continuity is lost and there is a lot in need of an explanation—these individuals must have felt a strong urge to ponder on the nature of their inner selves.

In terms of their content, the sexual life stories are about suffering, frustration, and thwarting, but sometimes also about surviving and surpassing. Some autobiographical case histories resemble romances in which the protagonist experiences difficulties, threats, and challenges, and engages in harsh struggles to overcome them, sometimes to emerge victoriously in the end. After a regressive phase of trials, terrors, and self-struggle in which life becomes increasingly problematic, there is a progressive phase or a catharsis, leading to the transformation of a negative self-image into a more or less positive identity. "I am now 38 years old, and, thanks to my abnormality, I look back on a life that has been so full of indescribable suffering that I am often astonished when I think of the extent of a man's capacity to endure suffering," wrote one urning in his self-confession.

My awareness of the suffering I have endured has recently become the source of a kind of self-respect, which, in itself, makes my life bearable, to a degree. . . . I am amazed by my ability to describe again here, in plain words, the feelings that stir about in my inner being. Anyway, I have been forced by the constant struggle to learn to conceal my inclination, and to smile when torn by pain. . . . Aside from this abnormality, I am

3. Letter of K (June 2, 1898), Nachlass Krafft-Ebing.

not insane, and I might ultimately be contented. However, I have, particularly in recent years, suffered again too much so that it is difficult not to look on the future with painful feeling. For the future will certainly not bring a fulfillment of the desire that constantly glows under the ashes: to have a lover who understands me and returns my love. Only such a relation would make me truly happy. . . . I might have long ago put an end to my misery, because I have no fear of death, and because in religion—which, strangely enough, has not departed from my impure heart—I find no warning against suicide. However, the awareness that I am not alone responsible that a worm has nipped my whole life in the bud, a certain resistance that has recently sprung up out of indescribable suffering, leads me in my endeavor to find, on an entirely new basis, some happiness in life. (1891h, 123, 125–26; cf. *Ps* 1999, 579)

Other autobiographers referred to the decisive (t)urning point in their lives. One of them, a thirty-seven-year-old technical engineer, remembered vividly how, fifteen years earlier, he had met an urning, who informed him about the nature of his leanings and introduced him to the subculture. His private suffering became part of a shared experience:

It was as if scales had fallen from my eyes, and I bless the day this enlightenment came to me. From that day I saw the world with different eyes; I saw that many others were cursed with the same fate, and I began to learn, as well as I could, to be content with my lot. (1891h, 128; cf. *Ps* 1999, 581–82)

For another correspondent, a twenty-seven-year-old homosexual, certain books had been the eye-opener:

By a fortunate coincidence I came across Plato's Symposium and Jäger's homosexual idiosyncrasy, something I cherish to this day. It was as if lighting had struck me—but in a very positive sense—and scales fell from my eyes. I recovered in a short time . . . and once again became a self-respecting person. . . . From that time I followed my leanings and, as far as possible, tried to arrange my life accordingly. (*Ps* 1887, 88)

From the perspective of moral justification, several autobiographical case histories belong to the genre that historian Thomas Laqueur (1989) has characterized as the "humanitarian narrative." The typical humanitarian narrative, which became current from the late eighteenth and early nineteenth century onward, is a story that describes concrete and particular personal suffering and that constructs this suffering so as to elicit sympathy and to offer a model for social action. Self-knowledge in itself was not enough: many of Krafft-Ebing's patients and correspondents also wanted to communicate their understanding of their "true" self to others in a credible, convincing way, writing their autobiographies explicitly for publication. An anonymous urning wrote in his autobiography:

> Even though I have nothing in my own conscience with which to re-proach myself and reject the judgment of the world, I suffer very much. To be true, I have done no one harm, and I consider my love, in its noblest expression, to be quite as holy as that of a normal man, but I often suffer, even to the extent of taedium vitae, because of the unfortu-nate lot that intolerance and ignorance cast upon us. No pen, no tongue can describe all the misery, all the unhappy situations, the constant fear of having this peculiarity revealed and of being cast from society. The thought that, with exposure, one's existence could be destroyed, that one could be cast away from all, is as terrible as any thought can be. . . . Par-don me, Professor, if I close without a signature. Do not try to find me. I could tell you nothing more. I give you these lines for the sake of future sufferers. In the interest of science, truth, and justice, publish what seems to you to be appropriate. (Ps 1890, 163; cf. Ps 1999, 569–70)

Some of them challenged the dominant moral discourse on sexuality and called for a fight against the injustice from which they suffered. The autobi-ography of the technical engineer, cited above, is a clear example of this:

> Writing down, as well as I can, the history of my suffering, I am driven only by the aspiration to clear up, to some extent, with this autobiogra-phy, the widespread misunderstandings and cruel errors concerning the "contrary sexual feeling." . . . That we do not feel as the crowd feels is not our fault, but a cruel trick of nature. Innumerable times I have racked my brains to figure out whether science, or any of her free and unpreju-diced devotees, could somehow think out a way to give us stepchildren of nature a more endurable position before the law and mankind. But I have always reached the same sad conclusion: if one enters the lists on behalf of anything, one must first thoroughly know and be able to ex-plain that for which one contends. And who is able today to perfectly explain and define contrary sexual feeling? Yet there must be some cor-rect explanation of it; there must be some way in which the mass of man-kind can be brought to a milder and more reasonable judgment of it. . . . With such a deed, a man could erect an immortal monument in his own honor, which would be justified by the gratitude of thousands of men of present and future generations; for there have always been, there are al-ways and there will always be urnings, perhaps in greater numbers than has been suspected. (1891h, 127, 129–30; cf. Ps 1999, 580, 583–84)

A thirty-one-year-old employee who sent Krafft-Ebing an extensive autobiography on his suffering as a homosexual stated that despite his pain he was not unhappy because of his love for young men, "but because the satisfaction of such love is considered improper, and therefore I cannot gratify it without restraint." He had gotten over his moral scruples and hoped for better times: "I am certain that one day prejudice will disappear, and . . . the right of unrestricted love will be acknowledged" (1891h, 108–9; *Ps* 1999, 555).

When we take Krafft-Ebing's case histories at face value, sexual identity appeared as a distinctive personal trait or essence, hidden from view and awaiting clearer recognition and expression. Given the narrative structures the case histories have in common, however, sexual identity can also be viewed as a script, on which individuals modeled their life history. The similarities in the narrative patterns of their case histories and autobiographies stand out. Again and again, the same elements appear in what was to become the standardized "coming out" narrative: descent, family background, the retrospective discovery of a peculiar way of feeling and acting during childhood and puberty, the conviction that one has always felt the same, the first sexual experiences, the struggle with masturbation that often raised more anxieties than did sexual contacts with other individuals, details about sexual fantasies, dreams and behavior, the exploration of one's health condition and gender identity in past and present, the sense of being overwhelmed by irresistible and "natural" drives for which one is not responsible, the (mostly failed) attempts to have "normal" sexual intercourse (usually with a prostitute) in order to "test" the constitutional character of one's sexual preference, the painful knowledge of being different and in conflict with society, the sense of isolation, the comforting discovery of not being alone, and the efforts at moral self-justification (cf. Müller 1991, 208–30).

Thus the "true self" appears less as the origin and center of meaning than as the point of reference by which then current models of self-understanding were reproduced. Identity is not just there to be discovered, but it has to be fashioned: it entails autobiographical narration, bringing together past and present experiences into a coherent *story* of the self. Much of autobiographical memory, selection, and narration is conditioned by the historical moment, the culturally available narratives that determine how people see themselves and interpret their lives. In the late nineteenth century, psychiatry was one of the cultural domains to offer a new configuration for looking at and making sense of one's intricate self. The psychiatric case history, as it was conceptualized by Krafft-Ebing and others, preeminently offered a fitting model for individuals feeling out of place and searching for clues to their apparently deviant nature. For many of his patients and correspondents, the medical model furnished them with a useful symbolic resource that could be employed to mitigate the feelings of anguish and guilt and help them to develop some sense of understanding and integrity in the face of confusion and despair.

Psychiatric theories of sexuality, such as those formulated by Krafft-Ebing, as well as the autobiographical accounts of his patients and correspondents, are a crucial part of what sociologist Anthony Giddens has characterized as the reflexivity of modernity: "the regularised use of knowledge about circumstances of social life as a constitutive element in its organisation and transformation" (Giddens 1991, 20; cf. Giddens 1992). In combination, psychiatric dissection and autobiographical self-scrutiny encouraged individual reflexivity; psychiatry especially offered a language that enabled detachment from the self, thus making it easier to observe and describe the self more or less objectively. The impulse to write down one's life history can be viewed as a heightened form of reflexive consciousness of the self. "The latent impulse became a conscious perversity," Krafft-Ebing said of one of his female patients who sent him her autobiography (1901a, 34; Ps 1999, 345). Such self-consciousness, shared by many individuals who read his work, was not only facilitated by his psychiatry, but even more presumed a reflexive awareness among individuals in society and an ability to modify sexual experience on the basis of an understanding of it. Each autobiographical text in Krafft-Ebing's work can be seen as a reflexive process, an ongoing deliberate (re)construction of the individual's relationship with his or her sexuality. The intertwining of psychiatric and autobiographical discourses not only described and gave meaning to human experiences, but also organized and shaped them. Since the modern reflexive project of the sexual self had to be undertaken in the absence of traditional social routines or moral certainties, self-contemplation was a cause for anxiety and uneasiness; yet, as many of Krafft-Ebing's case histories illustrate, it also created space for self-expression.

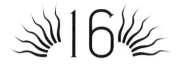

Romantic Love, Intimacy,
and the Sexual Self

Whereas the medical profession provided the specific role models and the conceptual frame in which sexual life stories were expressed, social developments from the eighteenth century onward had substantially transformed the experience of sexuality in society. To understand the privileging of sexuality as the quintessence of the individual self, the development of romantic love, privacy, and intimacy has to be taken into account.

Of course, as mere forms of (immoral) behavior and as libertine practices, or perhaps even as desires and fantasies, the perversions labeled in the late nineteenth century as homosexuality, fetishism, sadism, masochism, and exhibitionism were hardly new. Homosexual behavior—the "unmentionable vice," sodomy, pederasty, sapphism, tribadism, or whatever name was used for it—is probably as old as human history. Acts that could be taken for sadomasochism, fetishism, and exhibitionism, however, are more difficult to trace in the past. In his *Confessions*, Rousseau relates his desire to be dominated and maltreated by women and the way he exhibited himself to girls, although he did not yet use the terms *masochism* and *exhibitionism* to explain his leanings. The libertinist writer Restif de la Bretonne (1734–1806) described his erotic obsession with women's feet and shoes in his diaries and stories, a century before psychiatrists explained such leanings as a form of fetishism (Dekker 1980, Coward 1987). And as far as the cataloguing (but not the judgment) of the wide range of sexual behaviors is concerned, the literary and philosophical work of the Marquis de Sade might be considered as a precursor of Krafft-Ebing's *Psychopathia sexualis* and other late-nineteenth-century medical works on sexual deviance. Unconventional sexual behavior also received ample attention in many eighteenth- and nineteenth-century pornographic and semi-medical works (Marcus 1966; P. Wagner 1987; Kearney 1993).

The rising consumption of erotic literature and pornography as well as the growing attention to masturbation in the eighteenth century have been explained as related to an increasing privacy in social relations (P. Wagner 1987, 64). Both were associated with out-of-control fantasy and deemed dangerous for their solitary, antisocial character. From this perspective, authors like the Marquis de Sade and Restif de la Bretonne resembled some of Krafft-Ebing's masochistic and fetishistic correspondents. Although the Marquis de Sade's and Restif de la Bretonne's own sexual lives were far from conventional, the perversions and sexual cruelties they described in their work with such minute detail were largely a product of their imagination. By moving away from social reality and into their very personal universes, these authors seem to have derived pleasure from fantasizing and writing about sexuality. De Sade wrote his *Les cent vingt journées de Sodome* in solitude when he was in prison. Both the Marquis de Sade himself and some of the libertines who figure in his writings show an awareness of the idea that an unbridgeable gap exists between extravagant imagination and the natural restrictions of a limited reality. Even more than the sexual act or crime itself, fantasizing about it provided them with the utmost pleasure (Coward 1987; Heumakers 1988).

It is questionable, however, if these experiences, behaviors, and desires, whether they were expressed in a literary form or not, had a special meaning in the sense that they indicated that one was a certain kind of sexual person. In pornographic works and in those of the Marquis de Sade, the protagonists do not connect their behavior to some kind of inner being, nor do they reflect on motives or personal histories that could explain their leanings. Although the eighteenth century witnessed the beginnings of a psychological interpretation of sexuality, the conduct of individuals was generally more or less taken for granted, and when it was considered necessary to explain it, the most obvious cause one could think of was the impact of immediate circumstances and situational influences: moral corruption, seduction, hedonism, decadence, aristocratic frivolity and libertinism, the social environment, and power. Sexual aberration was seen as an ultimate form of more general debauchery and hedonism. Unlike nineteenth-century discourses, which stressed the biological and psychological origins of such behavior, eighteenth-century explanations focused on a moral condition that individuals acquired by their own doing. In the second half of the nineteenth century, however, sexual desires began to be conceived differently. In bourgeois circles, they became the focus of life stories that dealt with inner life (motives, character, memories, dreams, and fantasies) and that accentuated their continuity during the course of an individual's life. The subjects of the autobiographies published by Krafft-Ebing viewed and experienced their modes of behavior as inalienable components of their personality. They described their behavior and the things that had happened to them in order to make clear who they were and had been from an early age on.

Defining an individual's prime identity through his or her sexual taste is basically a nineteenth-century invention. The emergence of sexual identities, which reflect changes in the psychological habitus of people, can be explained as a consequence of the reconfiguration of the social function of sexuality. The modernization of sexuality was characterized by the linking of sexuality with privacy and intimacy, and the constitution of desire as the clue to the inner self. In premodern society, on the other hand, the regulation of sexual behavior was dominated to a large extent by a reproductive imperative, economic necessities, and traditional modes of communal organization. The essential differentiation was between reproductive sex within marriage and acts such as adultery and sodomy that interfered with procreation within marriage and thereby also with family interests, especially the inheritance of property. The decisive borderline was not so much the contrast between heterosexual intercourse and perverted sexual behavior, but the contrast between fruitfulness and barrenness, and between legal and illegal conduct (Porter 1987; Roodenburg 1988). Sexuality was perceived as part of a larger God-given and natural scheme. To a large extent, it could only be acknowledged in society as far as it was a function of social behavior: justifiable sexual activity was instrumentally integrated with reproduction, marriage, kinship, and the family's economic and social interests. Of course, sexual intercourse outside marriage did occur, and it could be solely inspired by love or mere pleasure and lust. The crucial point, however, is that such conduct threatened to upset the social order and could not be integrated into it, especially because of the risk that it might result in illegitimate children. Traditional society had to put drastic curbs on sexual behavior, because in subsistent economies one could not afford bastards.

The rise of the ideal of romantic love from the end of the eighteenth century onward entailed that sexuality was gradually dissociated from its embeddedness in fixed, putatively "natural" patterns of social behavior and, in the long run, also from the transcendental moral order that legitimized it. In his *Liebe als Passion* (1982), Niklas Luhmann explains the change in the experience of love around 1800 as a consequence of the increasing "functional differentiation" of society, especially the separation of public and private spheres (cf. Giddens 1992, 37–48; Featherstone 1999). Traditionally, the family was relatively open to the community, and family relations were generally more oriented toward material considerations and the preservation of social standing than toward intimacy. The rise of the ideal of romantic love entailed that the bond between the spouses came to be seen as a site of deep privacy. According to Luhmann, the essence of romantic love is the idea that intense emotional attraction between a man and woman is a legitimate basis, if not the only sincere ground, for marriage. Whereas traditional marriage was a contract, not only between partners, but also between families with strong legal and economic overtones, in the romantic view it is a lasting, intimate relationship between two individuals who are attached to each other, not by social interests but by mutual love. The choice of one's mate was transferred from parents and the family to the individual, and the experience of passionate love came to be valued as an essential part of a fulfilled life. In nineteenth-century bourgeois life, marriage became increasingly confined to a separate, private sphere, and man and woman were considered to be equal, at least in a formal sense.[1]

The ideal of romantic love, as it was conceptualized around 1800, gradually became part of social reality in the course of the nineteenth century, at least for a large part of the European and American middle class. To be sure, sexuality was more or less pushed to the background in the romantic ideal; it entailed a hierarchy between "true" spiritual love and "mere" physical sensuality. In the longer run, however, the sexual was to have its own domain and license in the wake of romantic love. Their connection undermined the traditionally restrictive pattern of sexuality based on social and familial demands and economic interests. In (marital) relationships based on free choice and mutual attraction and affection, it became possible to attach an autonomous and positive meaning to sexuality as an essential constituent of the emotional bond. Whereas in traditional society, justifiable sexual conduct was subservient to social and economic considerations, the elaboration of romantic love entailed that sexual passion was more and more recognized as an autonomous force in the separate and intimate sphere of dating, courtship, marriage, domesticity, and family. Romantic love presumed psychic communication and self-reflection: conceptualized as the desire directed toward one's partner, sex could be legitimized increasingly for a purpose other than procreation. In the course of the nineteenth century, the restraints on sexual behavior built into procreative sex gradually became less meaningful than they once had been, especially when contraception began to be employed on a wider scale.

Before the nineteenth century, the sexual conduct of individuals used to be determined by marital and procreative demands, social status,

1. Trumbach (1978) and Stone (1982) point out that "affective individualism" and a more egalitarian relationship between man and woman had already emerged from around 1700 in early capitalist countries like England and the Netherlands. Shorter (1975), using also French and central European sources, situates the making of the modern family on the basis of emotional relationships in the nineteenth century (cf. Eder 1999).

hierarchy, social responsibility, economic necessities and interests, and fixed gender roles; but in the context of romantic love and privacy, personal emotion and desire gained primacy. Sexuality became associated with profound and complex emotions and anxieties, and as such it achieved importance in self-reflection and self-understanding. In the wake of romantic love, sexuality was individualized and it grew into a separate, largely internalized, sphere in human life. This created the possibility for medical science to define sexuality as a distinct impulse—the sixth, genital sense, as Krafft-Ebing named this instinct—and to discover its internal physical and psychological laws. Whereas in premodern society, sexuality was more or less embedded in fixed social patterns of behavior, the emergence of a psychological conception of sexuality reveals that in modern experience the sexual domain developed into an autonomous sphere with its own structures of feeling and modes of expression, while the understanding of the goals of sexuality began to move beyond procreation and, to a certain extent, also beyond love (cf. Solomon 1987). The sexualization of what were previously nonsexual areas of life is clearly expressed in Krafft-Ebing's psychiatric diagnostics of perversions. The most diverse personality traits and activities took on a meaning in terms of one's sexual inclination: the kind of games one played as a child, hobbies, spending patterns, the preference for certain books and music, the handwriting, the motor system, the voice and the way of talking, the eye glance, clothing, the use of cosmetics and perfume, the talents, the smoking behavior, fondness of sweets, interest in art and science, the aesthetic taste, the way one furnished one's home, and the way in which one expressed one's religion. For some people even power relations and class differences had taken on a sexual dimension, as both sadomasochism and paranoia sexualis indicated.

However crucial psychiatric diagnosis was to the naming of new sexual categories and the public conception and visibility of perversion, the medical discovery of sexual deviants was prompted by longer-term social transformations outside the realm of medicine. Apart from the effects of the rise of the modern family and romantic love, more specific social developments might explain the appearance of particular, individualized sexual orientations in the second half of the nineteenth century. Voyeurism and exhibitionism, for example, could only appear in a society that drew strict boundaries between private intimacy and the more or less anonymous public sphere. Their emergence seems to be unthinkable without the increasing sensitivity to and intolerance in Western culture of physical closeness and nudity in public since the seventeenth century, which reached its zenith in the nineteenth (Van Ussel 1968; cf. Elias 1969). Nineteenth-century bourgeois culture especially placed unprecedented restraints on the exposition of naked human bodies; this applied to the male body even more than the female body. In early modern Europe, genital exposure was not taken all that seriously, and it would have been difficult to imagine that such an act in itself provided sexual pleasure to the one displaying himself. Such an experience appears to have been first reported by Rousseau in his *Confessions*. The more stress that was placed in society on hiding the nude body, the greater the possible sexual titillation in exposing one's genitals or observing someone else's uncovered body (McLaren 1997, 186–88). It is striking, however, that in Krafft-Ebing's work no self-conscious exhibitionists are given a voice. Most exhibitionists that he dealt with involved forensic cases, and almost without exception he interpreted this, in his words, "silly manner of obtaining sexual gratification" in terms of feeblemindedness, transitory insanity, and epilepsy (*Ps* 1903, 356; *Ps* 1999, 422). In *Psychopathia sexualis* voyeurism was only discussed in passing, and it was not illustrated by any individual case history.

Sexual flagellation had been a topic of medical and pornographic concern before Krafft-Ebing coined *masochism* as a form of sexual pathology (Marcus 1966; Davidson 1987; P. Wagner 1987, 50–52; Noyes 1997, 82–95). However, it used to be considered not so much as an individual aberration, but as a technique aimed at restoring sexual potency of men, something that frequently, with increasing age, left much to be desired. Physicians as well as laymen believed that the most effective way of bringing about an erection would be to stimulate the blood circulation by beating the buttocks. As such flagellation was not so much considered as a deviant alternative to, but as a more or less unusual preparation of the "normal" sexual act.[2] However, from the middle of the nineteenth century, the practice of men visiting brothels to have themselves flagellated by prostitutes more and more evoked suspicion. In the wake of general liberal attempts to maximize public well-being and civilize the lower classes, violence in general and sexual violence in particular came under increasing police scrutiny. As unbridled use of violence began to be considered uncivilized, the exercise of corporal punishment appeared problematic as well and was more and more removed from public view. Deriving pleasure from beatings

2. Emphasizing that flagellation and masochism were different phenomena, Krafft-Ebing referred to this practice in the case history of a patient who had himself regularly put in bondage and whipped by prostitutes: "The fact that he has put himself in bondage and disdains coitus shows that he resorts to flagellation simply as a means to gratify his masochistic inclination and not as a ruse to restore potency. In his masochistic imagination, the subjection staged and fantasized by him suffices to induce orgasm. Flagellation plays an important role, but only as an expression of the submissive position" (*Ps* 1901, 108; cf. *Ps* 1999, 129). One of Krafft-Ebing's informers wrote that prostitutes had told him that there was a difference between clients who had themselves whipped only to stimulate their libido and clients who wanted to be treated as a slave (1891h, 19).

or watching physical punishments administered could no longer be considered as a part of normal emotional life. Psychiatry redefined the possible connection between physical punishment and sexual stimulation as an individual psychological aberration: sadism and masochism. Typically, Krafft-Ebing, who coined these perversions, strongly opposed corporal punishment because of the possible "unhealthy" blurring of cruelty and sexual pleasure (1900c; Ps 1903, 29–30).

Thus the emergence of sadism and masochism as sexual preferences might be explained as a consequence of the disappearance from public view of violence and cruelty in civil society—in contrast to what the Marquis de Sade envisioned in his work. Blatant aggression could not be tolerated in bourgeois society, which was, at least formally, increasingly egalitarian. Whereas sheer force and power had once been part of social life, in civilized society a lustful fascination with cruelty and degradation had to be confined to fantasy—a privatization, as it were, of former public happenings— or it could only be enacted in self-controlled theatrical display (De Swaan 1982, 73–74). According to Krafft-Ebing, the *appearance* of subordination, not real violence, was the defining factor of masochism. Masochistic sexual behavior was characterized by elaborate private theatrical rituals, by "complicated comedy," as he and his correspondents phrased it. They conceptualized this perversion as a form of sexuality in which the exercise of power and violence was carefully delimited and characterized by utmost self-control. "If the friend, in his treatment of the weakly A, went beyond a certain limit and inflicted pain, the sexual excitement was destroyed instantly," Krafft-Ebing reported in the case history of A, a masochistic man who first played masochistic games with a male friend and later with a woman. In a letter, A stressed that it was of the utmost importance that his partner knew exactly where to draw the line. "The masochistic illusion is not realized immediately. . . . Neither did my dominatrix at first know where to draw the line. At first I only felt pain being punished by her" (1899d, 158).

Krafft-Ebing as well as some masochists themselves were perfectly aware of the parodic nature of masochism. In fact the submissive partner generally stipulated the rules of the game, especially when they instructed their dominatrices how to act. "The woman ordered to carry out the act," the psychiatrist wrote, "seems to be nothing more than the executive agent of his [the masochist's] own will" (Ps 1903, 108; Ps 1999, 128). To illustrate this, he referred in particular to Albert Moll's description of a masochistic urning sending "twenty paragraphs of written instructions to a man engaged for this purpose, and who was to treat and abuse him like a slave" (Ps 1903, 129; Ps 1999, 150). A thirty-five-year-old correspondent, who in his long

letter to Krafft-Ebing explained his views on masochism, stressed the contradictory nature of masochism by telling that in normal life he was not
submissive at all: "In my relations to the female sex that are not masochistic, the dominating position of the man is an indispensable condition, and
any attempt to change it would meet with my energetic opposition" (1891j,
20–21; Ps 1999, 134).

Sadism and masochism were not only about individual predilections,
but their meaning also articulated the perturbing awareness of the connection between sexuality and violence as well as the obsession with control
that characterized late-nineteenth-century bourgeois society. Western civilization in general and bourgeois liberalism in particular were haunted by a
fundamental tension between the scientifically backed recognition of the
inevitability of (male) aggression as being essential to the struggle for life
and the mastery of nature, on the one hand, and the necessity to restrain
this vital force for the sake of civilization, on the other. The individual was
the battlefield where civilization confronted inevitable biological drives.
The difficulty of differentiating between beneficial and harmful aggression,
and finding the appropriate balance between permitting the former and
checking the latter, bewildered liberal thinkers, including Krafft-Ebing. In
liberalism there was also a tension between the ideal of equality and the
social reality of inequality, between classes and races as well as between the
sexes. In the form of sadomasochism, sexuality was the very domain where
such preoccupations, veiled in parody and carefully delimited in time and
space, were expressed. Strikingly, most of Sacher-Masoch's stories and novels are situated in his native region of Galicia, one of the most backward
Slavic territories of the Habsburg Empire: his imagination was nourished
by the social and ethnic inequalities and harsh repression of peasants that
he had witnessed during his youth. In his historical works, Sacher-Masoch
focuses on the exertion of political power by female rulers (Koschorke
1988, 16–42; cf. Noyes 1997).

As indicated in part 3, fetishism was "invented" in the same period as
the psychiatric diagnosis of kleptomania became current: forensic experts
reported a strong rise in shoplifting, or more specifically, department-store
theft, by women from 1880 on (O'Brien 1983). There are some striking
similarities in the psychiatric conceptualization of these disorders. Both
were defined as an extreme obsession or mania for certain objects, and both
were associated with wasteful consumerism as well as with sexual excitement—kleptomaniac women were said to be sexually frustrated and experience sexual pleasure from the act of shoplifting. Kleptomania was defined
as a morbid impulse to steal things that were useless, such as luxury items
and objects of fashion, just like fetishism was viewed as a form of sexual

desire that was, above everything else, sterile and unproductive. In French psychiatry, fetishism was introduced as a master concept of sexual pathology: it referred to various behaviors that were not aimed at reproduction. Moreover, fetishists and kleptomaniacs both manifested an asocial proclivity: they derived emotional satisfaction from objects (or body parts) rather than from contacts with other humans.

Both psychiatric syndromes appeared in a period that witnessed the advent of mass consumption (Williams 1982). Kleptomania was especially associated with the new pattern of shopping in the newly created department stores, where goods were openly displayed and easy accessible. Although the merchandise itself was by no means available to all, consumption was more or less democratized and the vision of a seemingly unlimited profusion of commodities became more and more unavoidable. Advertising, appealing to the sensual pleasures of consumption and using visual stimulants, created artificial needs for goods and thus "seduced" buyers, especially by inciting their desire and fantasy. Commerce began to appeal to consumers by conjuring up before them a fantasy world of comfort, pleasure, and amusement: the needs of the imagination played as large a role as those of the body. Mass retailing provided a ceaseless introduction of new products, and acquisition of certain objects became a form of fulfillment in itself, irrespective of their usefulness. The new consumerist culture was characterized not so much by the utility of goods, as by the mere desire to possess them.

At the end of the nineteenth century, new economic theories reflected the shift in emphasis from production to consumption. Classical economic theory had focused on labor, production, and (re)investment, but from the 1870s on their primacy was challenged by the economists of the so-called marginalist and Austrian schools (Birken 1988, 22–39; Johnston 1972, 76–87). In their view, production was nothing more than a mere prerequisite for consumption: they postulated that the satisfaction of idiosyncratic desire was the end of human activity in the marketplace and that economic life was susceptible to psychological laws. Earlier, Karl Marx, introducing the term *commodity-fetishism*, had associated economics with religion and pointed to the irrational nature of economic transactions in capitalism. Thus, a new image of man as an irrational, desiring creature not only emerged in psychiatry but also in economics. Just like sexual desire, consumerism was viewed with ambivalence in bourgeois culture, which had traditionally nourished virtues of sobriety and rationality. Both sexual release and consuming were closely associated with "spending" energy, which was viewed as a scarce, nonreproducible natural resource. From this perspective, fetishism could be seen as the sexual equivalent of the new consumer behavior: fetishism was an idiosyncratic sexual desire that could only be satisfied by the "possession" of bodily or material objects, but that refrained from reproduction or even emotional investment in and involvement with a partner. In fetishism, lust was disconnected from social needs, just like in the emerging consumer culture "useless" spending was separated from constructive production and investment.

17

The Birth of the Modern Homosexual

Of all the perverts of whom Krafft-Ebing collected life histories so dili-
gently, homosexuals were best represented and also the most articulate (see
table 4). Although some masochists and fetishists displayed a self-conscious
and even militant attitude as well, a sense of individual or group identity
seemed most actively pursued among urnings. Whereas exhibitionism, sadomasochism, and fetishism may have been fairly new patterns of behavior
and specific for Western culture, same-sexual activity has probably existed
everywhere and always been practiced. However, as an individual property
of a minority, the concept of homosexuality is neither timeless nor universal, although historians fail to agree on when and how a homosexual social
category and identity came into being. Subcultures in the form of illicit
networks, clubs, and meeting places of sodomites have been documented
from the fifteenth century on in Italian towns and from the seventeenth
on in the urban centers of northwestern Europe. Although the legal and
religious definition of sodomy referred only to certain sexual acts, especially
anal intercourse, of which anyone, in theory, was regarded as being capable,
within urban subcultures in Britain, France, and the Netherlands, a more
specific sodomitical role evolved as early as the first half of the eighteenth
century. After 1700 the behavior of some sodomites began to be perceived
more and more as part of being "different," of effeminate proclivities, of a
sinful orientation, or of a particular hedonistic lifestyle.[1]

Randolph Trumbach has argued that the early eighteenth century saw
the birth of the modern homosexual as a third gender. This figure—the
sodomite who was effeminate in speech, manner, and clothing—was different from the traditional sodomite, who was considered as masculine, who

1. Trumbach 1986; 1989a; 1989b; 1998; Rey 1987; Gerard and Hekma 1989; Van der
Meer 1995.

had sex with adolescent boys as well as with women, and who only played
the active role in sexual intercourse. In the traditional pattern, same-sex
contacts were characterized by hierarchical social differences and active
versus passive behavior. The crucial distinction was not between hetero-
and homosexual activities, but between the adult masculine role, which
was active and insertive, and the effeminate or adolescent one, which was
passive and receptive. The new pattern, on the other hand, is characterized
by a majority of masculine men who exclusively desired women as sexual
partners and a minority of effeminate males who played the active as well
as the passive sexual role with other transvestite sodomites.

Trumbach finds an explanation for the shift from the old to the new
model of sodomy in the rise of the egalitarian family, characterized by the
companionate marriage, affective individualism, and domesticity. Formally
men and women were considered to be equal, but at the same time they
were assigned different, complementary social roles (economic and political versus domestic) and spheres (public versus private). The ideals of
the domesticated family entailed new gender roles, and these were increasingly legitimized by referring to the natural differences between men and
women. Normal men were supposed to be attracted only to women; a desire
for men, regardless whether they were adults or adolescents, resulted in a
loss of their masculine gender status. The new male gender identity depended on the avoidance of sodomy or even of being suspected of such
leanings. In fact, Trumbach enunciates, the very existence of a separate
deviant minority of effeminate sodomites boosted the heterosexual norm
for the majority of men. As far as women were concerned, he contends,
comparable hetero- and homosexual roles developed later in the second
half of the eighteenth century (Trumbach 1994). "Sapphists" appeared as
masculinized women, as another third gender and exclusively attracted to
the same sex, like transvestite sodomites. According to Trumbach, the sap-
phist role that emerged after 1750 was produced by the same cultural forces
responsible for the appearance of the sodomite role. For both men and
women, the third gender role of a (despised) minority served the purpose
of confirming a new heterosexual model that was characterized by equality
in difference: men and women were considered to fulfill complementary
roles.

Strongly opposing the Foucaultian thesis that the modern homosexual
was a medical invention, Trumbach argues that the late-nineteenth-
century homosexual man and woman, described and explained by physicians in biological and psychological terms, was not a new figure, but the
consequence of social roles that had been developed in the eighteenth century. Gender inversion, which took the place of the traditional hierarchical
form of same-sexual behavior before 1700, would constitute the dominant

homosexual pattern in the Western world to this day. Trumbach thus assumes a succession of two mutually exclusive variants in the Western history of homosexuality. It is questionable, however, whether this can be schematized so neatly. By and large, this theory is based on research of the patterns of sexual conduct in the London metropolitan area. His modern homosexual is based on a metropolitan subcultural model, but in the eighteenth and nineteenth century, other forms of homosexuality and homoeroticism can be traced, among men as well as among women (Hekma 1983; Everard 1994). Trumbach does not discuss the fact that in the past two centuries real changes have occurred in the fashioning of homosexuality and that several, older and newer, variants could exist alongside one another, whereby differences in class, gender, and status as well as geographical variation played an important role. (Trumbach himself admits that the modern model of gender and sexuality only came to full development in northwestern Europe and the United States, and that different patterns can be found in central, southern, and eastern Europe.)

The third sex model was neither the only nor a continuous form of homosexuality since the early eighteenth century. Myriam Everard (1994) has studied three forms of same-sex relationships among women in eighteenth-century Netherlands: the romantic friend, the passing woman, and the tribade in the world of prostitution. Her conclusion is that none of these figures can be identified as a historical precursor of the modern twentieth-century lesbian. In the eighteenth-century view of female sexuality, not so much the object of desire (the other or the same sex) was important, but the degree and intensity of lust; what was condemned was excess. Whereas men seem to have lost their masculine gender status when they indulged in homosexual behavior, be it actively or passively, same-sex activity of women was not so much considered as an infringement of their gender role. Thus, among women the relationship between homosexuality and gender inversion was less pronounced than among men. Until the end of the nineteenth century, masculine behavior and travesty of women were not always directly linked up with homosexuality, even if these cross-dressing women married other women. Women who passed for men in general did so because it would be to their benefit socially: greater freedom of movement, more job opportunities, and better pay. Women who passed for men supposedly just disguised themselves for social reasons and were not seen in a sexual light like cross-dressing men. In this respect, potential homosexual relationships between women were often more incidental or secondary (Mak 1997). Masculinity in women caused less aversion then femininity in men. This evaluative difference is related to the implicit hierarchy that, despite the formal equality, was still prevalent between men and women. As opposed to women, men had something to lose: effeminacy meant social degradation and stigmatization for them. Since they had nothing to win in a social sense, effeminacy in men tended to be sooner attributed to individual deviation than masculinity in women.

Also in another way, attitudes toward same-sex relationships between women differed from those toward male homosexuality. Contrary to men, women did not form an illicit subculture, and therefore they were not as visible and threatening to gender norms as sodomites. The homosexual activities of women are hidden from history to a much larger extent than those of men. One of the reasons for this is that male same-sex behavior has been prosecuted on a much larger scale—most of our information about sodomites before the middle of the nineteenth century comes from court records. Whereas the transvestite sodomite modeled himself on a semipublic subculture that overlapped with that of the promiscuous female prostitute, same-sex relationships among women, at least in bourgeois circles, were more geared to the ideal of the couple and realized in private emotional friendships. Because women, according to the new complementary gender ideology, would not possess an autonomous sexuality, intimate friendships between women were less likely to cause suspicion than those between men, even though erotic friendship traditions have also existed among men (Faderman 1981). Both traditions of romantic female friendships and passing women continued well into the twentieth century; inasmuch as it involved homosexual conduct, this was often left unarticulated. In comparison to male homosexuality, lesbian sexuality largely remained a muted discourse until the last decades of the nineteenth century, when physicians like Krafft-Ebing began to identify masculine women as lesbians (Vicinus 1989). It has been argued that increasing economic opportunities for women in the late nineteenth century facilitated the emergence of a lesbian identity. However, in Krafft-Ebing's work, homosexual women were far outnumbered by men, and the few of them who spoke for themselves were, apparently, not as self-conscious. In this sense, there was no parity between men and women.

A crucial difference between men and women was that from the eighteenth century on, some sodomites formed a social minority group on the basis of an exclusive same-sex desire. But this is not to deny that, in addition, other, nonexclusive forms of male homosexuality existed as well. For instance, there are indications that the hierarchical model, in which active, insertive homosexual behavior was not connected to an effeminate orientation and an exclusive social category, continued to be around far into the twentieth century (Marshall 1981; Hekma 1992). Many effeminate sodomites, and later urnings as well, were not looking for sexual contact with each other but with "real" men. As we have seen, various homosexuals in Krafft-Ebing's work acknowledged their preference for lower-class masculine men, such as soldiers, sailors, and workers. These sexual partners of urnings identified themselves not as homosexual, probably because in their experience the exclusively active part they played in same-sexual interaction was not at odds with their heterosexual conduct.

Another variant in which no specific homosexual role or identity is involved is what has been called "situational homosexuality" (or "pseudo-homosexuality" by sexologists and psychologists): more or less casual homosexual activities, especially in sex-segregated, all-male institutions: ships, prisons, the military, boarding schools, and monasteries. In the course of the nineteenth century, more attention was paid to sexual extravagances in these institutions and, increasingly, strong measures were taken against it in the form of a stricter control on moral conduct in general and the introduction of solitary confinement in prisons and coeducation at schools in particular. The bourgeois civilization offensive contributed to the increase of physical distance between men; men sleeping together in one bed, customary in the houses of the working class and guest houses, was more and more perceived as immoral and uncivilized. Regarding the prevention of homosexuality, Krafft-Ebing advanced that hereditarily tainted boys and girls must not be admitted to boarding schools and warned against private tutors, who often became their pupils' object of love. In this respect, he advocated coeducation and cautioned that military training facilities, seminaries, and prisons were breeding grounds of homosexuality (*Ps* 1903, 317, 326, 429).

In addition to the incidental, situational homosexual contacts and the sodomitic subculture, attention should be called to same-sex arrangements that were, to be sure, not so much homo*sexual* as homo*erotic* or homo*social:* the cultural tradition of intimate friendships between men, which flourished in academic and literary circles, and in schools, in Great Britain as well as in Germany (Rousseau 1987; Oosterhuis and Kennedy 1991, 8–12). Grasping the significance of this tradition may contribute to an understanding of the development of the modern homosexual identity in intellectual bourgeois circles in the second half of the nineteenth century. This identity was built not only on the subcultural third sex model dating from the early eighteenth century, but also on the tradition of emotional friendship that mirrored the ideal of romantic love. This type of friendship, which will be exemplified in the following paragraphs on the basis of developments in Germany, could be erotic but did not imply sodomy. Sodomy and friendship can be seen as two extremes on a sliding scale of same-sex relationships, the first representing the sexual and the second the affective pole.

In the literary Sturm und Drang and Romantic movements, friendship was held in high esteem as a bond of intimate feelings. In such circles, the personal character of friendship was closely related to an awareness of the gulf that existed between one's true self and the role one played in society. The Romantic ideal of friendship was based on a bond between kindred spirits and provided the exclusive atmosphere in which one could give expression to one's deepest and most personal emotions. True friendship was reserved for an intellectual elite consisting principally of men. Referring to Plato, friendship between men was sometimes seen as superior to the excited, unpredictable love relationships between men and women. But male bonds were also seen as a form of love that could be passionate and sensual. The German expression *Freundesliebe* (love between friends) originated from the Sturm und Drang period, when in many university towns, literary "societies of friends" were founded in which men wrote each other passionate letters, dedicated real love poems to one another, embraced and kissed each other warmly, and shed many tears when they had to take leave of one another or met again after a long absence. To many of the Romantics, love between men and women and friendship between men were on one and the same level. They proceeded from the idea that the ideal emotional and intellectual relationship went hand in hand with physical sensations.

The renewed interest in Greek culture and art in the eighteenth century contributed in no small measure to the appreciation of the physical side of male friendship. According to the art historian Johann Joachim Winckelmann (1717–1768), Greek sculpture, which strongly concentrated on male beauty, was unsurpassable, and under his influence, various writers and poets (including Goethe, Johann Gottfried Herder, Friedrich Schiller, Hölderlin, Heinrich von Kleist, Jean Paul, and August von Platen) expressed more or less positive views about Greek male love and pedagogical Eros (Derks 1990; Kuzniar 1996). The first apologies of "Socratic love" in the German language before that of Ulrichs, Heinrich Zschokke's *Eros oder über die Liebe* (1821) and Heinrich Hössli's two-volume *Eros: Die Männerliebe der Griechen* (1836, 1838), were part of this cultural tradition. The Platonic or Socratic model, by which passionate friendships between men were justified until the middle of the nineteenth century, did indeed emphasize the importance of intellectual and moral sympathy, but it confirmed at the same time the sensual element. Although some literary men were criticized from time to time for being too sentimental or for allowing themselves to be carried away by their emotions, friendships could be sensual without suspicions of sodomy far into the nineteenth century. The difference between sensual friendship and sodomite lust was apparently still so great in the middle of the nineteenth century that the composer Richard Wagner (1813–1883), speaking of his friendship with Franz Liszt (1811–1886), could say quite unconcernedly that he could not imagine any friendship without love. In his *Kunstwerk der Zukunft* (1850) about Greek art, he stated that friendship was sensual because it came from sensitivity to physical beauty (Fuchs 1903, 133–35).

It was only later in the nineteenth century that such open-mindedness concerning erotically-tinted friendship—which is also found, for example, in Friedrich Nietzsche's work—gave way to a certain distrust. Whereas in the eighteenth and early nineteenth century, passion-filled romantic friendships could flourish between members of the same sex without fear of the sexual, such relationships became more and more suspect in the second half of the nineteenth century. A book about the friendship between Goethe and Schiller, written by the philosopher Gustav Portig (1894), is symptomatic of the mixed feelings with which close relationships between men were perceived at the end of the nineteenth century. Portig anxiously asks to what extent the lack of a clear distinction between love and friendship brought with it moral decline. According to Portig, male friendship in ancient Greece had, after all, under the influence of figures like Plato and Socrates, degenerated into pederasty. Although German Romantic friendship found itself, he continues, on an altogether higher plane than the Greek "pollution" and fulfilled an important cultural function, expressions of friendship from that "effeminate" period had something ridiculous and objectionable about them. True enough, he still saw an important social role for male friendship, but its range should be restricted so that no harm was done to the institution of marriage. Whereas the Greeks used the same word for love and friendship, he advocates a clear division between the two concepts (Portig 1894, 13–24).

One of Krafft-Ebing's forensic reports illustrates the changing evaluation of intimate friendships between men. It concerns two German men whose close friendship had raised suspicion: they had embraced and kissed each other, and the one had declared his love to the other. They were accused of "unnatural vice" because of this behavior. After they had indeed been convicted, they appealed to a higher court, and Krafft-Ebing was asked to explore their case from a psychological viewpoint. On the basis of extensive conversations with the men and observations of their mutual interaction, he concluded that their friendship was indeed very intimate and that it was understandable that it raised eyebrows, but that homosexuality was not involved at all (Ps 1890, 283–90). Although Krafft-Ebing as a medical expert differentiated between emotional friendship and contrary sexual feeling in this case, it was precisely the increasing medical interest in homosexual behavior, desire, and disposition from 1870 on that made no small contribution to situations in which emotional friendships between men aroused suspicion. Earlier, close relationships between men were generally not connected to sexuality, because the latter was mainly understood as behavior aimed at coitus; its sphere was fairly clearly delineated and limited to certain physical activities. The traditional equation of sexuality with coitus implied that a variety of intimate contacts not involving penetration were not always thought of as sexual and might pass as more or less permissible (Katz 1995, 47). However, under the influence of medical theorizing as well as the ideal of romantic love, the definition of sexuality broadened in the course of the nineteenth century: it was more and more related to emotional life and intimacy between two partners. With the upgrading of romantic love as the foundation of marriage, physical and emotional intimacy were exclusively associated with the heterosexual bond. Among the bourgeoisie, emotional security was confined more and more to marriage and the nuclear family at the expense of close relationships outside the family. For intimate same-sex friendships, there was, so to speak, no "safe" borderland anymore between marriage and family on the one hand and the underworld of sodomy on the other. Close friendship between men was not taken for granted anymore and lost its innocence. Passionate friendship was sexualized; as such, it was marginalized. However, at the same time it was incorporated in the emerging modern homosexual identity.

The individualization of male homosexuality and its attendant polarization of homo- and heterosexuality were advanced by the marginalization of close emotional friendships, on the one hand, and the ever stronger discouragement of diffuse and casual forms of homosexual behavior, on the other. The homosexual identity, which crystallized at the end of the nineteenth century and which was very much a product of bourgeois culture, was characterized by three new features. First, before the nineteenth century, there was hardly an awareness of homosexual desire as a psychological category, as a central feature of the inner self—a state of mind that is so striking in many autobiographies of Krafft-Ebing's homosexual patients and correspondents. The psychological criterion of self-awareness made the crucial difference between modern homosexual identity and the sodomitical role: the orientation existed independently of the conduct and frequently preceded it (at least, in the retrospective stories of homosexuals); one could be homosexual without necessarily showing homosexual behavior. As I have tried to explain, modern autobiographical self-reflection has contributed substantially to this mind-set. On the one hand, the modern homosexual was tormented by guilt and struggled with the question of how he could give shape to his sexuality in a responsible way. On the other hand, the awareness of the gap between the social order and his individual leanings, whereby the first was an impediment to self-fulfillment, signals the emergence of a critical mind that would foster the emergence and growth of emancipation movements. Some of Krafft-Ebing's patients and correspondents clearly manifested such awareness. Already before Hirschfeld founded the Wissenschaftlich-humanitäres Komitee in 1897, in the 1870s Ulrichs and H. Marx, author of the pamphlet "Urningsliebe" (1875), called on urnings to organize themselves (Herzer 1997, 28–29; Brunner and Sulzenbacher 1998, 49). In the early 1890s homosexual societies were said to exist in Vienna (Klub der Vernünftigen), Rome (Club degli Ignoranti), and Brussels (Réunion philantropique) (De Joux 1893, 128).

Secondly, modern homosexual identity linked two aspects that were formerly perceived as distinct until the late nineteenth century: sexual activity previously associated with sodomy and the feeling of deep friendship that could be put on a par with (romantic) love. Many homosexuals who expressed themselves in Krafft-Ebing's work stressed that a love relationship was as important to them as sexual gratification. A thirty-one-year-old employee who was in love with a soldier stated that he felt quite happy with him, although he was of lower class: "the sexual satisfaction is merely the crowning of our love" (1891h, 106; Ps 1999, 552). Although many of them participated in the homosexual subculture—which, from the eighteenth century on, was founded on sexual promiscuity and geared to the demimonde of prostitution—urnings jumped at the ideal of romantic love as a more respectable model to justify themselves. This aspect in particular turned the modern homosexual identity, in addition to the subculture, into an organizational principle at the level of personal life and in part at the level of social life as well. While previously sodomites were often married, the new homosexual identity was hard to reconcile—in the experience of those involved—with marriage and family life. The men who thought they could combine marriage and homosexual contacts constituted a minority in Krafft-Ebing's casuistry. Precisely because of the increasing effect of the romantic love ideal in marriage, it became more difficult for individuals with homosexual desires to meet the modern marital demands.[2] One of Krafft-Ebing's homosexual correspondents, who looked back on an un-

2. The same was sometimes true for other perverts as well. Heterosexual fetishists, masochists, and sufferers of sexual anesthesia called on Krafft-Ebing because they wanted to marry but doubted whether that was a good decision or because they felt they did not live up to the expectations of marriage. For instance, a thirty-year-old civil servant who was excited sexually only by women who limped with the left foot doubted whether he could marry a lame woman: "Unfortunately, because he could not love the soul of such a wife, but only her defect of lameness, he considered such a union a profanation of matrimony and an unbearable ignoble existence" (Ps 1898, 155; Ps 1999, 201). Another fetishist, a thirty-two-year-old aristocrat who failed to satisfy his wife sexually, was tormented by the idea that he had made her unhappy (Ps 1892, 180). The man, who felt urges to masochism, fetishism, and coprolagnia and who—much to Krafft-Ebing's surprise and dismay—satisfied his perversions in marriage, was exceptional: "The end of this cynical but scientifically important exposition was: marriage, a decision B took after his mistress had run away. B, who is already fathering a child, assures me that he does the same thing with his wife as with his mistress, and that both were completely satisfied by this kind of conjugal intercourse!!" (1899d, 131).

happy marriage that had lasted four years, wrote to him that if he had read the psychiatrist's book earlier and known for sure that he was an urning, then he would never have married (Ps 1889, 135). A married homosexual civil servant told Krafft-Ebing that he rarely engaged in sexual intercourse with his wife, especially because emotionally it was not satisfying (Ps 1898, 239). Others indicated as well that, if already physically capable of having sexual intercourse with a woman, they felt a lack in a psychological respect. A correspondent who was diagnosed with psychic hermaphroditism and who had sex with women as well as men explained why, in the end, he preferred men:

> I could easily dispense with women if I had regular satisfaction with a male, but I think that occasionally I would like to embrace a woman for the sake of variety, as my nature is absolutely hermaphroditic in a psychosexual sense. (Whereas I can only sensually desire women, I can love as well as sensually desire youths.) If marriage between men would be possible, I think I would not avoid a lifelong union, while marriage with a woman seems to me to be something impossible. . . . [T]rue love for a wife would be absent, that is, it would lack the attraction that I feel toward the young men I love. . . . A constant association with a youth who is physically pleasing and in mental harmony with me, who could understand all my feelings and share my intellectual opinions and endeavors, would, it seems to me, be the greatest happiness. (1891h, 107; cf. Ps 1999, 553)

Urnings could only simulate heterosexual love and that was at odds with the romantic love ideal, which dictated that partners have to be fully open to one another. Thus a homosexual woman renounced marriage: "The patient seriously considered whether a marriage might save her, but her conscience objected against it: her children might inherit her misfortune or she might make a sincere husband unhappy" (Ps 1894, 286; cf. Ps 1999, 334). In fact, many projected the romantic love ideal onto the homosexual relationship they craved. "He declared that his love for his own sex developed just as the love affairs between men and women do in novels," Krafft-Ebing noted in the case history of a forty-one-year-old urning (Ps 1901, 265; cf. Ps 1999, 308). A thirty-eight-year-old man revealed that his ideal was "a marriage-bond with a male lover," and a twenty-seven-year-old man also made it clear that he did not desire a wife and children: "I, for my part, would prefer to spend all time and care on my lover" (Ps 1890, 153; Ps 1887, 91). "Of course, I shall never marry," another one confided to Krafft-Ebing. "To me, this seems not a misfortune. . . . I live in the hope that some day I shall have a steady lover; I must have one, otherwise the future seems dark and barren to me, and all the aspirations usually cherished—honor, career, etc.—empty and unattractive" (1890j, 108–9; cf. *Ps* 1999, 555).

In addition to the mental and affective aspects, the third feature of the new model is the shift from gender inversion to object-choice as the core of homosexual identity (cf. Chauncey 1982–83). Although Krafft-Ebing conceptualized homosexuality as a form of inversion, several of his patients and autobiographers classified under contrary sexual feeling stated that they did not consider themselves effeminate: apart from their sexual leanings, they were men like other normal men. In his subclassification of contrary sexual feeling, these urnings formed a group that he labeled as homosexual. Although others, classified under other subgroups, did emphasize their feminine inclination, this indicated a shift in the conceptualization of the desire for the same sex as a form of gender inversion (the man who feels attracted to men because of his feminine mind-set) toward a sexual object-choice (the man who feels masculine and has a sexual preference for men). In the latter case, there is no longer a polarity between masculinity and femininity as a precondition for sexual attraction. In the course of the twentieth century, this has led to both a delimitation and an extension of the homosexual category. First, it was distinguished much more clearly from forms of gender inversion like androgyny, travesty, and transsexuality, phenomena that Krafft-Ebing also categorized under contrary sexual feeling. Second, it became possible that men who in homosexual interaction assumed a male gender role and who could not identify themselves with an identity that was based on gender inversion now began to identify themselves as homosexual.

All three features matched with the effort of bourgeois men to voice their same-sex desire in respectable terms—the frequent references to ancient Greece and famous historical figures who had supposedly been homosexual also fit into this strategy—and it met with some success. Krafft-Ebing adopted the first two features completely and the last one partly in his theory of contrary sexual feeling. He stressed that homosexuals were different from sodomites or pederasts, not only because most of them recoiled from anal intercourse and preferred other, in Krafft-Ebing's eyes less offensive, sexual activities, but even more because of their homosexual state of mind, which had expressed itself already from early childhood on independently of their conduct. In this way he also differentiated along a rigid line between contrary sexual feeling, be it inborn or acquired, and "irregular" same-sex behavior of normal men, which he continued to condemn as immoral. He also concurred with his bourgeois patients and correspondents that homosexual love was equivalent to heterosexual love and that therefore it was legitimate in a moral sense. In his last article on contrary sexual feeling, Krafft-Ebing admitted that Ulrichs's striving for the recognition of homosexual marriage proved that this kind of love was genuine and profound (1901a, 2). Finally, the claim that contrary sexual feeling did not necessarily involve effeminacy in men was partly confirmed by Krafft-Ebing, especially when he diagnosed some of them as psychosexual hermaphrodites or just as homosexuals. In his taxonomy, psychosexual hermaphroditism and homosexuality were subcategories of the larger category of contrary sexual feeling, in which, except for the sexual preference for men that was characterized as effeminate, there was no physical or mental femininization, as opposed to those who fell under the subcategories effeminatio, androgyny, and sexual metamorphosis. Only the last three categories were, in Krafft-Ebing's words, "intermediates," "neither fully male nor female" (Ps 1903, 310). This differentiation was especially relevant in the light of Krafft-Ebing's judgment of urnings: he judged the masculine characters clearly more positively than the effeminate types, with whom the degeneration process would have been more advanced. Only the first were superior degenerates; not only were they more respectable, according to the psychiatrist, they were also more sincere and their information was deemed more reliable (Ps 1903, 309; 1901b, 130).

From a social perspective, the historical development of sexual identities, homosexual as well as masochistic and fetishistic, depended for a large part on the modernization of society at large. Most of Krafft-Ebing's private patients and correspondents were economically independent, often living in large cities and outside of the traditional family. Sexual identities could only come into being when more and more individuals could pursue their idiosyncratic desires, not as short-term, random diversions from fixed social roles and family responsibilities, but on a more regular basis as part of their lifestyle. To follow one's sexual tastes in such a way depended on being able to live and support oneself outside of the rather close-knit communities and productive family units that dominated living space and oversaw the conduct of each of its members before the rise of wage labor in cities. The market economy advanced social openness and affected sexual relations. Industrialization broadened access to premarital sexual intercourse; demographic statistics show a remarkable increase of illegitimacy, especially between 1750 and 1850 (Shorter 1975). Large-scale industrialization and urbanization entailed vast displacements of individuals and the loss of the control of the family and community censorship that had existed in a more encapsulated universe. Many nineteenth-century observers feared that capitalism, the amoral economic market, and urban life, which loosened up "natural" distinctions between ranks and the sexes, facilitated promiscuity (Laqueur 1992). The pursuit of sexuality outside the con-

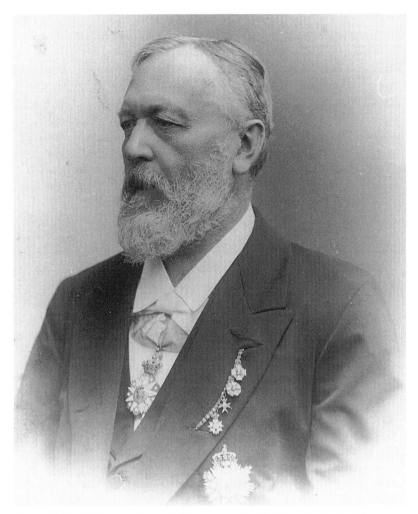

Figure 15. Krafft-Ebing at the end of his career. (Krafft-Ebing Family Archive, Graz, Austria)

straints of the family indeed became possible, especially in cities, big and anonymous enough to shelter and support a "sexual market" as well as deviant subcultures.

In the expanding metropolitan areas of the nineteenth century, where various segments of the population mingled, sexuality became more visible. They became sites of sexual dangers (especially for women) as well as of sexual adventures (mainly for men) (Wilson 1991; Walkowitz 1992; Bech 1999). With the growing concentration of population in big cities, not only the numbers of prostitutes increased, but they also offered more variation to satisfy specific desires; masochists, for example, could find gratification with prostitutes who specialized in role-playing and had the necessary equipment at their disposal. Also city life made it easier for men desiring other men to find each other and to realize that they were not alone in the world. Previously isolated individuals, who might have felt their desires to be odd and unique, found others with similar predilections in the crowded cities. Covert networks and specialized meeting places gradually came into existence: private circles, certain cafés, restaurants, parks, swimming pools, bathhouses, railway stations, shopping malls, theaters; all these could foster a sense of community. Some homosexual gatherings were not even hidden but widely publicized, such as the fancy balls of urnings in Berlin that were considered big social events.[3]

It was in the context of an emerging consumer culture that sexual desire became significant in a new way. For members of the middle class, capitalism entailed not only increasing opportunities to enter into free economic relations with other individuals, but also, as living standards rose at the end of the nineteenth century, to place more stress on individual choice, taste, and pleasure. In the late eighteenth and early nineteenth century, the middle class had differentiated itself from the aristocracy by stressing its extravagant consumption, but from the 1870s on the bourgeoisie began to set aside its scruples against comfort and luxury. As free labor and free exchange were the hallmarks of productive capitalism, consumer capitalism depended on the satisfaction of boundless desire—for goods, services, distinction, sophistication, leisure, and entertainment. Consumerism stood in opposition to a society of scarcity in which convention and sumptuary legislation were meant to keep desire in check. The need to assure the absorption of a greatly increased mass production of consumer goods entailed a positive stress on desire and impulse. Once the dynamics of desire was given free play, it was difficult to restrain it when it drew in sexuality (Birken 1988; Laqueur 1992).

Sexual themes were emerging as topics for novels, the stage, and the visual arts; sexual scandals were discussed in newspapers, and in some newspapers, personal ads began to appear in which individuals with specific sexual desires looked for partners. Technical innovations and reforms in taxations facilitated the production and the spreading of the printed word as well as images, including pornography; the tightening of moral censorship around 1900 was in fact a reaction to the increase of titillating printed matter in the fin de siècle. The first commercial illustrated homosexual magazine, *Der Eigene*, appeared around 1900 in Berlin, and the erotic pho-

---

3. For the homosexual subculture in Vienna, see Hacker and Lang 1986; Brunner and Sulzenbacher 1998; for Berlin, Theis and Sternweiler 1984; Krafft-Ebing 1903, 418–20.

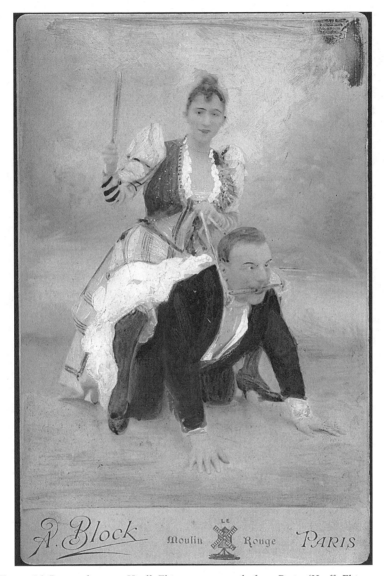

Figure 16. Postcard sent to Krafft-Ebing anonymously from Paris. (Krafft-Ebing Collection, Wellcome Institute Library, London)

tos of Wilhelm von Gloeden, Guglielmo Plüschow, and several others found many eager buyers. Krafft-Ebing's work reached a public that was getting familiar with literary, pornographic, and popular medical works on the subject of sexuality in its various forms. Like several of his patients and correspondents, Krafft-Ebing referred to literature as an important source

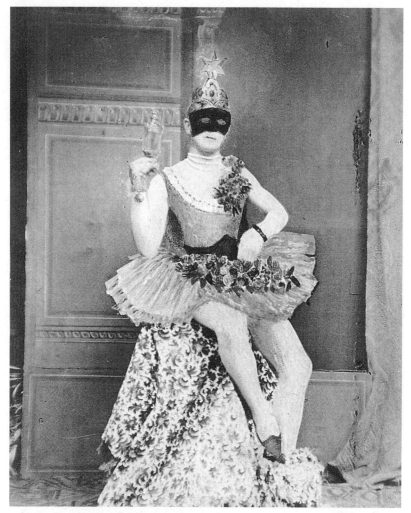

Figure 17. Postcard sent to Krafft-Ebing anonymously from Paris. (Krafft-Ebing
Collection, Wellcome Institute Library, London)

for understanding sexual pathology. His model of sexuality began to center
on desire instead of reproduction, and many subjects of his case histories
appeared as sexual consumers. They were more or less able to pursue their
sexual desires as part of a lifestyle, as they also formed the clients of a newly
emerging market for a psychologically oriented psychiatry that responded
to the need for self-knowledge.

Several of Krafft-Ebing's patients and correspondents made it clear that
for them the city represented freedom and an expansion of experience. For

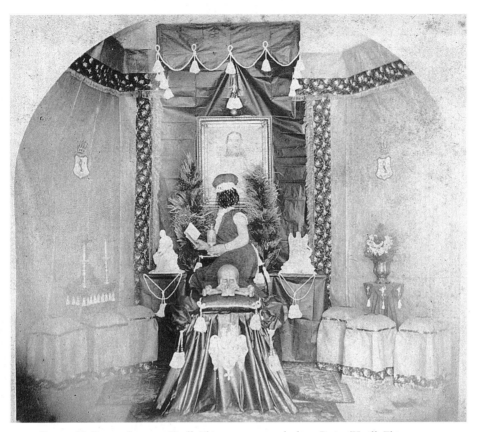

Figure 18. Postcard sent to Krafft-Ebing anonymously from Paris. (Krafft-Ebing Collection, Wellcome Institute Library, London)

those who could afford it, cities like Paris, Vienna, Budapest, and Berlin were centers of pleasure, excitement, and consumption. Cultivating an expansive public life in restaurants, cafés, hotels, theaters, concert halls, opera, parks, department stores, and promenades, such as Vienna's famous Ringstrasse, these metropolises offered a spectacle and invited voyeurism, a play of gazes and glances. "Seeing so many beautiful men thrilled me," remembered a thirty-three-year-old homosexual the moment when, as a young man of sixteen, he visited a big city for the first time in his life (*Ps* 1887, 75). Such cities opened the way to sexual exploration, and the fulfillment of fantasies. At the end of the nineteenth century, Vienna was well-known for its pleasure-seeking lifestyle; Paris became a tourist and consumerist mecca, and also the city of erotic amusement—or vice, as it was experienced by a man who informed Krafft-Ebing about what one could find in certain "art shops" in decadent Paris.

Highly honored Hofrath! In the Rue Rivoli, opposite of the Louvre, I found the enclosed picture displayed in a shop window, in between religious images and pictures of political figures and crowned heads!! Since I presume you will be interested in this picture, I hereby send it to you. In the same store they showed me numerous other photographs of "artists" of the very popular establishment "Moulin Rouge"—and what kind of pictures and acts these were! I hesitate to describe them; put briefly, they were showing all kinds of sexual abnormalities, between men and women as well as between women, and between women and dogs! They ensured me that this was nothing special, because "c'est usuel à Paris"! Children, girls, women, the old and young, all may look at these pictures, without insulting the "noble" French soul![4]

Paris and Vienna not only enjoyed a reputation for lax morals; both cities were the centers of cultural modernism as well. Elsewhere, too, sexual themes were receiving much attention during the fin de siècle, but especially in Vienna intellectuals and modernist artists were obsessed with sexuality and gender. In Vienna—where Krafft-Ebing lived and worked from 1889 until 1902—the various incompatible forces, stifling sexual repression, and more or less freely displayed libertinism not only seem to have engendered disturbing psychological insights: the confluence of all these incongruent and contradictory forces also contributed to the modern understanding of sexuality.

4. Postcard to Krafft-Ebing, anonymous (undated), Nachlass Krafft-Ebing. In Krafft-Ebing's estate I found three such postcards: a woman riding horseback on a man, a masked man in a ballet dress, a woman sitting on a coffin. See figures 16, 17, and 18.

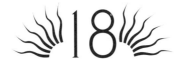

Pressure-Cooker Vienna

Krafft-Ebing's work reflected the cultural anxieties and the inconsistencies involving sexuality, in particular the preoccupation of the Viennese bourgeoisie with its pleasures as well as its dangers. In his autobiographical *Die Welt von Gestern*, Viennese author Stefan Zweig (1881–1942) observes a striking parallel between the prevailing sexual morality and the flowering artistic climate of fin de siècle Vienna. In his eyes, both were symptomatic of the disingenuousness and the lack of a sense of reality that were characteristic of Vienna's bourgeois culture as a whole. While the monomaniac attention to art and aestheticism kept the social and political changes that were undermining the seemingly stable Habsburg monarchy from view, the hypocrisy and double morality veiled the truth about sexuality. On the outside a sense of public morality prevailed, but behind the façades much was possible, at least for men. Like Paris and Budapest, Vienna was a major center for the production of pornography, and prostitution—despite its illegality—was also practiced widely; it was regulated by means of police monitoring and mandatory medical testing to counter the extreme proliferation of venereal diseases. While bourgeois women's sexuality was basically denied and their virginity had to be safeguarded until marriage (which was often an arranged one), bourgeois men engaged in paid sexual interaction with lower-class prostitutes or they kept mistresses. Although sexual interaction with girls under the age of consent (fourteen years old in Austria) was officially severely punished, even younger prostitutes could be found. The sense of discretion was normally at odds with the scandals and morality trials that were widely covered by the sensation-seeking press. Whereas the authoritative liberal newspaper *Neue Freie Presse* would preach the blessings of family life on its front page, on the back page the reader could find all kinds of personal ads and paid sex offers, involving the whole spec-

trum of sexual variance, including fetishism, homosexuality, and masochism.

Victorian moralism and religious conformity coexisted with blatant
erotic displays. The mixture of prudery and curiosity, of disguising and dis-
closing, reflected the continual confrontation between semblance and reality in Viennese society. Precisely in this tension between rigid morality and
transgression of boundaries, Zweig suggests, an eroticized climate came into
existence in which wild fantasies continued to provoke and titillate the
senses in unnatural and unhealthy ways. His diagnosis, which is basically
supported by many of his contemporaries as well as by recent historical
scholarship, makes it to some extent understandable why the articulation
and representation of sexuality in Viennese modernism was of great significance.[1] The modernist discourse of sexuality, in fact, expressed important cultural messages and meanings. Freud was not the first and only one
who extended the analysis of sexual relations into a critique of civilization
as a whole by suggesting that the antagonisms of public life were associated
with unresolved tensions in the private, hidden world of instincts. Sexuality became a symbolic territory for debates on the discrepancy between
public role and private self, personal identity, and the conflicts between
reason and irrationalism.

The innovative élan with which the young Viennese artists and intellectuals from bourgeois families reacted against the world of their fathers
was not so much aimed at the prevailing social and political climate but at
bourgeois morality and lifestyle (Pynsent 1989, 148, 153, 164; cf. Mosse
1991, 574, 578). For authors from the literary movement *Jung Wien*, such
as Arthur Schnitzler (1862–1931) and Hugo von Hofmannsthal (1874–
1929), and for the visual artists belonging to *Sezession*, led by Gustav Klimt
(1862–1918), and expressionism, notably Oskar Kokoschka (1886–1980)
and Egon Schiele (1890–1918), sexuality was an intriguing subject that
could be deployed to unveil bourgeois society's sense of security as a façade,
full of empty conventions. To counter the false, merely outward conformity
of bourgeois culture, these artists pretended to uncover the true yet suppressed and invisible nature of man. True life could only be fully lived by
rejecting artificial social conventions. Inspired by the philosophies of Arthur Schopenhauer and Friedrich Nietzsche, the rediscovery of the archaic
Dionysian Greek culture, and the insights of psychiatry, the younger generation posited that the deeper truths of humans could be found in their bewildering experience of urges and feelings. Thus they disputed the enlight-

---

1. Zweig 1942, 87–114; Forel 1935, 64–65; Johnston 1972, 118–19; Janik and Toulmin
1973, 46, 61; Gilman 1985, 39–58; Timms 1986, 21–29; Pynsent 1989, 188–89; Eder 1993;
1990, 20–28; Jusek 1992.

ened values of liberal bourgeois society: the belief in reason, the control of nature, social harmony, and economic, scientific, and technological progress. Female sexuality was especially associated with true life, which did not let itself be restricted by the limits of rigid rational knowledge and which would enable social regeneration.

Sexuality was a major subject not only in modernist art, but also in Viennese cultural critique, philosophy, and science. The witty cultural critic Karl Kraus (1874–1936), editor of *Die Fackel*, aimed his shots at bourgeois hypocrisy, the double standard, and the legal and medical involvement with sexuality. The discrepancy between appearance and reality, pinpointed by Zweig, is the central theme in Kraus's biting satire. In several essays he attacked moralistic attitudes toward sex and efforts to enforce them through courts of law and psychiatric interference. Thus Kraus also fired his shots at Krafft-Ebing because the psychiatrist had yielded to the efforts of the duke of Sachsen-Coburg-Gotha to have his adulterous wife declared insane and have her placed under legal restraint (Kraus 1970, 75–93). Kraus idealized the "otherness" of women, their supposed unspoiled, natural sensuousness and spontaneity, which were constricted by male civilization. In his view, the prostitute especially embodied emotional liberation (Timms 1986; N. Wagner 1987).

Kraus admired the philosopher Otto Weininger (1880–1903), who, in his monumental *Geschlecht und Charakter* (1903), also pictured the strongest possible contrast between masculinity and femininity, although Weininger, contrary to Kraus, despised femininity. *Geschlecht und Charakter*, a book of ill repute because of its misogynist and anti-Semitic tenets, became an even bigger best-seller than Krafft-Ebing's *Psychopathia sexualis*; between 1903 and 1922, it was reprinted twenty-four times and also appeared in numerous translations.[2] Masculinity and femininity are such pervasive forces, according to Weininger, that they exert their influence at all levels of human life, from the protoplasm cells are made of to the most sublime cultural expressions. Although he starts from the assumption that there are no absolute differences between men and women and that every individual possesses, both in a physical and mental sense, masculine and feminine qualities to various degrees, Weininger's study is concerned with the philosophical-psychological characteristics of the so-called absolute man and the absolute woman, ideal types that do not exist in reality, but that still function as the basis of his cultural critique. In his book, Weininger posited a dualistic worldview that he carried to its extremes and in which the masculine-feminine opposition coincides with classical dichoto-

2. On Weininger, see Le Rider and Leser 1984; Janik 1985; Le Rider 1985; and Sengoopta 1992 & 2000.

mies such as body-mind, reason-instinct, conscious-unconscious, idea-matter, subject-object, freedom-determinism, culture-nature, order-chaos, morality-immorality, and, ultimately, good-evil. Woman embodies, above all, sexuality, associated by Weininger with breaking the fixed boundaries between self and outside world, interiority and exteriority, and body and soul. He not only considered masculinity and femininity as biological or psychological categories, but also as philosophical and cultural categories. Thus, he distinguished between masculine and feminine periods in history and asserted that his own era was marked by an effeminization of culture. To support his theory, Weininger referred to the countless biomedical and psychological studies about gender and sexuality that had appeared in the closing decades of the nineteenth century, including Krafft-Ebing's *Psychopathia sexualis*. The young philosopher, who shortly after the publication of *Geschlecht und Charakter* committed suicide, had taken Krafft-Ebing's classes on psychiatry.

The scientific attention to sexuality in Vienna was inspired by the combination of a positivist scientific climate and the popularity of neo-Romantic views on life—quite a paradoxical combination at first sight (McGrath 1974; Luft 1990). By the end of the nineteenth century, Vienna had become one of the leading centers of modern scientific medicine and psychiatry, with prominent medical scholars like Carl von Rokitansky (1804–1878), Ernst Brücke (1819–1892), Theodor Billroth (1829–1894), Theodor Meynert, and Krafft-Ebing (Lesky 1965). Next to Darwinism, the reductionist experimental physiology of Hermann von Helmholtz and Brücke set the tone for the materialist approach of the Vienna medical school. But, at the same time, Viennese intellectuals were deeply impressed by the philosophies of Schopenhauer and Nietzsche, Johann Jakob Bachofen's depiction of matriarchy, and Richard Wagner's music and conception of the world. All these views and philosophies stressed subjective feeling, the physical instincts, and the unconscious as the driving forces in humans.

Together, the intellectual trends of positivism and neo-Romanticism combined an objective biological view of physical reality with a notion of human subjectivity as fundamentally irrational. Humans were determined by instincts and hidden motives rather than by a machine-like predictability and rational calculation. Psychiatry especially—drawing attention to the impact of instincts, heredity, neurophysiological reflexes, compulsive behavior, and unconscious urges and motives—sought to incorporate this irrational view of man in the positivist system of thought. Whereas in the first half of the nineteenth century it was psychiatry's aspiration to cure a relatively small group of lunatics, in the fin de siècle many psychiatrists were concerned with the fundamental irrationality of the human mind in general and the omnipresence of abnormality within society. Their interest extended from pervasive dysfunction to mental states that fell within the range of normal human experiences but that might lead to mental disorders. We have seen how Krafft-Ebing turned away from the insane in the asylum and concentrated on his career in academia, his private practice, and his psychiatric writing. Especially in his work on sexuality and neurasthenia, he frequently hinted that the very boundary between the normal and the insane, which psychiatry had originally helped to institute, was fragile. This psychiatric awareness was a source of inspiration to many artists. Hermann Bahr, the major representative of Viennese modernism, labeled the new art as "nerve art." Vienna's fin de siècle culture in general has been characterized as a Gefühlskultur and also as Nervenkultur (Luft 1990, 95; cf. Schorske 1980; Worbs 1983). In both art and psychiatry, particular value was attached to the nerves—as the connecting link between the external physical reality and the subjective inner world. Scientific as well as literary descriptions of the nervous system were scattered with metaphorical images juxtaposing "higher" and "lower" tendencies, control and disinhibition, harmony and struggle, equilibrium and destabilization, and economy and excess.

Thus, both in art and science, there was a move away from the rationalist view of human nature that characterized classical liberalism. The attention to feelings and the inner self, characteristic of Vienna's late-nineteenth-century cultural climate, cannot be properly understood without taking into account the crisis of liberalism. Throughout Europe, liberalism was under pressure, but in Austria its failure was even more evident than elsewhere. The liberal reforms increasingly met with resistance, not only from the conservative establishment—since the 1880s the liberal hegemony was disputed by various mass movements that were guided by Christian-social, socialist, nationalist, or anti-Semitic views. The liberals lost much of their political power, not only in the Austrian parliament but also in the city administration of Vienna. A growing discrepancy had become evident between liberal values and social reality. The liberal ideals of freedom, progress, and equality had become a façade, not only for the property interests of capitalist entrepreneurs, but also to gloss over the gross social injustices and violent repression of ethnic groups in the eastern, Slavic parts of the Habsburg Empire.

In the period 1870–1900, the central European bourgeoisie was confronted with rapid economic, social, and political transformations. Many disturbing changes in norms and values, occurring in the process of modernization, forced changes in people's self-conceptions. In reaction to the cold objectivities of natural science and disorderly, alienating mass society, many turned to self-concern, personal values, and emotional life. In Vienna the young generation of artists and intellectuals, who were raised in an atmosphere of bourgeois liberalism, turned themselves against its optimistic worldview, which seemed securely anchored in Enlightenment values. The sense of alienation and powerlessness caused them to look for new certainties in art, the realm of feeling, and the cultivation of the individual self. Aestheticization—partly building on aristocratic and ecclesiastical traditions as well as the bourgeois cultivation of theater and opera—and psychologizing were two sides of the same coin: art and introspection served as refuges from unpleasant social and political realities (Schorske 1980; cf. Janik and Toulmin 1973, 48; Pynsent 1989, 120, 144).

The anti-bourgeois ethos of the modernist artists and intellectuals might give one the impression that they favored a liberation of the drives, but, as a matter of fact, the artistic, intellectual, and scientific cultivation of sexuality, masculinity, and femininity was quite ambiguous. The attention to the inner self contributed little to a liberation from the suffocating bourgeois morality; sexuality became the subject of endless psychological reflection and as such it was considered highly problematic. This ambivalence is particularly expressed in the unusually strong tension between opposing cultural tendencies of setting and transgressing boundaries. Sexuality was deployed to both delineate and undermine the boundaries between normal and abnormal, health and disease, masculine and feminine, purity and impurity. The work of Krafft-Ebing, of course, provides a clear illustration of this effort.

Psychopathia sexualis gave a strong impetus to sexual awareness, self-knowledge, and identity formation, but these involved all but unequivocal matters. On the one hand, the autobiographical confessions frequently had a redeeming effect, while the case histories reinforced a sense of self-awareness: many patients and correspondents were relieved by the book because they felt acknowledged. But, on the other hand, the study confirmed that they were not normal, and this painful realization often resulted in endless and compunctious self-reflection, which only reinforced the unbridgeable gap between private desire and social role and between fantasy and reality. Although some arrived at the insight that it was not their inclination itself that made them unhappy, but rather the prevailing Christian-bourgeois morality, sustained self-scrutiny did not always offer a way out of the uncertainties and inner conflicts that weighed them down. "I was aware of the inborn nature of my anomaly, but I felt myself in opposition with the whole world," one of them articulated this dilemma (*Ps* 1888, 75). Many oscillated between social rejection and the conviction that they could not belie their desire, for it constituted the core of their personality. "I was appalled by it, since I considered the love for my own sex as immoral and as something which deserves contempt," wrote a thirty-four-year-old urning.

I was painfully aware that I could not follow the course of nature, despite a moral upbringing and good will, and I was tormented by anguish. On the other hand I began to assume more and more that my feeling was rooted in a natural disposition, especially because the desire for a beautiful, strong man made itself felt frequently, although I made every effort to fight the urge. . . . Since I know that many men feel the same as I do and satisfy their urge, my desire is even stronger than before. I suffer physically and morally a lot and I feel that my nerves are completely shattered. . . .

"The patient complains," Krafft-Ebing noted in his case history, "that he cannot bring himself to follow his natural drives, although he feels that his moral and physical suffering would then disappear" (Ps 1888, 80). "It is terrible," another urning confided to Krafft-Ebing,

if one cannot enjoy the simple pleasure of associating with friends, and if every tough soldier or butcher boy makes one tremble and throb. It is frightening when the night comes, to watch at the window for someone to urinate against a wall across the street offering me the opportunity to see his genitals. Such hang-ups are terrible and also the awareness that my disposition and desire is immoral and criminal. . . . Thus I vacillate between hopeful gaiety and frightening hopelessness, neglecting my occupation and family. (Ps 1892, 244; cf. Ps 1999, 547)

A woman who had been seduced by another woman and who had fallen in love with her was, like several others, tormented by contradictory feelings:

What I felt immediately after this occurrence defies description: worry over the broken resolutions, which I had made such strenuous efforts to keep; fear of detection and subsequent contempt, but also exuberant joy to be rid at last of the tortured watchings and longings of the single state; unspeakable sensual pleasure; and wrath against the unfortunate companion mingled with feelings of the deepest tenderness toward her. (Ps 1894, 287; cf. Ps 1999, 335)

A thirty-eight-year-old man agonized because he could accept his feelings of love for a friend but not the sexual desire connected to those feelings:

I long for the closest, most complete relationship that can be conceived of between two human beings—always together, common interests, unlimited confidence, sexual union. . . . Just now I am fighting the battle again: I forcefully stifle the insane passion that has enthralled me for so long. All night long I toss and turn, haunted by the image of the man for whose love I would give up all I possess. How very sad it is that the

noblest feeling given to man, friendship, is sullied by common sensual
feeling! (1891h, 126; cf. *Ps* 1999, 580)

The capricious sexual urges were difficult to capture in univocal categories
because of their transgressive character, while they offered no stable footing
for a fixed, socially sanctioned identity. "Until this very day I have not been
able to grasp my nature," wrote a thirty-six-year-old homosexual man. "In
the past I imagined that I knew myself, but since then I have come across
all kinds of contradiction" (1890e, 53).

Such inner conflict was somehow encouraged by the contradictory tenor
of Krafft-Ebing's work. It gave way to confirmation and acceptation of
sexual variance. The boundaries between normal sexuality and abnormal
sexuality—including sadism, masochism, fetishism, and contrary sexual
feeling—were not so much qualitative and absolute but rather quantitative
and flexible. The positivist and liberal-minded Krafft-Ebing countered the
biases of church, government, and the legal system with a more scientific
approach, aimed at understanding, and he even espoused, to a certain extent, a favorable view of sexuality. In the actual descriptions of sexual activities that he used in his work, it was not so much reproduction he invoked,
but pleasure, orgasm, and mental satisfaction as the "aim" of lust. Yet his
writings also betray pessimism regarding the irresolvable contradiction between the rational, moral cultural order and the fickle and frequently bizarre sexual urges. Already on the first pages of *Psychopathia sexualis*, Krafft-
Ebing depicted uncontrollable lust as a swamp in which human beings were
sinking under, as a yawning chasm that devoured honor, promise, and
health, and as a volcano eruption that scorched everything that provided
dignity to human beings. The control and refinement of primitive, aggressive, and promiscuous urges constituted a precondition for the progress of
culture. Basically, human history was an ongoing struggle between sensu-
alness and morality. As is true of Freud's work, that of Krafft-Ebing is per-
fused with a huge dilemma. On the one hand, the human is largely driven
by sexual urges and suppressing these urges causes nervous complaints and
mental disorders (only a minority of Krafft-Ebing's patients did not suffer
from nervousness or neurasthenia). On the other hand, it is impossible to
freely surrender or give way to lust, because, as a transgressive force that
constantly undermines the distinction between normal and abnormal, it is
simultaneously a great threat to social life.

In this way, Krafft-Ebing voiced a profound pessimism about human nature, which was characteristic of the intellectual fin de siècle climate. Man
seemed to be caught in an unending and unpredictable struggle between
unruly passions and the need to tame them. Especially worrisome, for instance, was Krafft-Ebing's claim that sadomasochism formed the foun-

dation of the sexual relationship of man and woman, because it readily invited associations with overpowering, rape, murder for lust, and even cannibalism (1877, 301; *Ps* 1903, 69–70, 161–62). One of his masochistic patients, for instance, told him that in his youth he had been roused by the sight of a woman slaughtering an animal. "From that time, for many years, he had reveled in the lustfully colored fantasy of being stabbed and cut, and even killed, by women with knives" (1891h, 25; cf. *Ps* 1999, 141). Krafft-Ebing commented that the desire to be killed was indeed the ultimate consequence of masochism, just as murder for lust was the ultimate form of sadism. His casuistry also suggested that masochism was mainly found among men. Because Krafft-Ebing reasoned that these men assumed the female role, male masochism was a rudimentary form of sexual inversion. Sadism in women would be related to their masculinization. In this way, *Psychopathia sexualis* made its contribution to further the nightmare of many men regarding man's increasing subjection to woman (Aarts 1981; Showalter 1991; Verplaetse 1999).

Although Krafft-Ebing was hardly influenced by modernist art, his psychiatry has much ground in common with the artistic imagination of erotics, not just because of a shared attention for perversion. Wavering between the old familiar bourgeois values and the lure of emotional life, both Krafft-Ebing's patients and the modernist artists were looking to find new expressions of the self. Many of Krafft-Ebing's homosexual correspondents reported that they liked literature, art, and especially music; some of them mentioned Wagner in particular. One of them noted that most of his homosexual friends were devotees of Wagner: "I find that this music is perfectly in tune with our nature" (1891h, 129; cf. *Ps* 1999, 582). Another clearly referred to modernist art when he wrote: "Among poets and novelists, I typically prefer those who describe refined feelings, peculiar passions, and farfetched impressions; an artificial or hyperartificial style pleases me. Likewise, in music, it is the nervous, exciting music of a Chopin, a Schumann, a Schubert, or a Wagner, etc. that is in most perfect harmony with me. Everything in art that is not only original, but also bizarre, attracts me" (1891, 108; cf. *Ps* 1999, 554).

The ambiguous attitude regarding sexual diversity in Krafft-Ebing's work can also be traced in the literature and painting of the Viennese avantgarde. Although at first these artists tended to idealize female sexuality especially as a counterforce to the rigid, fossilized bourgeois culture, around the turn of the century they began to display more sensitivity as well for the dark sides of the diffuse life of the sexual urges. Author and physician Arthur Schnitzler, whose evocative descriptions of the psychological life of his characters were unsurpassed, felt just as ambivalent about human instinctual life as his fellow traveler Freud. Schnitzler, who reviewed vari-

ous works of Krafft-Ebing, was convinced that sexuality needed acknowledgment as a decisive influence on individuals and therefore he criticized
the prevailing morality, but he also concluded that sexuality's liberation
provided no solace for the emptiness of bourgeois social life.[3] He described
sexuality without love as a mechanistic ritual, as an expression of pleasure-
seeking egotism, and even as a form of cruelty versus the other.

Visual artists like Gustav Klimt, Oskar Kokoschka, and Egon Schiele,
who pictured woman as a sensuous creature embodying the fullness of natural life, also evoked the fear caused by her unfettered sexuality. Women's
sexuality not only connoted harmonious unification with unspoiled nature
and a beneficial confluence of male and female: it was also associated with
egotism, cruelty, destruction, and death; the reverse of unsparing female
lust—frequently symbolized by the snake—was the male fear of impotence
and the ruthless, amoral femme fatale, the embodiment of evil. Sexuality
proved to be an anarchistic, demonic, and transgressive force that undermined the established self and could hardly provide a suitable basis for a
delimited identity and stable social relationships. Both in Krafft-Ebing's casuistry and in the work of modernist artists, it was emphasized that the gap
between the inscrutable depths of the true self and a social identity based
on an artificial social order was hard to close. Moreover, the psychological
quest for a new certainty of the authentic self not only led to liberation but
also to all sorts of discontents, to inward conflict, nervousness, feelings of
guilt, solitude, and isolation. In an intellectual climate in which the power
of the irrational loomed large, many bourgeois had good reasons to be anx-
ious about the stability of their self. It soon turned out that a subjectivity
that was rooted in feelings was built on sandy ground and lacked a stable
center.

Not just in art but also in positivist science and philosophy, the common
idea of a self that existed independently of time and place as a solid foundation of personal identity was subverted. Theorists in the biomedical sciences, psychiatry, and experimental psychology argued that human beings
were not guided by an autonomous rational mind, but that they were at
the mercy of instincts, mechanistic reflexes, hereditary qualities, and the
random circumstances of their immediate environment. The self could not
be saved, thus argued the Viennese physicist and philosopher Ernst Mach
(1838–1916), who in his epistemology questioned the distinction between
reality and perception and in his Die Analyse der Empfindungen (1885) expounded that consciousness was not much more than a succession of fleet-

3. He reviewed Neue Forschungen auf dem Gebiet der Psychopathia sexualis, Psychopathia
sexualis, Hypnotische Experimente and Der Conträrsexuale vor dem Strafrichter in Internationale
Klinische Rundschau 5 (1891), 69–70; 7 (1893), 1247, 1399; 8 (1894), 1030.

ing, constantly changing individual impressions, feelings, sensations, and
memories. The autonomous self proved an illusion; it was not more than,
as Otto Weininger described it, "a *waiting room* of emotions" (Weininger
1912, 199). Freud too showed that, psychologically speaking, identity was
not a given but something that could only be acquired in a long process of
conflictive identifications.

When, at the end of the nineteenth century, scientific and literary attention for the irrational side of man increased, self-dissection appeared
to be as risky as it was seductive. Modern psychological individualism, as
conceived in fin de siècle Viennese culture, evoked so much insecurity and
discontent that it may be referred to as a crisis of identity, whereby male
identity was at issue in particular (Le Rider 1990). The fear and defense
that this identity crisis triggered in some men caused a transformation
within Viennese modernism, which took the form of a revaluation of a
clear demarcation between masculinity and femininity, including a rejection of cross-bordering sexual urges and feelings and an argument in favor
of moral purity.

This rejection of sexuality and femininity was articulated most clearly
by Weininger. His analysis entails a sharp critique of the tendency toward
intermingling that would be characteristic of female sexuality and a plea
for a pure masculinity as a way to safeguard culture and morality. Although
in *Geschlecht und Charakter* femininity, next to Jewishness, represented everything that Weininger despised in modern society, science, and art, he
claimed in the introduction of his book that his argument was equally directed against men. After all, it was the male sexual urge that again and
again degraded woman to a sexual object, thus reconfirming her lack of
freedom. The bourgeois ideal of romantic love was criticized by Weininger
because it disguised that the man used woman as a means to satisfy his own
lust and that he could dominate and exploit her. He considered marriage
founded on love an illusion: there could be no true respect for woman
among men. Bringing some of Krafft-Ebing's views to a head, he argued
that, by definition, heterosexuality was based on inequality and on a sadomasochistic relationship, which easily degenerated into cruel lust and rape;
he even compared heterosexual intercourse with murder. Only when man
did not see woman as a sexual object any longer might he be able to love
and respect her. As long as lust prevailed, however, neither man nor
woman could be liberated and love based on equality was impossible.

Weininger was not only concerned with the opposition between individual men and women: the conflict between male and female was played
out within each human being. Femininity was also part of men, and therefore the integrity of the subject was constantly undermined. A close reading of Weininger's book reveals that his attitude regarding masculinity and

femininity was ambivalent and that his ideal type of woman was constructed on the tottery basis of fear and wishful thinking. The "absolute" woman, who is fully one with nature and inhabits a sensuous realm, embodied the desire for a blissful unlimitedness that had been lost in Western culture. But this woman also threatened the safe armor of man, which had taken him so much trouble to put on and which he could not do without anymore if he wanted to control nature.

In his *Geschlecht und Charakter*, Weininger referred to a remarkable case history in Krafft-Ebing's *Psychopathia sexualis* (Weininger 1912, 494). It involves the self-analysis of a physician who described in detail how he thought he had undergone a gradual metamorphosis from a man into a woman and how, in the process, he felt more and more dominated by sexuality:

> I feel like a woman in a man's form, and even though I am often sensible of this male form, the body part concerned always feels feminine. Thus, for example, I feel my penis as a clitoris, my urethra as a urethra and vaginal orifice . . . my scrotum as a labia majora; in short, I always feel a vulva. . . . The skin all over my body feels feminine; it receives all impressions, whether a warm touch, or an unfriendly touch, as feminine, and I have the sensations of a woman. . . . It almost seems to me as if feeling like a woman is like being entirely controlled by the vegetative system. . . . The overwhelming natural instinct of the female concupiscence overcomes my feeling of modesty, so that indirectly coitus is desired. . . . Sometimes it causes me such great pleasure that there is nothing to compare it to: it is the most blissful and powerful feeling in the world, for which everything can be sacrificed—at that moment the woman in me is simply a vulva that has devoured my whole person. . . . I almost feel like a prostitute. My reason does not help; the imperative feeling of femininity dominates and rules everything. (1890e, 73–75; cf. *Ps* 1999, 261–63)

The physician articulated what for Weininger must have been a haunting nightmare: the all-swallowing female sexuality that annulled the integrity of the personality as well as its autonomous mind. After the distinction between masculine and feminine was relativized in biomedical science—and, notably, in Krafft-Ebing's work—and the authors of *Jung Wien* and the artists of *Sezession* had represented femininity as a counterbalance to instrumental masculine reason, Viennese modernism responded ascetically. As opposed to the nervous and sensual sensibility of Krafft-Ebing's patients and the immersion in aestheticism and sensuality by *Jung Wien* and *Sezession* artists, Weininger and representatives of Viennese modernism like Ludwig Wittgenstein (1889–1951), Adolf Loos (1870–1933), and Arnold

Schönberg (1874–1951) opted for maintaining clearly demarcated bound-aries and moral purity in the form of rigid logical and rational forms. Witt-genstein's quest for an authentic, mathematical language, Schönberg's ra-tional twelve-tone system, and Loos's declaration of war to the ornament, to the "feminine" adornment that he felt was superfluous and devoid of content, suggested the general atmosphere in which Weininger formulated his uncompromising defense of (male) purity (Le Rider 1990, 157–62). In their modernism, no room was left for ambivalence, multi-interpretability, and endless psychological self-reflection, which characterized both Krafft-Ebing's *Psychopathia sexualis* and the art of *Jung Wien* and *Sezession*. How-ever, in the longer term, it was Krafft-Ebing and his articulate clients, rather than Weininger and his admirers, who anticipated twentieth-century attitudes toward sexuality and identity.

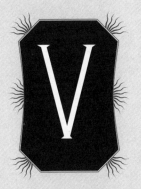

Krafft-Ebing's
Legacy

AFTER KRAFFT-EBING'S DEATH, *PSYCHOPATHIA SEXUALIS* CONTINUED TO enjoy popularity. Numerous new editions were published in the twentieth century: his pupil Alfred Fuchs edited three (1907, 1912, 1918) and the German sexologist Albert Moll brought out another one (1924). In 1937 an adapted version of the book was published by the Viennese psychiatrist Alexander Hartwich under the title *Die Verirrungen des Geschlechtslebens*. This edition was reprinted twelve times between 1937 and 1962. In 1984 the fourteenth edition was republished in a facsimile version, with introductions by, among others, Georges Bataille, Salvador Dali, and Julia Kristeva.

Already during Krafft-Ebing's lifetime, *Psychopathia sexualis* was translated into several languages: Russian, Japanese, Italian, French, Hungarian, Dutch, and English. Especially in the Anglo-Saxon world, Krafft-Ebing's reputation among the general public was exclusively based on this book. The British medical establishment, however, was not happy at all about the publication of an English translation and distanced itself explicitly from it again and again. "Better if it had been written entirely in Latin, and thus veiled in the decent obscurity of a dead language," the editors of the *British Medical Journal* commented when the second edition of the first authorized English translation appeared in 1893.[1] Although physicians could not do without studying "many morally disgusting subjects," as a reviewer phrased it in the same journal, at the same time these subjects should not be brought before the public (Porter and Hall 1995, 158; Hall 1994, 355). The board of the British Medico-Psychological Association was so displeased with the success of the book that it even considered canceling Krafft-Ebing's honorary membership (Benedikt 1906, 163). By the time the English translation of the tenth edition of *Psychopathia sexualis* appeared in

1. Quoted in the introduction of *Ps* 1965.

1902, the *British Medical Journal* voiced the opinion that it was "the most repulsive of a group of books of which it is the type," not sparing "the minutest and the most nauseous detail" (Porter and Hall 1995, 163). And the author of Krafft-Ebing's obituary in the *British Medical Journal* spoke of his "somewhat unfortunate prominence" because of *Psychopathia sexualis*. Its "questionable popularity" was due "rather to the curiosity of the public than to the appreciation of the medical profession."[2]

In general the American medical establishment was as reluctant as the British one to deal with sexuality and acknowledge the existence of variant sexual behavior. Although some medical scientists were active in this field—for instance, Frank Lydston and James Kiernan, whose biogenetic theory was adopted by Krafft-Ebing—such research was viewed with suspicion and considered unrespectable. As Vern Bullough writes, in the American medical world "a more or less official prudery" was enforced (Bullough 1994, 93). In 1893 a reviewer of the *American Journal of Insanity* questioned the popularity of *Psychopathia sexualis*:

> How much of its sales has been due to professional interest, how much to the interest of sufferers in what concerns their own cases, and how much to a morbid and prurient curiosity, it would not be easy to determine. Surely, it would be an extraordinary appetite for nastiness that would not be satiated by the records which it contains of the inconceivable depths of degradation into which human beings, often in some respects highly endowed, may be plunged by the vagaries and perversions of the sexual passion. (Cited by Rosario 1997, 10)

In a review of Havelock Ellis's *Sexual Inversion*, published in 1897, it was also regretted that the book was widely distributed for popular reading. The reviewer criticized not only Havelock Ellis, but also Krafft-Ebing, who was reproached for putting "unnecessary emphasis and importance" on sexual perversion (Bullough 1994, 94). Probably in order to protect himself against such accusations beforehand, the publisher of the American translation of the twelfth edition of *Psychopathia sexualis* wrote in the book's preface that it was not intended for the general public and that its sale was "rigidly restricted to the members of the medical and legal professions" (Ps 1906, ix).

Official public discourse was more prudish in Britain and America than in France and central Europe, and the moral climate in Anglo-Saxon countries was less receptive to psychiatric thinking on sexuality. Although British and American physicians also presented themselves as specialists in the field of sexuality, they took a rather reserved stance: few of them really

2. *British Medical Journal* 1 (1903): 53.

wanted to have much to do with this shady subject or participate in public debates (Hall 1999). Havelock Ellis was the exception that proved the rule. Too obvious an interest in sex was associated with commercially motivated quackery. Physicians acknowledged the urgency of the need to warn the public of impending dangers, but at the same time they believed that sexual knowledge ought to be discussed only with due caution and was not to be disseminated outside the established respectable medical circles. The medical establishment in Britain and the United States viewed German and French works on sexual perversion, these "turbid continental out-pourings," as dubious (Hall 1994, 355). Most of them scarcely attained any scientific respectability before the 1920s, and, under British law, they could even be prosecuted as "obscene," as happened to Havelock Ellis's works.

In the Anglo-Saxon world, Krafft-Ebing's *Psychopathia sexualis* gained a reputation as little more than a work of scientific pornography. Yet, despite this disqualification by professional medicine, if not because of it, the book was at least as popular in Britain and the United States as on the Continent. In fact, most foreign editions of the book have appeared in English; between 1892 and 1978 at least thirty-four editions of authorized English translations have been counted (Hauser 1992, 450–52). The most recent American edition dates from 1999. Even more than the German ones, several English and American editions show that publishers did not only cater to the scientific interest of readers. The dividing line between scientific vulgarization and pornography is difficult to draw. The preface of the 1939 edition states that in his professional life Krafft-Ebing encountered

a succession of the undersexed and the hypersexed, rapists, stranglers, rippers, stabbers, blood-sucking vampires and necrophiliacs, sadists who hurt their partners, masochists who thrilled at the sight of the whip, males in female clothes, stuff-fetishists dominated by a shoe or handker-chief, lovers of fur and velvet, slaves of scatology, defilers of statues, de-spoilers of children and animals, frotteurs and voyeurs, renifleurs and stercoraires, pageists and exhibitionists, paedophiliacs and gerontophili-acs, satyriasists and nymphomaniacs, and again and again male-craving males and female-craving females, and the endless army of men who lusted after Woman in perverse ways, but had no desire for her vagina. The ability to enjoy and perform the sexual act, in the normal manner, appeared to be the most difficult of the arts. (*Ps* 1939, vi)

Advertisements noting that all "important phrases and paragraphs in Latin or French [sic]" had been translated into English betray that publishers were consciously offering *Psychopathia sexualis* as a saucy book. In 1969 an American mail order company promoted the book explicitly as pornography:

Krafft-Ebing's *Psychopathia Sexualis*. 624 pages. Startling case histories
of unnatural sex practices, weird auto-erotic methods, sex—lust—tor-
ture—much, much more! Many of the hundreds of case histories are
from secret files and hushed-up court proceedings. Monstrous strange,
almost unbelievable sex acts! For mature adults only! (Brecher 1969, 60)

Today, fully three decades after the sexual revolution of the 1960s, it is
difficult to imagine that *Psychopathia sexualis* is still read because of its titillating qualities. For the general public, Krafft-Ebing is not a household
name anymore, and among professionals his fame has been superseded by
that of Freud, Kinsey, and Masters and Johnson. Considering his work as a
specimen of an outdated pre-Freudian view on sexuality, several historians
added him to the curiosity cabinet of repressive Victorianism. Yet the historical significance of Krafft-Ebing's work should not be underestimated. It
marks a central moment in the constitution of the modern conception of
sexuality. Part of his vocabulary—such as *sadism, masochism,* and *pedophilia*—is still with us; both terms *homosexuality* and *heterosexuality* first entered the English language in the 1892 translation of *Psychopathia sexualis*.
And, even more importantly, his understanding of sexuality retains its influence to this day. In his work, the sexual lost its fixed place in reproduction, and the old distinction between procreative and nonprocreative acts
gave way to a new fundamental differentiation between heterosexual and
homosexual preferences, which, together with their stepchild bisexuality,
are still our basic sexual categories.

Late-nineteenth-century French psychiatrists tended to consider fetishism as the "master perversion" that included all the aberrations by which
sexual desire had fixed itself on the wrong (nonreproductive) goal, be it an
object, a body part, a certain act or physical type, a person of the same sex,
an unusual age category, or an animal. By contrast, Krafft-Ebing, as his career progressed, highlighted the dichotomy of heterosexuality and homosexuality more and more. Although the pathological was his lens, his use of
the term *heterosexual,* meaning sexual attraction between a male and a female free from a reproductive goal, marked a shift away from the centuries-
old procreative norm. By pushing reproduction aside and stressing the emotional and affective dimension of sexuality, it became possible to character-
ize heterosexuality and homosexuality as equivalents. In one of his last publications on sexual perversion, a rendering of lectures for students, Krafft-
Ebing indeed distinguished two basic categories: contrary sexual feeling
and heterosexual perversions (1901b). Other perversions he identified—
such as sadism, masochism, and fetishism—have generally become subvari-
ations of the more fundamental heterosexual-homosexual division. In this
way, Krafft-Ebing underlined that the gender of one's sexual partner—the

other (hetero), the same (homo), or both sexes (bi)—became the distinctive feature of the modern sexual order.

In yet another way Krafft-Ebing's work heralded a decisively new phase in Western conceptions of sex and sexuality. Whereas previously the main criterion was the distinction between male and female anatomy, while the congruence between a man's or a woman's body and their sexual desire was seldom questioned, the late-nineteenth-century psychiatric model of sexuality postulated a complicated interaction between mind and body. It embraced physiology and psychology, imagination and real bodily sensations, fantasy and concrete behavior. Sexuality emerged as a concept that pointed to both internal and external phenomena. The physical dimension of sexuality affected the mental and its psychological dimension affected the body. The satisfaction of the sexual urge was not only made up of physical release, Krafft-Ebing pointed out, but also of emotional fulfillment. In his work the sexual took on a strong meaning, especially because physical sensations and experiences played such a significant role in the intrapsychic lives of individuals. This very interaction between mental and physical experience, which is so central in his understanding of sexuality, might explain why sexuality itself has become such a meaningful experience in modern Western culture: the emphasis on sexual experience is an expression of the preoccupation with the interplay between the body and the inner self. As such, sexuality has become a sensitive issue giving cause to an array of emotional problems: fears of being abnormal, endless self-scrutiny, anxieties about erotic attractiveness and sexual achievement, and conflicts between sexual fantasies and the realities of everyday life.

The modern concept of sexuality, crafted around the turn of the century not only in the work of Krafft-Ebing but also in that of scholars like Alfred Binet, Albert Moll, Henry Havelock Ellis, and Sigmund Freud, was not just a reaction against Victorian prohibitions, but also, and even more so, it brought along an ideological transformation, namely the psychologizing and individualization of sexuality. Late-nineteenth-century psychiatric interference with sexuality was largely based on a biographical (or autobiographical) model, forging a strong link between sexual desire and personal identity. What is striking in Krafft-Ebing's study of sexuality is not only that case studies and life histories were so prominent, but even more that the confessions of his patients and correspondents were not forced into the straitjacket of existing psychiatric explanations. As we have seen, many of the self-observations were submitted voluntarily, supporting as well as challenging medical discourse, and although the subjects of these observations thought of themselves as fundamentally different from average people, this did not necessarily mean that they considered themselves to be immoral, vicious, or ill. The case history method was not just a means of categorizing and pathologizing deviant sexualities; it also offered a space in which uncertain individuals could articulate their predicament in the form of personal narrative.

Their stories were not only told by the expert voices "from above" but also "from below," by those who had lived or were living them in their role of the story's protagonist. In a way, Krafft-Ebing and his most articulate private patients and correspondents closely cooperated with each other: perverts who wanted to make their voice heard in public depended on sympathetic physicians like him because medical science was the only respectable forum available, while, conversely, the psychiatrist had to rely on their confessions and stories to validate his own discourse, thus giving his theoretical considerations an empirical basis. To a large degree he did not pretend to know better than some of his clients. He considered their narrations seriously as crucial material to support his psychiatric analysis. Lay views and medical views of sexuality overlapped, so that shared knowledge and judgments tended to structure and mediate interactions between the psychiatrist and the pervert. This facilitated medical treatment and other forms of restraint or intervention, but it also stimulated self-awareness and, in the longer term, emancipation.

With the exception of psychoanalysis, after the turn of the century the psychologically and biographically oriented approach to sexuality was partly replaced by the more specialist and scientific endocrinological model. This (re)confirmed the belief in the biological basis of sexuality and cut off the world of lived experience from the world of medical science. Biomedical research of sexuality tended to abstract from direct human behavior and experience, and it increasingly became an experiment-based scientific study of chemical compounds and animals in the laboratory. But in some of the experiments, people were used as guinea pigs as well. Within twenty years of Krafft-Ebing's death, the Viennese physician Eugen Steinach (1861–1944), after experimenting on animals, attempted to cure homosexuals by transplanting testicles of heterosexual men. It seems that the understanding of the physiology of sexuality was largely based on animal models in general. Both Albert Moll and Alexander Hartwich, who edited Krafft-Ebing's *Psychopathia sexualis* in the first half of this century, updated the book by discussing biological research of sexuality, especially endocrinology. Strikingly, Hartwich also replaced the forensic part with a chapter on therapy.

Yet, as far as the diagnosis and treatment of human sexual problems was concerned, psychoanalysis developed into a strong rival of the biomedical model. After World War II, the center of sexology shifted from central Europe to North America. Especially in the United States, psychoanalysis found many adherents among psychiatrists. Stressing the impact of sexuality on personality formation, it was in line with Krafft-Ebing's psychological approach, although Freud's theory was, of course, more sophisticated. Freud showed that sexual identity was not given by nature but the unstable product of an intricate psychical development, yet his theory established a much more normative-developmental scheme than Krafft-Ebing's relatively simple and open case history method. An influential American alternative to the Freudian theory was the more empirically-based research of the biologist Alfred Kinsey (1894–1956). Interviewing large numbers of people, Kinsey focused on human sexual behavior and its statistical measurement. Like Kinsey, the practice-oriented sex therapists William Masters and Virginia Johnson also adopted a behaviorist approach, which, contrary to psychoanalysis, downplayed the importance of sexual psychology and identities.

More recently, postmodern social and cultural theorists have undermined the idea that sexual identities are fixed in nature or the psyche. However, in the popular commonsense understanding of sexuality, this notion is still paramount. Sexual identities may be debunked or "deconstructed" at a theoretical level; they are nevertheless "real" in a historical sense, a product of social life itself, and as such they have become an inalienable part of the self-experience of modern man. Continuity over time as well as differentiation, something to set oneself off from others, are still essential functions of identity formation. It casts individuals into their own structure of values and priorities, which enable them to make choices in a steady and purposive fashion; identity gives the individual self-esteem and a sense of potentiality as well. However many varying patterns of sexual behavior may be chosen under the influence of immediate and accidental circumstances and subtle situational influences, these preferences are still very much regarded as expressing something deep and fixed from within the inner self. In the West, sexual identity is still experienced or conceptualized as a psychological essence that is already there, waiting to be discovered, explored, understood, or enjoyed. Sexologists, psychotherapists, self-help groups and manuals, and emancipation movements have only intensified the preoccupation with the true self. Scanning their own past life for clues to their sexual being, people still tell each other "sexual stories" to foster a sense of identity, even more perhaps since the 1960s, because sexuality has become a focal point of personal awareness, individual growth, self-actualization, and emancipation (Plummer 1995). Moreover, the idea that it is wholesome to transform one's (sexual or other) pleasure or suffering into a personal, authentic story is generally approved of in modern Western culture. What Krafft-Ebing's patients and correspondents did in the privacy of the psychiatric consulting room or in their correspondence has become public property: nowadays such candid stories are told not only on the couch of the analyst, but also in popular magazines, on television, and on the Internet all the time.

Foucault rightly understood the continuity of nineteenth-century psychiatric interference with sexuality and the present-day craving for self-expression: both are based on the confessional model, which proclaims sexuality as the key to personality. In this sense, Krafft-Ebing's case histories and the self-observations of his clients are a foreshadowing of the post-1960s sexual liberation. However, I would argue that Foucault's assessment of this confessional and psychological model of sexuality as a limitation of possibilities is one-sided. In this book I have tried to make clear that Krafft-Ebing's psychiatry was more than an instrument of professional power and social control. The formation and articulation of sexual identities became only possible in a self-conscious, reflexive bourgeois society, in which there was a dialectic between humanitarian reform and emancipation, on the one hand, and efforts to enforce social integration, on the other. The elaboration of psychological explanations of various sexual tastes in the last decades of the nineteenth century was advanced by professional psychiatry as well as by the long historical development of individualism and democratization.

Individual autonomy and self-determination have been two of the crucial values of modernity. However, in the actual social process of modernization, these rights were not granted on the basis of equality. The larger part of the nineteenth century was dominated by a narrow, restricted liberalism: the applicability of individual self-determination was largely limited to the "normal" and "responsible" male members of the bourgeoisie. In fact the liberal bourgeoisie subordinated the Enlightenment ideal of equality to a more hierarchical system of different scales of social integration and adjustment. The various forms of evolutionism, especially degeneration theory, can be seen as scientific mirrors of liberal ideology, which stressed civilized morality and, above all, self-control as necessary preconditions for individual rights and liberties. The male bourgeois elite tended to identify other social groups—women, the working class, children, colonized people, the insane, perverts and other deviants—with the unruly passions. The evolutionist argument for excluding these outsiders from the liberal social contract was that they had not (yet) reached the stage of development necessary to be in control of themselves.

At the end of the century, however, it became increasingly difficult to justify some of these exclusions, and more and more they were contested by the rising tide of socialism, feminism, and also, as we have seen, by some articulate perverts and sexual reform movements. The established social and sexual boundaries were shaken by the call of outsiders for further democratization. Using the respectable forum of medical science, perverts be-

gan to voice experiences and desires that, until then, had been unknown
or denied existence in public discourse. Krafft-Ebing's writings reflected
and also promoted the emergence of a new experience of sexuality that is
intrinsically bound up with the appearance of new kinds of individuals and
their aggregation into rudimentary communities. Some of them expressed
a critical awareness of the social suppression of deviant sexualities. Although they were still few in number, they prominently figured among
Krafft-Ebing's correspondents: in some of his autobiographical case histories, the seeds of sexual emancipation were sown.

Viewed in this context, Krafft-Ebing's own understanding of sexuality
was ambivalent and transitional. The psychiatric interference with sexual
deviance aiming at medical treatment can be viewed as an effort to create
a new, scientifically backed, sexual order to replace traditional morality.
From the beginning, however, there was a mismatch between the intent of
Krafft-Ebing and the effects of his writings. Driving at the heart of a major
anxiety in Western culture, he not only enabled sexuality to be debated
more widely and seriously in society; he also offered perverts an opportunity
to express themselves in public and even to apply medical insights for their
own purposes. The reception of medical thinking on sexuality in society,
especially by those concerned, set in motion a dynamic that was difficult
to keep in check. The way some of them read Krafft-Ebing's work illustrates
that the sexual domain became a contested field and that it was but one
step from the admission of the right of perverts to express themselves. The
psychiatric understanding of perversions was trapped between scientific
control and the realization of the liberal ideals of individual self-expression
and self-realization. Whether the scale tipped to one side or the other depended to a large extent on the social position and gender of the psychiatrist's clients. Upper- and middle-class men capitalized on psychiatric models and knowledge in order to become conscious of themselves and realize
their desires. But lower-class men, prosecuted sexual offenders, and most
women were generally not in a position to escape the coercion that undeni-
ably was part of psychiatric practice as well.

Thus Krafft-Ebing's psychiatry had two faces. As more and more private
patients and correspondents came up with life histories that did not fit the
established perception of psychiatry and bourgeois morality, the more
Krafft-Ebing's approach became enmeshed in contradictory views and interests. On the one hand, he propagated the current idea that the sexual
urge posed a persistent threat to the moral order because of its explosive
and barely controllable nature; especially because of the violent and de-
structive manifestations of the sexual impulse, it had to be repressed by
outside regulation and self-control. At the same time, however, he stressed
that sexuality also played a constructive role in personal and social life. He

attached great value to having a gratifying, harmonious sexual life, believing it to be crucial in the development of personality and affective relations. Love was sexualized by Krafft-Ebing; he replaced negative attitudes
toward sexuality with a positive evaluation of it within the context of romantic love. In this way he anticipated the increasing sexualization of marriage and love in the course of the twentieth century, which after World
War I was widely propagated in marriage manuals like Marie Stopes's *Married Love* (1918) and *Enduring Passion* (1928) and Theodoor van de Velde's
Ideal Marriage (1926).

Sexual desire was not only inevitable, according to Krafft-Ebing; its fulfillment was also necessary for mental health, personal happiness, and social harmony. One of the abnormalities he discussed in his work was sexual
anesthesia, the absence of sexual feeling. One of its characteristic symptoms was a lack of altruism and sociability. Strikingly, one of his patients,
a masochist who declared that he was impotent and not sensual, worried
about the weakness of his sexual desire: it "was painful to him . . . because
he acknowledged that the sexual element played an important role in social life and he was not sure whether one could live a sexless life in society"
(1899e, 156). Whereas usually too much sex or uncontrollable passion was
viewed as the problem, in this and other cases a new worry came to the
fore: was the absence or weakness of sexual desire normal and healthy? In
most cases, Krafft-Ebing's reply would have been an unequivocal "no." For
one thing, he had shown that forced sexual abstinence often resulted in
mental and nervous complaints. Acknowledging that sexual abstinence indeed could be detrimental to one's mental health, he also anticipated today's assumption that sexual restraint is unhealthy repression. From his
viewpoint, it was only a small step to the idea that every man and woman
had a right to sexual fulfillment.

Another striking feature of Krafft-Ebing's approach to sexuality was that
he vacillated between the absolutism of the normal/abnormal dichotomy
and an increasing relativization of this differentiation. His approach fluctuated between the stigmatization of sexual variations as mental illness and
the recognition of the individual's particular and unique desires. Like that
of Freud, his understanding of sexuality began to center on desire instead
of reproduction. The perverse sexual impulse was in fact a pleasure wish
that yearned innately neither for generation nor for intercourse per se, but
only for fulfillment. Homosexuality, which was earlier explained in terms
of degeneration, gradually came to be viewed as variation. Fetishism and
sadomasochism, though labeled as perversions, also served Krafft-Ebing's
efforts to understand sexual attraction in general. In this way *Psychopathia
sexualis* began to incorporate perversion into the normal and, significantly,
made sexual variance imaginable. With his approach, Krafft-Ebing created

the possibility of enlarging the sphere allotted to idiosyncratic desire. The acknowledgment of desire, irrespective of its "natural" goal, is central to the modern sexual ethos.

Influenced by his predominantly bourgeois patients and correspondents, Krafft-Ebing's work anticipated twentieth-century attitudes toward sexuality. Many of his patients and correspondents expressed a desire for self-actualization. Their self-confessions marked a transition in the urban bourgeois milieu from a Christian and productivist ethos, dictating self-denial and control of the passions, to a consumerist culture of abundance, one that valued the expression of the inner self and the satisfaction of individual desire. Just like democratization, the shift in capitalism from production to consumption entailed a rejection of collective constraints and a disembedding from traditional social contexts. Together with the spread of contraception, better nutrition, and health, it was the coming of affluence and consumer capitalism's promotion of pleasure and leisure that in the twentieth century would thrust sex to the forefront of our society.

BIBLIOGRAPHY

ARCHIVES

Autograph 146/38–1, 146/38–2, 213/61–2, 213/61–3, 469/16–2. Österreichische Nationalbibliothek, Vienna.

Exhibiten-Protokoll 1872/1873–1888/1889 der medizinischen Fakultät der k. k. Universität Graz. Archiv Karl Franzens Universität Graz.

Nachlass Richard von Krafft-Ebing. Krafft-Ebing Family Archive, Graz; The Wellcome Institute for the History of Medicine, London.

Personalakt Krafft-Ebing. Allgemeines Verwaltungsarchiv des Österreichischen Staatsarchivs, Vienna.

Personalakt Krafft-Ebing. Archiv Karl Franzens Universität Graz.

Personalakt Krafft-Ebing. Archiv Universität von Wien.

"Richard von Krafft-Ebing," Manuskript Nr. 854. Institut für Geschichte der Medizin der Universität von Wien.

Stransky, E. 1938. "Aus einem Gelehrtenleben um die Zeitenwende." Manuskript. Institut für Geschichte der Medizin der Universität von Wien.

Verlagsverträge. Archiv Ferdinand Enke Verlag, Stuttgart.

Wagner-Jauregg, J. Festrede zur Enthüllung der von Krafft-Ebing-Büste. Manuskript. Obersteinerbibliothek des neurologischen Instituts, Universität von Wien.

WORKS OF RICHARD VON KRAFFT-EBING

1864. *Die Sinnesdelirien. Ein Versuch ihrer physio-psychologischen Begründung und klinische Darstellung.* Erlangen: Ferdinand Enke.

1865. *Die Lehre von der Mania transitoria für Aerzte und Juristen dargestellt.* Erlangen: Ferdinand Enke.

1867a. Ueber einige Grundirrthümer in der forensischen Beurtheilung Seelengestörter. *Friedreichs Blätter für gerichtliche Medizin* 18:321–36.

1867b. *Beiträge zur Erkennung und richtigen forensischen Beurtheilung krankhafter Gemüthszustände für Aerzte, Richter und Vertheidiger.* Erlangen: Ferdinand Enke.

1867c. Ein Besuch in Gheel vom 27.–29. November 1866. *Allgemeine Zeitschrift für Psychiatrie* 24:665–88.

1867d.　Review of Morel, *De l'hérédité progressive ou des types dissemblables et disparates dans la famille* Paris 1867. *Allgemeine Zeitschrift für Psychiatrie* 24: 777–79.

1868a.　*Die transitorische Störungen des Selbstbewusstseins. Ein Beitrag zur Lehre vom transitorischen Irresein in klinisch-forensischer Hinsicht für Aerzte, Richter, Staatsanwälte und Vertheidiger.* Erlangen: Ferdinand Enke.

1868b.　Die Erblichkeit der Seelenstörungen und ihre Bedeutung für die forensische Praxis. *Friedreichs Blätter für gerichtliche Medicin* 19:188–211.

1868c.　*Ueber die durch Gehirnerschütterung und Kopfverletzung hervorgerufenen psychischen Krankheiten.* Erlangen: Ferdinand Enke.

1868d.　Die Gelüste der Schwangeren und ihre gerichtlich-medizinische Bedeutung. *Friedreichs Blätter für gerichtliche Medicin* 19:52–61.

1869a.　Über die prognostische Bedeutung der erblichen Anlage im Irresein. *Allgemeine Zeitschrift für Psychiatrie* 26:438–56.

1869b.　Zur therapeutischen Casuistik 2. Sexuelle Verrücktheit. Traitement moral nach Leuret. Dauernde an Genesung grenzende Besserung. *Allgemeine Zeitschrift für Psychiatrie* 26:326–28.

1869c.　Zur therapeutischen Casuistik 3. Mehrjährige Onanie durch Oxyuris vermicularis mit folgender Psychose. Beseitigung der Madenwürmchen mittelst Kali picronitricum. Aufhören der Onanie und Genesung der dadurch bedingten Psychose. *Allgemeine Zeitschrift für Psychiatrie* 26:556–57.

1869d.　Ein Beitrag zur Kenntnis der Heilwirkung des konstanten galvanischen Stromes. *Ärztliche Mitteilungen aus Baden* 23:77–80.

1869e.　Zur allgemeinen Diagnostik der Seelenstörungen in foro. *Deutsche Zeitschrift für Staatsarzneikunde* 27:192–223.

1871a.　*Beobachtungen und Erfahrungen über Typhus abdominalis während des deutsch-französischen Kriegs 1870/71 in den Lazarethen der Festung Rastatt.* Erlangen: Ferdinand Enke.

1871b.　Die Lehre vom moralischen Wahnsinn und ihre Bedeutung für das Forum. *Friedreichs Blätter für gerichtliche Medicin* 22:360–84.

1871c.　Ueber Heilung und Heilbarkeit der Tabes dorsalis durch den constanten galvanischen Strom. *Deutsches Archiv für klinische Medizin* 9:274–82.

1872a.　Verbrechen und Wahnsinn. Ein Beitrag zur Criminalpsychologie. *Allgemeine Deutsche Strafrechtszeitung* 12:354–61.

1872b.　*Grundzüge der Criminalpsychologie auf Grundlage des Strafgesetzbuchs des deutschen Reichs für Aerzte und Juristen.* Erlangen: Ferdinand Enke.

1872c.　Beischlaf an Willenlosen, Bewusstlosen und Geisteskranken. *Allgemeine Deutsche Strafrechtszeitung* 12:537–40.

1872d.　Zur Classifikation der Psychosen. *Der Irrenfreund* 14:129–37.

1873a.　*Die Zweifelhaften Geisteszustände vor dem Civilrichter für Aerzte und Juristen.* Erlangen: Ferdinand Enke.

1873b.　Irrenheil- und Gefängnisskunde. *Allgemeine Zeitschrift für Psychiatrie* 29: 242–45.

1873c.　Rede zur Eröffnung der psychiatrischen Klinik in Strassburg am 17. Mai 1872. *Allgemeine Zeitschrift für Psychiatrie* 29:378–90.

1873d.　Ueber Missbrauch willenloser, bewusstloser oder geisteskranker Frauenspersonen zur Wollust. (Paragraph 176 des dt. Strafgesetzbuches.) *Friedreichs Blätter für gerichtliche Medicin* 24:95–100.

1873e. Zur Frage der Unterbringung geisteskrank gewordene Verbrecher. *Friedreichs Blätter für gerichtliche Medicin* 24:301–9.

1874. *Die Melancholie. Eine klinische Studie.* Erlangen: Ferdinand Enke.

1875a. Castrirungsversuch an einem Knaben. Zweifelhafte Geistesstörung. Psychischer Degenerationszustand mit Perversion des Geschlechtstriebs. Facultätsgutachten. *Friedreichs Blätter für gerichtliche Medizin* 26:161–70.

1875b. Ueber Irresein durch Onanie bei Männern. *Allgemeine Zeitschrift für Psychiatrie* 31:425–40.

1875c. *Lehrbuch der gerichtlichen Psychopathologie mit Berücksichtigung der Gesetzgebung von Österreich, Deutschland und Frankreich.* Stuttgart: Ferdinand Enke.

1877. Ueber gewisse Anomalien des Geschlechtstriebs und die klinischforensische Verwerthung derselben als eines wahrscheinlich functionellen Degenerationszeichens des centralen Nervensystems. *Archiv für Psychiatrie und Nervenkrankheiten* 7:291–312.

1878a. Ueber primäre Verrücktheit auf masturbatorischer Grundlage bei Männern. *Der Irrenfreund* 20:129–46.

1878b. Untersuchungen über Irresein zur Zeit der Menstruation. Ein klinischer Beitrag zur Lehre vom periodischen Irresein. *Archiv für Psychiatrie und Nervenkrankheiten* 8:65–107.

1878c. Zweifelhafter Geisteszustand einer Frauensperson zur Zeit eines an ihr unternommenen Beischlafs. Facultäts-Gutachten. *Der Irrenfreund* 20: 177–88.

1879. *Der Stand der Irrenpflege in Steiermark. Ein Nothstand.* Graz: Leuschner & Lubensky.

1879–80. *Lehrbuch der Psychiatrie auf klinischer Grundlage für practische Ärzte und Studierende.* 3 vols. Stuttgart: Ferdinand Enke.

1881. Ueber Nutzen und Ausführbarkeit der eigenen Regie in österreichischen Irrenanstalten. *Jahrbücher für Psychiatrie und forensische Psychologie* 2: 23–26.

1882. Zur "conträren Sexualempfindung" in klinisch-forensischer Hinsicht. *Allgemeine Zeitschrift für Psychiatrie* 38:211–27.

1883a. *Lehrbuch der Psychiatrie auf klinischer Grundlage für practische Ärzte und Studirende.* 2d ed. Stuttgart: Ferdinand Enke.

1883b. Schändung. Zweifelhafter Geisteszustand. Keine Geisteskrankheit. *Friedreichs Blätter für gerichtliche Medizin* 34:100–7.

1884a. *Ueber Nervosität. Vortrag gehalten am 25 Jänuar 1884 zu Gunsten des Mädchen-Lyceums in Graz.* Graz: Selbstverlag des Mädchen-Lyceums.

1884b. Unzuchtsdelicte mit Kindern in einem Zustande von Bewusstlosigkeit (wahrscheinlich auf Grund traumatisch entstandener Reflexepilepsie). Gerichtärztliches Gutachten. *Friedreichs Blätter für gerichtliche Medizin* 35:81–90.

1884c. Zur Lehre von der conträren Sexualempfindung. *Der Irrenfreund* 26:1–14.

1884d. Diebstahl und socialistische Umtriebe. Moralischer Irrsinn und moralische Verkommenheit. Gerichtärztliches Gutachten. *Friedreichs Blätter für gerichtliche Medicin* 35:216–23.

1885a. Die conträre Sexualempfindung vor dem Forum. *Jahrbücher für Psychiatrie und forensische Psychologie* 6:34–47.

1885b.   *Über gesunde und kranke Nerven*. Tübingen: H. Laupp'schen.

Ps 1886.   *Psychopathia sexualis. Eine klinisch-forensische Studie*. Stuttgart: Ferdinand Enke.

1886.   Ein Fall von originärer Paranoia vor Gericht. (Betrug. Hysterismus. Conträre Sexualempfindung. Hypnotismus.) Gerichtärztliches Gutachten. *Friedreichs Blätter für gerichtliche Medizin* 37:36–59.

Ps 1887.   *Psychopathia sexualis. Mit besonderer Berücksichtigung der conträren Sexualempfindung. Eine klinisch-forensische Studie*. 2d ed. Stuttgart: Ferdinand Enke.

1887a.   Originäre geistige Schwächezustände in foro criminali. VIII. Unzuchtsdelicte mit Kindern. Schwachsinn. Trunkenheit. *Jahrbücher für Psychiatrie und forensische Psychologie* 7:131–37.

1887b.   Ueber Neurasthenia sexualis beim Manne. *Wiener medizinische Presse* 28:161–65, 201–5.

Ps 1888.   *Psychopathia sexualis. Mit besonderer Berücksichtigung der conträren Sexualempfindung. Eine klinisch-forensische Studie*. 3d ed. Stuttgart: Ferdinand Enke.

1888a.   Biss in die Nase der Geliebten. Fragliche Sinnesverwirrung zur Zeit der That. Gerichtärztliches Gutachten. *Friedreichs Blätter für gerichtliche Medizin* 39:415–22.

1888b.   *Eine experimentelle Studie auf dem Gebiete des Hypnotismus*. Stuttgart: Ferdinand Enke.

1888c.   Perversion of the Sexual Instinct—Report of Cases. *Alienist and Neurologist* 9:565–81.

1888d.   Ueber Neurosen und Psychosen durch sexuelle Abstinenz. *Jahrbücher für Psychiatrie und forensische Psychologie* 8:1–6.

1888e.   Ueber pollutionsartige Vorgänge beim Weibe. *Wiener medizinische Presse* 14:1–7.

Ps 1889.   *Psychopathia sexualis. Mit besonderer Berücksichtigung der conträren Sexualempfindung. Eine klinisch-forensische Studie*. 4th ed. Stuttgart: Ferdinand Enke.

1889a.   Die Entwicklung und Bedeutung der Psychiatrie als klinischer Wissenschaft. Antrittsvorlesung gehalten am 21. October 1889. *Wiener klinische Wochenschrift* 2:817–20, 843–45.

1889b.   Kritik des Eherechts nach dem Entwurf des bürgerlichen Gesetzbuchs. *Allgemeine Zeitschrift für Psychiatrie* 45:548–61.

1889c.   Bemerkungen zur hypnotischen Heilmethode. *Wiener medizinische Presse* 30:1185–87.

1889d.   Dementia paralytica oder progressive Paralyse. *Wiener medizinische Presse* 30:1801–5, 1847–54, 1889–99.

1889/   Angeborene konträre Sexualempfindung. Erfolgreiche hypnotische
1890a.   Absuggerierung homosexualer Empfindungen. *Internationales Centralblatt für die Physiologie und Pathologie der Harn- und Sexualorgane* 1: 7–11.

1889/   Ueber psychosexuales Zwittertum. *Internationales Centralblatt für die Physi-*
1890b.   *ologie und Pathologie der Harn- und Sexualorgane* 1:55–65.

Ps 1890.   *Psychopathia sexualis. Mit besonderer Berücksichtigung der conträren Sexual-*

empfindung. Eine klinisch-forensische Studie. 5th ed. Stuttgart: Ferdinand Enke.

1890a. Gynandrie. Ein Beitrag zur conträren Sexualempfindung. *Wiener medizinische Blätter* 13:451–53.

1890b. *Der klinische Unterricht in der Psychiatrie. Eine Studie.* Stuttgart: Ferdinand Enke.

1890c. Körperverletzung. Paranoia. Gerichtärzliches Gutachten. *Friedreichs Blätter für gerichtliche Medizin* 41:1–9.

1890d. Misshandlungen. Paranoia persecutoria ex masturbatione. Gerichtärztliches Gutachten. *Friedreichs Blätter für gerichtliche Medizin* 41:10–14.

1890e. *Neue Forschungen auf dem Gebiet der Psychopathia sexualis. Eine medicinisch-psychologische Studie.* Stuttgart: Ferdinand Enke.

1890f. Ueber Masochismus. Aus einer neuen medizinisch-psychologischen Studie des Verfassers. *Wiener medizinische Blätter* 13:817–20.

1890g. Die Psychiatrie und das medizinische Studium. *Internationale klinische Rundschau* 4:1801–6.

1890h. Psychiatrie und Staatsexamen. *Wiener klinische Wochenschrift* 3:776–78.

1890i. Ueber psychiatrische Kliniken. *Wiener klinische Wochenschrift* 3:872–75.

Ps 1891. *Psychopathia sexualis. Mit besonderer Berücksichtigung der conträren Sexualempfindung. Eine klinisch-forensische Studie.* 6th ed. Stuttgart: Ferdinand Enke.

1891a. Ueber Fetischismus eroticus. *Wiener medizinische Blätter* 14:400–2, 432–34.

1891b. Ueber das Zustandekommen der Wollustempfindung und deren Mangel (Anaphrodisie) beim sexuellen Akt. *Internationales Centralblatt für die Physiologie und Pathologie der Harn- und Sexualorgane* 2:94–106.

1891c. Vorwort. In *Conträre Sexualempfindung. Mit Benutzung amtlichen Materials,* by A. Moll. Berlin: Fischer's Medicinische Buchhandlung, H. Kornfeld.

1891d. Zur Verwerthung der Suggestionstherapie (Hypnose) bei Psychosen und Neurosen. *Wiener klinische Wochenschrift* 4:795–99; Seperatabdruck, 1–15.

1891e. Die Suggestion und die Dichtung. *Deutsche Dichtung* 9:251–52.

1891f. Zur conträren Sexualempfindung. Autobiographie und strafrechtliche Betrachtungen über den Paragraphen 175 des deutschen Strafgesetzbuchs von einem Conträr-Sexualen. *Friedreichs Blätter für gerichtliche Medicin* 42:385–400.

1891g. Zur Therapie der Geisteskrankheiten. Klinischer Vortrag. *Wiener medizinische Presse* 32:489–94, 529–32, 573–75, 623–24, 700–4, 780–82, 827–30, 864–68.

1891h. *Neue Forschungen auf dem Gebiet der Psychopathia sexualis. Eine medicinisch-psychologische Studie.* 2d ed. Stuttgart: Ferdinand Enke.

Ps 1892. *Psychopathia sexualis. Mit besonderer Berücksichtigung der conträren Sexualempfindung. Eine klinisch-forensische Studie.* 7th ed. Stuttgart: Ferdinand Enke.

1892a. Die Bedeutung der Menstruation für das Zustandekommen geistig unfreier Zustände. *Jahrbücher für Psychiatrie und Neurologie* 10:232–54; Separatabdruck, 1–24.

1892b. Bemerkungen über "geschlechtliche Hörigkeit" und Masochismus. *Jahrbücher für Psychiatrie und forensische Psychologie* 10:199–211.

1892c. Nachwort zu: Paragraph 175 des deutschen Strafgesetzbuches und die Urningsliebe. Von Dr. iur ***. *Zeitschrift für die gesammte Strafrechtswissenschaft* 12:34–54.

1892d. Zur Differentialdiagnose der Dementia paralytica und der Neurasthenie cerebralis. In *Festschrift zur Feier des 50.jährigen Jubiläums der Anstalt Illenau*, edited by H. Schüle et al., pp. 65–77. Heidelberg: C. Winter.

1892e. Ueber Eifersuchtswahn beim Manne. *Jahrbücher für Psychiatrie und forensische Psychologie* 10:212–31.

1892f. Ueber eine seltene Form von Neurasthenia sexualis mit Zwangsvorstellungen. *Allgemeine Zeitschrift für Psychiatrie* 40:368–79.

1892g. Ueber Exhibitionismus. Verletzung der Sittlichkeit in Form des Exhibitionierens. *Wiener medizinische Blätter* 15:229–31, 248–50.

1892h. *Ueber "Gesittung." Volkstümliche Vorträge 14*. Vienna: Volksbildungsverein Wien und Umgebung.

1892i. Zur conträren Sexualempfindung. Autobiographie und strafrechtliche Betrachtungen von einem conträr Sexualen. *Wiener medizinische Blätter* 15:7–9, 42–44.

1892j. Paranoia politica. *Wiener medizinische Blätter* 15:757–58, 775–77.

Ps 1893. *Psychopathia sexualis. Mit besonderer Berücksichtigung der conträren Sexualempfindung. Eine klinisch-forensische Studie*. 8th ed. Stuttgart: Ferdinand Enke.

1893a. *Hypnotische Experimente*. Stuttgart: Ferdinand Enke.

1893b. Taschentuch-Fetischismus. (Fortgesetzte Diebstähle von Weibern gehörigen Taschentüchern.) *Wiener medizinische Blätter* 16:209–10.

Ps 1894. *Psychopathia sexualis. Mit besonderer Berücksichtigung der conträren Sexualempfindung. Eine klinisch-forensische Studie*. 9th ed. Stuttgart: Ferdinand Enke.

1894a. *Der Conträrsexuale vor dem Strafrichter. De sodomia ratione sexus punienda. De lege lata et de lege ferenda. Eine Denkschrift*. Leipzig: Franz Deuticke.

1894b. Neuropathia sexualis feminarum. In *Klinisches Handbuch der Harn- und Sexualorgane*, edited by W. Zülzer, vol. 4, pp. 80–103. Leipzig: F.C.W. Vogel.

1894c. Ueber Zoophilia erotica, Bestialität und Zooerastie. *Allgemeine Zeitschrift für Psychiatrie* 50:761–65.

1894d. Unzuchtsdelikte, begangen von einem Schulleiter an seinen Schülerinnen. Alkoholismus chronicus. Fragliche Zurechnungsfähigkeit. *Friedreichs Blätter für gerichtliche Medizin* 45:321–30.

1894e. Zur Aetiologie der conträren Sexualempfindung. *Jahrbücher für Psychiatrie und Neurologie* 12:338–65.

1894f. Zur Psychopathia sexualis. *Jahrbücher für Psychiatrie und neurologie* 12:84–93.

1894g. Ueber Zunahme und Ursache der progressiven Paralyse. *Internationale klinische Rundschau* 8:1273–79.

1895a. *Nervosität und neurasthenische Zustände*. Wien: Alfred Hölder.

1895b. Ueber die Zunahme der progressiven Paralyse, im Hinblick auf die sociologischen Factoren. *Jahrbücher für Psychiatrie und Neurologie* 13:127–43.

1895c. Zur Erklärung der conträren Sexualempfindung. *Jahrbücher für Psychiatrie und Neurologie* 13:1–16.

1895d. Ueber Dementia paralytica. *Allgemeine Wiener medizinische Zeitung* 40: 395–96, 405–6, 415–16, 426–27.

1896a. Paranoia sexualis persecutoria einer Ehefrau. Grundlose Denunciationen des Ehemanns im Sinne der Schändung des eigenen Kindes. Fakultäts- gutachten der Wiener medicinischen Fakultät. *Friedreichs Blätter für gerichtliche Medizin* 47:1–10.

1896b. Ueber Unzucht mit Kindern und Pädophilia erotica. *Friedreichs Blätter für gerichtliche Medizin* 47:261–83.

1896c. Zur Suggestivbehandlung der Hysteria gravis. *Zeitschrift für Hypnotismus* 4:27–31.

1897a. Gerichtliches Gutachten über ein von dem Techniker Paul Gassen erfun- denes Instrument zur Behebung der Impotenz, genannt Erector. *Fried- reichs Blätter für gerichtliche Medizin* 48:217–21.

1897b. Unzucht wider die Natur. Psychische Hermaphrodisie. Fragliche Anfälle krankhafter Bewusstlosigkeit epileptoider Art tempore delicti. *Jahrbücher für Psychiatrie und Neurologie* 14:312–20.

1897c. Gutachten des k. k. Obersten Sanitätsrathes bezüglich der gesetzlichen Regelung des Hypnotismus in Oesterreich. In *Arbeiten aus dem Gesammt- gebiet der Psychiatrie und Neuropathologie*, vol. II, pp. 153–60. Leipzig: Barth.

1897d. Gutachten des k. k. Obersten Sanitätsrathes über die Berechtigung des spiritistischen Vereines zur Anwendung des Hypnotismus. In *Arbeiten aus dem Gesammtgebiet der Psychiatrie und Neuropathologie*, vol. II, pp. 161–64. Leipzig: Barth.

1897e. *Lehrbuch der Psychiatrie auf klinischer Grundlage für practische Ärzte und Studirende.* 6th ed. Stuttgart: Ferdinand Enke.

Ps 1898. *Psychopathia sexualis. Mit besonderer Berücksichtigung der conträren Sexu- alempfindung. Eine klinisch-forensische Studie,* 10th ed. Stuttgart: Ferdi- nand Enke.

1898a. Tabes dorsalis. Klinische Vorlesung. *Allgemeine Wiener medizinische Zei- tung* 43:337–38, 347–48, 359–60, 369–70.

1898b. Ueber Dämmer- und Traumzustände. In *Arbeiten aus dem Gesammtgebiet der Psychiatrie und Neuropathologie*, vol. III, pp. 20–46, 47–68, 69–95. Leipzig: Barth.

1899a. Vorwort. In *Therapie der Anomalien Vita sexualis bei Männern. Mit specieller Berüchsichtigung der Suggestivbehandlung,* by A. Fuchs, pp. 3–4. Stuttgart: Ferdinand Enke.

1899b. *Zur Geschichte der Pest in Wien 1349–1898.* Leipzig: Barth.

1899c. Ueber Unzucht mit Kindern und Pädophilia erotica. In *Arbeiten aus dem Gesammtgebiet der Psychiatrie und Neuropathologie*, vol. IV, pp. 117–27. Leipzig: Barth.

1899d. Beiträge zur Kenntniss des Masochismus. In *Arbeiten aus dem Gesammt- gebiet der Psychiatrie und Neuropathologie*, vol. IV, pp. 127–60. Leipzig: Barth.

1899e. Zum Sadismus. In *Arbeiten aus dem Gesammtgebiet der Psychiatrie und Neu- ropathologie*, vol. IV, pp. 160–69. Leipzig: Barth.

1899f. Zum Fetischismus. In *Arbeiten aus dem Gesammtgebiet der Psychiatrie und Neuropathologie*, vol. IV, pp. 169–74. Leipzig: Barth.

1899g.   Ueber Anaesthesia sexualis congenita. In *Arbeiten aus dem Gesammtgebiet der Psychiatrie und Neuropathologie*, vol. IV, pp. 175–80. Leipzig: Barth.

1899h.   Ueber Hyperaesthesia sexualis. In *Arbeiten aus dem Gesammtgebiet der Psychiatrie und Neuropathologie*, vol. IV, pp. 175–89. Leipzig: Barth.

1899i.   Zur Castratio virorum. In *Arbeiten aus dem Gesammtgebiet der Psychiatrie und Neuropathologie*, vol. IV, pp. 189–92. Leipzig: Barth.

1899j.   Ueber das Zustandekommen der Wollustempfindung und deren Mangel (Anaphrodisie) beim sexuellen Akt. In *Arbeiten aus dem Gesammtgebiet der Psychiatrie und Neuropathologie*, vol. IV, pp. 193–203. Leipzig: Barth.

1900a.   Die Aetiologie der progressiven Paralyse. *Comptes-rendus du XII congrès international de médecine. Moscou, 7 (19)(14 (26) Aout 1897*. Moscow: I. N. Kouchnerev.

1900b.   Drei Conträrsexuale vor Gericht. *Jahrbücher für Psychiatrie und Neurologie* 19:262–82.

1900c.   Flagellatio puerorum als Ausdruck des larvirten Sadismus eines paedophilen Conträrsexualen. Fragliche rechtliche Verantwortlichkeit. *Zeitschrift für Psychiatrie* 58:545–57.

1900d.   Ueber sexuelle Perversionen, welche, in Gestalt von Zwangsvorstellungen und Zwangshandlungen sich äussernd, gerichtlich-medizinisch von Bedeutung sind. *Wiener Medizinische Blätter* 23:584–85.

Ps 1901.   *Psychopathia sexualis. Mit besonderer Berücksichtigung der conträren Sexualempfindung. Eine medicinisch-gerichtliche Studie.* 11th ed. Stuttgart: Ferdinand Enke.

1901a.   Neue Studien auf dem Gebiete der Homosexualität. *Jahrbuch für sexuelle Zwischenstufen* 3:1–36.

1901b.   Ueber sexuelle Perversionen. In *Die deutsche Klinik am Eingang des 20. Jahrhunderts in akademischen Vorlesungen*, edited by E. von Leyden and F. Klemperer, vol. 6, pp. 113–54. Berlin: Urban und Schwarzenberg.

1902a.   *Psychosis Menstrualis. Eine klinisch-forensische Studie.* Stuttgart: Ferdinand Enke.

1902b.   Zur "Vera"-Literatur. *Die Zeit*, 29 oktober.

Ps 1903.   Edited by H. Gugl and A. Stichl. *Psychopathia sexualis. Mit besonderer Berücksichtigung der konträren Sexualempfindung. Eine medicinisch-gerichtliche Studie für Ärzte und Juristen.* 12th ed. Stuttgart: Ferdinand Enke.

Ps 1906.   Edited by F. J. Rebman. *Psychopathia Sexualis. With especial reference to the Antipathic Sexual Instinct. A Medico-Forensic Study.* New York: Medical Art Agency.

Ps 1907.   Edited by A. Fuchs. *Psychopathia sexualis. Mit besonderer Berücksichtigung der konträren Sexualempfindung. Eine medicinisch-gerichtliche Studie für Ärzte und Juristen.* 13th ed. Stuttgart: Ferdinand Enke.

Ps 1912.   Edited by A. Fuchs. *Psychopathia sexualis. Mit besonderer Berücksichtigung der konträren Sexualempfindung. Eine medicinisch-gerichtliche Studie für Ärzte und Juristen.* 14th ed. Stuttgart: Ferdinand Enke.

Ps 1918.   Edited by A. Fuchs. *Psychopathia sexualis. Mit besonderer Berücksichtigung der konträren Sexualempfindung. Eine medicinisch-gerichtliche Studie für Ärzte und Juristen.* 15th ed. Stuttgart: Ferdinand Enke.

Ps 1924.   Edited by A. Moll. *Psychopathia sexualis. Mit besonderer Berücksichtigung der konträren Sexualempfindung. Eine medicinisch-gerichtliche Studie für Ärzte und Juristen.* 16th and 17th eds. Stuttgart: Ferdinand Enke.

Ps 1937. Edited by A. Hartwich. *Die Verirrungen des Geschlechtslebens (Perversionen und Anomalien).* Zürich: A. Müller, Rüschlikon.

Ps 1939. Edited by F. J. Rebman. *Psychopathia Sexualis. A Medico-Forensic Study.* New York: Pioneer Publications.

Ps 1965. Edited by F. S. Klaff. *Psychopathia sexualis.* New York: Bell Publishing Company.

Ps 1999. Edited by B. King. *Psychopathia Sexualis.* Burbank: Bloat.

WORKS CITED

Aarts, J. 1981. Hyena's, panters en andere vrouwen. Duitse seksuologen in het fin-de-siècle en hun receptie van Sade. *Bzzlletin* 83:29–36.

Ackerknecht, E. H. 1986. Private institutions in the genesis of psychiatry. *Bulletin of the History of Medicine* 60:387–95.

Akademisches Jubiläum des Hofrathes Freiherrn von Krafft-Ebing. 1902–03. *Psychiatrisch-neurologische Wochenschrift* 40:1–2.

Allerhand, J. 1903. Nekrolog R. v. Krafft-Ebing. *Ärztliche Central-Zeitung,* 17–22.

Barker-Benfield, G. J. 1973. The Spermatic Economy: A Nineteenth-Century View of Sexuality. In *The American Family in Social-Historical Perspective,* edited by M. Gordon, pp. 374–402. New York: St. Martin's Press.

Baumeister, R. F. 1986. *Identity: Cultural Change and the Struggle for Self.* New York: Oxford University Press.

Bech. H. 1999. Citysex. Representing Lust in Public. In *Love and Eroticism,* edited by M. Featherstone, pp. 215–41. London: Sage.

Benedikt, M. 1894. *Hypnotismus und Suggestion. Eine klinisch-psychologische Studie.* Leipzig: Breitstein.

————. 1906. *Aus meinem Leben. Erinnerungen und Erörterungen.* Vienna: Carl Konegen, Ernst Stülpnagel.

Berger, P. 1892. *Führer durch die Privatheilanstalten Deutschlands, Österreichs und der Schweiz. Mit ausführliche Darstellungen der modernen Behandlungsmethoden zum Hausgebrauch für Ärzte und Laien.* Berlin: Steinitz.

Berner, P. et al. 1983. *Zur Geschichte der Psychiatrie in Wien.* Vienna: Christian Brandstätter.

Berrios, G. E. 1995. Mood Disorders. In *A History of Clinical Psychiatry. The Origin and History of Psychiatric Disorders,* edited by G. E. Berrios and R. Porter, pp. 384–420. London: Athlone.

Berrios, G. E. and R. Porter, eds. 1995. *A History of Clinical Psychiatry: The Origin and Histories of Psychiatric Disorders.* London: Athlone.

Birken, L. 1988. *Consuming Desire: Sexual Science and the Emergence of a Culture of Abundance, 1871–1914.* Ithaca, N.Y.: Cornell University Press.

Bleys, R. C. 1996. *The Geography of Perversion: Male-to-Male Sexual Behavior Outside the West and the Ethnographic Imagination, 1750–1918.* London: Cassell.

Brecher, E. M. 1969. *The Sex Researchers.* Boston: Little and Brown.

Bristow, J. 1997. *Sexuality.* London: Routledge.

Brunner, A., and H. Sulzenbacher. 1998. Donauwalzer—Herrenwahl. Schwule Geschichte der Donaumetropole vom Mittelalter bis zur Gegenwart. In *Schwules*

Wien. Reiseführer durch die Donau-metropole, edited by A. Brunner and H. Sulzenbacher, pp. 9–108. Vienna: Promedia.

Buckley, J. H. 1984. *The Turning Key: Autobiography and the Subjective Impulse Since 1800*. Cambridge: Harvard University Press.

Bullough, V. L. 1994. *Science in the Bedroom: A History of Sex Research*. New York: Basic Books.

Bullough, V. L., and B. Bullough. 1977. *Sin, Sickness, & Sanity: A History of Sexual Attitudes*. New York: Garland, New American Library.

Carr, D. 1997. Narrative and the Real World: An Argument for Continuity. In *Memory, Identity, Community: The Idea of Narrative in the Human Sciences*, edited by L. P. Hinchman and S. K. Hinchman, pp. 7–25. Albany: State University of New York Press.

Castel, R. 1976. *L'ordre psychiatrique. L'age d'or de l'aliénisme*. Paris: Minuit.

Chauncey, G. 1982–83. From Sexual Inversion to Homosexuality: Medicine and the Changing Conceptualization of Female Deviance. *Salmagundi* 58–59: 114–46.

Comité für Befreiung der Homosexualen vom Strafgesetz. 1899. *Aufruf an alle Gebildeten und edelgesinnten Menschen!* Berlin: Comité für Befreiung der Homosexualen vom Strafgesetz.

Coward, D. 1987. The Sublimations of a Fetishist: Restif de la Bretonne (1734–1806). In *'Tis Nature's Fault: Unauthorized Sexuality During the Enlightenment*, edited by R. B. Maccubbin, pp. 98–108. Cambridge: Cambridge University Press.

Darnton, R. 1990. Don Juanism from Below. In *Don Giovanni: Myths of Seduction and Betrayal*, edited by J. Miller, pp. 20–35. New York: Schocken.

Davidson, A. I. 1987. Sex and the Emergence of Sexuality. *Critical Inquiry* 14:16–48.

———. 1990. Closing Up the Corpses: Diseases of Sexuality and the Emergence of the Psychiatric Style of Reasoning. In *Meaning and Method: Essays in Honor of Hilary Putnam*, edited by G. Boolos, pp. 295–325. Cambridge: Cambridge University Press.

Degler, C. N. 1973. What Ought to Be and What Was: Women's Sexuality in the 19th Century. In *The American Family in Social-Historical Perspective*, edited by M. Gordon, pp. 403–25. New York: St. Martin's Press.

de Joux, O. 1893. *Die Enterbten des Liebesglücks. Ein Beitrag zur Seelenkunde*. Leipzig: Max Spohr.

Dekker, R. M. 1980. De fatale voet in de literatuur van de negentiende eeuw. *De Gids* 143:420–28.

Delon, M. 1987. The Priest, the Philosopher, and Homosexuality in Enlightenment France. In *'Tis Nature's Fault: Unauthorized Sexuality During the Enlightenment*, edited by R. B. Maccubbin, pp. 122–31. Cambridge: Cambridge University Press.

Derks, P. 1990. *Die Schande der heiligen Päderastie. Homosexualität und Öffentlichkeit in der deutschen Literatur 1750–1850*. Berlin: rosa Winkel.

de Swaan, A. 1982. Historische psychopathologie en de sociogenese van het moderne karakter. In *Geschiedenis, psychologie en mentaliteit*, edited by D. Damen, pp. 63–76. Amsterdam: Skript.

Dornblüth, O. 1902. Richard von Krafft-Ebing. *Frankfurter Zeitung* (25 december).

Dörner, K. 1969. *Bürger und Irre. Zur Sozialgeschichte und Wissenschaftssoziologie der Psychiatrie*. Frankfurt am Main: Europäische Verlagsanstalt.

Dowbiggin, I. 1991. *Inheriting Madness: Professionalization and Psychiatric Knowledge in Nineteenth-Century France*. Berkeley: University of California Press.

Duc, A. [M. Wettstein-Adelt]. 1976. *Sind es Frauen?* Berlin: Amazonen Frauen-Verlag.

Eder, F. X. 1990. Erotisierendes Wissen. Zur Geschichte der 'Sexualisierung' im Wiener Fin de Siècle. In *Erotik, Versuch einer Annäherung. Ausstellungskatalog des Historischen Museums der Stadt Wien*, pp. 20–28. Wien: Historisches Museum.

———. 1993. "Diese Theorie ist sehr delikat . . ." Zur Sexualisierung der Wiener Moderne. In *Die Wiener Jahrhundertwende. Einflüsse, Umwelt, Wirkungen*, edited by J. Nautz and R. Vahrenkamp, pp. 159–78. Vienna: Löcker Verlag.

———. 1999. Sexual Cultures in Germany and Austria, 1700–2000. In *Sexual Cultures in Europe: National Histories*, edited by F. X. Eder, L. A. Hall, and G. Hekma, pp. 138–72. Manchester: Manchester University Press.

Egan, S. 1984. *Patterns of Experience in Autobiography*. Chapel Hill: University of North Carolina Press.

Elias, N. 1969. *Über den Prozess der Zivilisation*. Bern: Francke.

Ellenberger, H. F. 1970. *The Discovery of the Unconscious: The History and Evolution of Dynamic Psychiatry*. New York: Basic Books.

———. 1993. Moritz Benedikt (1835–1920): An Insufficiently Appreciated Pioneer of Psychoanalysis. In *Beyond the Unconscious: Essays of Henri F. Ellenberger in the History of Psychiatry*, edited by M. S. Micale, pp. 104–18. Princeton: Princeton University Press.

Eulenburg, A. 1903. Nekrologe. Krafft-Ebing. *Deutsche medicinische Wochenschrift* 29:39.

Everard, M. 1994. *Ziel en zinnen. Over liefde en lust tussen vrouwen in de tweede helft van de achttiende eeuw*. Groningen: Historische Uitgeverij.

Faderman, L. 1981. *Surpassing the Love of Men: Romantic Friendship and Love between Women from the Renaissance to the Present*. New York: Morrow.

Farley, J. 1982. *Gametes and Spores: Ideas about Sexual Reproduction, 1750–1914*. Baltimore: John Hopkins University Press.

Featherstone, M., ed. 1999. *Love and Eroticism*. London: Sage.

Festschrift Freiherr von Krafft-Ebing. 1902. *Psychiatrisches Centralblatt* 20.

Fischer, M. 1935. Richard von Krafft-Ebing. In *Badische Biographien*, edited by A. Krieger and R. Obser, vol. IV, pp. 317–25. Heidelberg: Winter.

Fleishman, A. 1983. *Figures of Autobiography: The Language of Self-Writing in Victorian and Modern England*. Berkeley: University of California Press.

Forel, A. 1935. *Rückblick auf mein Leben*. Zürich: Europaverlag.

Fossel, V. 1913. *Geschichte der medizinischen Fakultät in Graz. Festschrift zur Feier des 50-jährigen Bestandes 1863–1913*. Graz: Leuschner und Lubinsky.

Foucault, M. 1961. *Folie et déraison. Histoire de la folie a l'âge classique*. Paris: Plon.

———. 1975. *Surveiller et Punir. Naissance de la prison*. Paris: Gallimard.

———. 1976. *Histoire de la sexualité I. La volonté de savoir*. Paris: Gallimard.

———. 1978. About the Concept of the "Dangerous Individual" in 19th Century Legal Psychiatry. *International Journal of Law and Psychiatry* 1:1–18.

Fout, J. C., ed. 1992. *Forbidden History: The State, Society, and the Regulation of Sexuality in Modern Europe*. Chicago: University of Chicago Press.

Freiheit, Liebe Menschlichkeit. Ein Manifest des Geistes von hervorragenden Zeitgenossen. 1893. Berlin: J. van Groningen.

Fuchs, A. 1902. Richard Freiherr v. Krafft-Ebing. Ein Beitrag zur Geschichte der Psychiatrie und Neurologie in Wien. *Wiener klinische Rundschau* 17:243–46, 263–65, 281–84.

———. 1903. Hofrat Richard Freiherr von Krafft-Ebing. *Münchener medizinische Wochenschrift* 50:167.

———. 1921. Richard Freiherr von Krafft-Ebing. In *Deutsche Irrenärzte. Einzelbilder ihres Lebens und Wirkens*, edited by Th. Kirchhoff, vol. II, pp. 173–83. Berlin: Springer.

Fuchs, H. 1903. *Richard Wagner und die Homosexualität*. Berlin: Barsdorf.

Gauld, A. 1992. *A History of Hypnotism*. Cambridge: Cambridge University Press.

Gay, P. 1984. *Education of the Senses*. Vol. 1, *The Bourgeois Experience: Victoria to Freud*. New York: Oxford University Press.

———. 1986. *The Tender Passion*. Vol. 2, *The Bourgeois Experience: Victoria to Freud*. New York: Oxford University Press.

———. 1988. *Freud. A Life for Our Time*. New York: Norton.

———. 1995. *The Naked Heart*. Vol. 4, *The Bourgeois Experience: Victoria to Freud*. New York: Norton.

Geertz, C. 1973. Thick Description: Toward an Interpretive Theory of Culture. In *The Interpretation of Cultures: Selected Essays*, pp. 3–30. New York: Basic Books.

Gerard, K., and G. Hekma, eds. 1989. *The Pursuit of Sodomy: Male Homosexuality in Renaissance and Enlightenment Europe*. New York: Harrington Park Press.

Gergen, K. J., and M. M. Gergen. 1997. Narratives of the Self. In *Memory, Identity, Community: The Idea of Narrative in the Human Sciences*, edited by L. P. Hinchman and S. K. Hinchman, pp. 161–84. Albany: State University of New York Press.

Giddens, A. 1991. *Modernity and Self-Identity: Self and Society in the Late Modern Age*. Cambridge: Polity Press.

———. 1992. *The Transformation of Intimacy: Sexuality, Love and Eroticism in Modern Times*. Cambridge: Polity Press.

Gilbert, A. N. 1985. Conceptions of Homosexuality and Sodomy in Western History. In *The Gay Past: A Collection of Historical Essays*, edited by S. J. Licata and R. P. Petersen, pp. 57–68. Binghamton, N.Y.: Harrington Park Press.

Gilman, S. L. 1985. *Difference and Pathology. Stereotypes of Sexuality, Race, and Madness*. Ithaca, N.Y.: Cornell University Press.

Gilman, S. L., and E. Chamberlain, eds. 1985. *Degeneration: The Dark Side of Progress*. New York: Columbia University Press.

Goldstein, J. E. 1987. *Console and Classify: The French Psychiatric Profession in the Nineteenth Century*. Cambridge: Cambridge University Press.

Gosling, F. G. 1987. *Before Freud: Neurasthenia and the American Medical Community 1870–1910*. Urbana: University of Illinois Press.

Grazer Tagesblatt. 1902. (December 24).

Greenberg, D. F. 1988. *The Construction of Homosexuality*. Chicago: University of Chicago Press.

Gröger, H., E. Gabriel, and S. Kasper, eds. 1997. *On the History of Psychiatry in Vienna*. Vienna: Christian Brandstätter.

Gugl, H., R. von Krafft-Ebing, and A. Stichl. 1886. *Prospect des Sanatoriums "Maria-grün" nächst Graz*. Graz: Verlag des Sanatoriums "Mariagrün."

Gugl, H., and A. Stichl. 1892. *Neuropathologische Studien*. Stuttgart: Ferdinand Enke.

Güse, H. G., and N. Schmacke. 1976. *Psychiatrie zwischen bürgerliche Revolution und Faschismus*. Kronberg: Athenäum.

Haberda, A., ed. 1927. *Eduard von Hoffmanns Lehrbuch der gerichtlichen Medizin*. Berlin: Urban & Schwarzenberg.

Hacker, H. 1987. *Frauen und Freundinnen. Studien zur "weiblichen Homosexualität" am Beispiel Österreich 1870–1938*. Weinheim: Beltz Verlag.

Hacker, H., and M. Lang. 1986. Jenseits der Geschlechter, zwischen ihnen. Homosexualitäten im Wien der Jahrhunderwende. In *Das lila Wien um 1900. Zur Ästhetik der Homosexualitäten*, edited by N. Bei et al., pp. 8–18. Vienna: Promedia.

Hacking, I. 1995. *Rewriting the Soul: Multiple Personality and the Sciences of Memory*. Princeton: Princeton University Press.

Hahn, A. 1982. Zur Soziologie der Beichte und anderer Formen institutionalisierter Bekenntnisse: Selbstthematisierung und Zivilisationsprozess. *Kölner Zeitschrift für Soziologie und Sozialpsychologie* 34:408–34.

Hall, L. A. 1992. "Forbidden by God, Despised by Men: Masturbation, Medical Warnings, Moral Panic and Manhood in Britain, 1850–1950." *Journal of the History of Sexuality* 2:365–87.

———. 1994. "The English Have Hot-Water Bottles": The Morganatic Marriage between Medicine and Sexology in Britain Since William Acton. In *Sexual Knowledge, Sexual Science: The History of Attitudes to Sexuality*, edited by R. Porter and M. Teich, pp. 350–66. Cambridge: Cambridge University Press.

———. 1999. Sexual Cultures in Britain: Some Persisting Themes. In *Sexual Cultures in Europe: National Histories*, edited by F. X. Eder, L. A. Hall, and G. Hekma, pp. 29–52. Manchester: Manchester University Press.

Hansen, B. 1992. American Physician's "Discovery" of Homosexuals, 1880–1900: A New Diagnosis in a Changing Society. In *Framing Disease: Studies in Cultural History*, C. E. Rosenberg and J. Golden, pp. 104–33. New Brunswick: Rutgers University Press.

Harris, R. 1991. *Murders and Madness: Medicine, Law, and Society in the Fin de Siècle*. Oxford: Oxford University Press.

Hauser, R. I. 1989. Richard von Krafft-Ebing. Hypnose als Intervention. In *Wunderblock. Eine Geschichte der modernen Seele*, edited by J. Clair, C. Pickler, and W. Pircher, pp. 317–20. Vienna: Löcker Verlag.

———. 1992. *Sexuality, Neurasthenia and the Law: Richard von Krafft-Ebing (1840–1902)*. London: Dissertation University College, University of London.

———. 1994. Krafft-Ebing's Psychological Understanding of Sexual Behaviour. In *Sexual Knowledge, Sexual Science: The History of Attitudes to Sexuality*, R. Porter and M. Teich, pp. 210–27. Cambridge: Cambridge University Press.

Hekma, G. 1983. Social Philosophies, Social Practices: Some Preludes to the Homosexual. In *Among Men, Among Women*, edited by M. Aerts et al., pp. 258–67. Amsterdam: University of Amsterdam.

———. 1985. Geschiedenis der seksuologie, sociologie van seksualiteit. *Sociologische Gids* 5–6:352–70.

————. 1987. *Homoseksualiteit, een medische reputatie. De uitdoktering van de homo-seksueel in negentiende-eeuws Nederland.* Amsterdam: SUA.

————, ed. 1992. *Honderd jaar homoseksuelen. Documenten over de uitdoktering van homoseksualiteit.* Amsterdam: Het Spinhuis.

Herzer, M. 1997. Opposition im 19. Jahrhundert. In *Goodbye to Berlin? 100 Jahre Schwulenbewegung*, pp. 27–34. Berlin: rosa Winkel.

Heumakers, A. 1988. Sade, een pessimistische libertijn. In *Van Sappho tot de Sade. Momenten in de geschiedenis van de seksualiteit*, edited by J. Bremmer, pp. 100–14. Amsterdam: Wereldbibliotheek.

Hill, A. 1994. "May the Doctor Advise Extramarital Intercourse?": Medical De-bates on Sexual Abstinence in Germany, c. 1900. In *Sexual Knowledge, Sexual Science: The History of Attitudes to Sexuality*, edited by R. Porter and M. Teich, pp. 284–302. Cambridge: Cambridge University Press.

Hinchman, L. P., and S. K. Hinchman, eds. 1997. *Memory, Identity, Community: The Idea of Narrative in the Human Sciences.* Albany: State University of New York Press.

Hirschmüller, A. 1989. *The Life and Work of Joseph Breuer: Physiology and Psychoan-alysis.* New York: New York University Press.

————. 1991. *Freuds Begegnung mit der Psychiatrie. Von der Hirnmythologie zur Neu-rosenlehre.* Tübingen: Diskord.

Höflechner, W. 1975. Leopold Sacher-Masoch Ritter von Kronenthal und die Universität Graz. In *Publikationen aus dem Archiv der Universität Graz*, edited by H. Wiesflecker, vol. 4, pp. 125–38. Graz: Akademische Druck und Verlagsan-stalt.

Honegger, C. 1991. *Die Ordnung der Geschlechter. Die Wissenschaften vom Menschen und das Weib.* Frankfurt: Campus Verlag.

Hutter, J. 1993. The Social Construction of Homosexuals in the Nineteenth Cen-tury: The Shift from the Sin to the Influence of Medicine on Criminalizing Sod-omy in Germany. *Journal of Homosexuality* 24(3–4):73–93.

Jacyna, L. S. 1982. Somatic Theories of Mind and the Interests of Medicine in Brit-ain, 1850–1879. *Medical History* 26:233–58.

Jahresbericht Wissenschaftlich-humanitäres Komitee 1902–1903. 1903. *Jahrbuch für sexuelle Zwischenstufen* 5:1292–97.

Janik, A. 1985. *Essays on Wittgenstein and Weininger.* Amsterdam: Rodopi.

Janik, A., and S. Toulmin. 1973. *Wittgenstein's Vienna.* New York: Simon & Schuster.

Johnson, W. S. 1979. *Living in Sin: The Victorian Sexual Revolution.* Chicago: Nelson-Hall.

Johnston, W. 1972. *The Austrian Mind: An Intellectual and Social History, 1848–1938.* Berkeley: University of California Press.

Jordanova, L. J. 1986. Naturalizing the Family: Literature and the Bio-Medical Sci-ences in the Late Eighteenth Century. In *Languages of Nature: Critical Essays on Science and Literature*, edited by L. J. Jordanova, pp. 86–116. London: Free Association Books.

Jusek, K. 1992. *Auf der Suche nach der Verlorenen. Die Prostitutionsdebatten im Wien der Jahrhundertwende.* Groningen: Dissertatie Rijksuniversiteit Groningen.

Karplus, [J. P.] 1903. Nekrologe Krafft-Ebing. *Wiener klinische Wochenschrift* 16: 21–22.

Kaschuba, W. 1993. German Bürgerlichkeit After 1800: Culture as Symbolic Practice. In *Bourgeois Society in Nineteenth-Century Europe*, edited by J. Kocka and A. Mitchell, pp. 392–422. Oxford: Berg.

Katz, J. N. 1995. *The Invention of Heterosexuality*. New York: Penguin.

Kearney, P. J. 1993. *A History of Erotic Literature*. London: Dorset Press.

Keilson-Lauritz, M. 1997. *Die Geschichte der eigenen Geschichte. Literatur und Literaturkritik in den Anfängen der Schwulenbewegung*. Berlin: rosa Winkel.

Keilson-Lauritz, M., and F. Pfäfflin. 1999. "Unzüchtig im Sinne des Paragraphen 184 des Strafgesetzbuchs." Drei Urteilstexte und ein Einstellungsbeschluss. *Forum. Homosexualität und Literatur* 34:33–98.

Kennedy, H. 1988. *Ulrichs: The Life and Works of Karl Heinrich Ulrichs. Pioneer of the Modern Gay Movement*. Boston: Alyson.

Kerby, A. P. 1997. The Language of the Self. In *Memory, Identity, Community: The Idea of Narrative in the Human Sciences*, L. P. Hinchman and S. K. Hinchman, pp. 125–42. Albany: State University of New York Press.

Kershner, R. B. 1986. Degeneration: The Explanatory Nightmare. *The Georgian Review* 40:416–44.

King, D. 1981. Gender Confusions: Psychological and Psychiatric Conceptions of Transvestism and Transsexualism. In *The Making of the Modern Homosexual*, edited by K. Plummer, pp. 155–83. London: Hutchinson.

Klabundt, P. 1994. Psychopathia sexualis—die ärztliche Konstruktion der sexuellen Perversionen zwischen 1869 und 1914. *MedGG* 13:107–30.

Kohl, F. 1997. Die "Illenauer Psychiater-Schule"—Zur Bedeutung der Modellanstalt als Ausbildungsstätte. *Psychiatrische Praxis* 24:10–14.

Kornfeld, S. 1903. Nekrolog R. von Krafft-Ebing. *Klinisch-therapeutische Wochenschrift*, 22–25.

Koschorke, A. 1988. *Leopold von Sacher-Masoch. Die Inszenierung einer Perversion*. Munich: Piper.

Kraepelin, E. 1983. *Lebenserinnerungen*. Heidelberg: Springer Verlag.

Krafft-Ebing, R[ainer]. 2000. *Richard von Krafft-Ebing. Eine Studienreise durch Sudeuropa 1869/70*. Graz: Leykam Buchverlag.

Kraus, K. 1970. Irrenhaus Österreich. In *Sittlichkeit und Kriminalität*, pp. 75–93. Munich: Kösel.

Kuzniar, A. A., ed. 1996. *Outing Goethe & His Age*. Stanford: Stanford University Press.

Laehr, H. 1882. *Die Heil- und Pflege-Anstalten für Psychisch-Kranke des deutschen Sprachgebietes*. Berlin: Reimer.

———. 1907. *Die Anstalten für Psychisch-Kranke in Deutschland, Deutsch-Österreich, der Schweiz und den baltischen Ländern*. Berlin: Reimer.

Laehr, H., and M. Lewald. 1899. *Die Heil- und Pflege-Anstalten für Psychisch-Kranke des deutschen Sprachgebietes am 1 Januar 1898*. Berlin: Reimer.

Lanteri-Laura, G. 1979. *Lectures des perversions. Histoire de leur appropriation médicale*. Paris: Masson.

Laqueur, T. 1989. Bodies, Details, and the Humanitarian Narrative. In *The New Cultural History*, edited by L. Hunt, pp. 176–204. Berkeley: University of California Press.

———. 1990. *Making Sex: Body and Gender from the Greeks to Freud*. Cambridge: Harvard University Press.

———. 1992. Sexual Desire and the Market Economy During the Industrial Revolution. In *Discourses of Sexuality: From Aristotle to AIDS*, edited by D.C. Stanton, pp. 185–215. Ann Arbor: University of Michigan Press.

Laurence, J. R., and C. Perry. 1988. *Hypnosis, Will, and Memory*. New York: The Guilford Press.

Le Rider, J. 1985. *Der Fall Otto Weininger. Wurzeln des Antifeminismus und Anti-Semitismus*. Vienna: Löcker Verlag.

———. 1990. *Modernité viennoise et crises de l'identité*. Paris: Presses Universitaires de France.

Le Rider, J., and N. Leser, eds. 1984. *Otto Weininger. Werk und Wirkung*. Vienna: Österreichische Bundesverlag.

Lesky, E. 1965. *Die Wiener medizinische Schule im 19. Jahrhundert*. Graz: Hermann Böhlhaus.

Luft, D. S. 1990. Science and Irrationalism in Freud's Vienna. *Modern Austrian Literature* 23:89–97.

Luhmann, N. 1982. *Liebe als Passion. Zur Codierung von Intimität*. Frankfurt am Main: Suhrkamp Verlag.

Lynch, M. 1985. "Here Is Adhesiveness": From Friendship to Homosexuality. *Victorian Studies* 29:67–96.

Lyons, J. O. 1978. *The Invention of the Self: The Hinge of Consciousness in the Eighteenth Century*. Carbondale: Southern Illinois University Press.

MacIntyre, A. 1997. The Virtues, the Unity of a Human Life, and the Concept of a Tradition. In *Memory, Identity, Community: The Idea of Narrative in the Human Sciences*, edited by L. P. Hinchman and S. K. Hinchman, pp. 241–63. Albany: State University of New York Press.

Mak, G. 1997. *Mannelijke vrouwen. Over grenzen van sekse in de negentiende eeuw*. Amsterdam: Boom.

Marcus, S. 1966. *The Other Victorians: A Study of Sexuality and Pornography in Mid-Nineteenth-Century England*. New York: Meridian.

Marshall, J. 1981. Pansies, Perverts and Macho Men: Changing Conceptions of Male Homosexuality. In *The Making of the Modern Homosexual*, edited by K. Plummer, pp. 133–54. London: Hutchinson.

Marx, O. 1970. Nineteenth-Century Medical Psychology. *Isis* 61:355–70.

Mason, M. 1994. *The Making of Victorian Sexuality*. Oxford: Oxford University Press.

Matlock, J. 1993. Masquerading Women, Pathologized Men: Cross-Dressing, Fetishism, and the Theory of Perversion, 1882–1935. In *Fetishism as Cultural Discourse*, edited by E. Apter and W. Pietz, pp. 31–61. Ithaca, N.Y.: Cornell University Press.

Maudsley, H. 1874. *Body and Mind*. New York: Appleton.

McGrath, W. 1974. *Dionysian Art and Populist Politics in Austria*. New Haven: Yale University Press.

McGuire, W., ed. 1989. *Analytical Psychology: Notes of the Seminar Given in 1925 by C. G. Jung*. New York: Routledge.

McLaren, A. 1983. *A History of Contraception from Antiquity to the Present Day*. Oxford: Blackwell.

———. 1997. *The Trials of Masculinity: Policing Sexual Boundaries 1870–1930*. Chicago: University of Chicago Press.

Micale, M. S. 1990. Hysteria and Its Historiography: The Future Perspective. *History of Psychiatry* 1:33–124.

———. 1995. *Approaching Hysteria: Disease and Its Interpretations*. Princeton: Princeton University Press.

Moll, A. 1903a. Nekrolog. Krafft-Ebing. *Deutsche Medizinische Press* 2:14–15.

———. 1903b. Krafft-Ebing. *Die Zukunft* 43:463–68.

———. 1936. *Ein Leben als Arzt der Seele. Erinnerungen*. Dresden: Carl Reissner.

Mort, F. 1987. *Dangerous Sexualities: Medico-Moral Politics in England Since 1830*. London: Routledge, Kegan Paul.

Morton, F. 1980. *A Nervous Splendour: Vienna 1888/1889*. London: Weidenfeld and Nicolson.

Mosse, G. L. 1985. *Nationalism and Sexuality. Respectability and Abnormal Sexuality in Modern Europe*. New York: Howard Fertig.

———. 1988. *The Culture of Western Europe: The Nineteenth and Twentieth Centuries*. Boulder, Colo.: Westview Press.

———. 1991. Fin-de-siècle. Challenge and Response. *Bijdragen en mededelingen betreffende de geschiedenis der Nederlanden* 4:573–80.

Müller, K. 1991. *Aber in meinem Herzen sprach eine Stimme so laut. Homosexuelle Autobiographien und medizinische Pathographien im neunzehnten Jahrhundert*. Berlin: rosa Winkel.

Novitz, D. 1997. Art, Narrative, and Human Nature. In *Memory, Identity, Community: The Idea of Narrative in the Human Sciences*, L. P. Hinchman and S. K. Hinchman, pp. 143–60. Albany: State University of New York Press.

Noyes, J. 1997. *The Mastery of Submission: Inventions of Masochism*. Ithaca, N.Y.: Cornell University Press.

Nye, R. A. 1984. *Crime, Madness, and Politics in Modern France: The Medical Concept of National Decline*. Princeton: Princeton University Press.

———. 1989. Sex Difference and Male Homosexuality in French Medical Discourse, 1830–1930. *Bulletin of the History of Medicine* 63:32–51.

———. 1991. The History of Sexuality in Context: National Sexological Traditions. *Science in Context* 4:387–406.

———. 1993. The Medical Origins of Sexual Fetishism. In *Fetishism as Cultural Discourse*, edited by E. Apter and W. Pietz, pp. 13–30. Ithaca, N.Y.: Cornell University Press.

———. 1999. Sex and Sexuality in France Since 1800. In *Sexual Cultures in Europe: National Histories*, edited by F. X. Eder, L. A. Hall, and G. Hekma, pp. 91–113. Manchester: Manchester University Press.

Obituary Freiherr Von Krafft-Ebing, MD. 1903. *British Medical Journal*, 53.

O'Brien, P. 1983. The Kleptomania Diagnosis: Bourgeois Women and Theft in Late Nineteenth-Century France. *Journal of Social History* (fall): 65–77.

Oosterhuis, H., and H. Kennedy, eds. 1991. *Homosexuality and Male Bonding in Pre-Nazi Germany: The Youth Movement, the Gay Movement, and Male Bonding Before Hitler's Rise*. New York: Hayworth Press.

Pagel, J. 1902. Richard Freiherr von Krafft-Ebing. *Jahresbericht über die Leistungen und Fortschritte in der gesamten Medizin* 37:418.

Perrot, M. ed. 1990. *From the Fires of Revolution to the Great War*, Vol. IV, A History of Private Life. Cambridge: The Belknap Press of Harvard University Press.

Peterson, L. H. 1986. *Victorian Autobiography: The Tradition of Self-Interpretation*. New Haven: Yale University Press.

Pettinger, A. 1993. Why Fetish? *New Foundations. A Journal of Culture/Theory/Politics* 19:83–93.

Pick, D. 1989. *Faces of Degeneration: A European Disorder 1848–1918*. Cambridge: Cambridge University Press.

Pilkington, A. E. 1986. "Nature" as Ethical Norm in the Enlightenment. In *Languages of Nature: Critical Essays on Science and Literature*, edited by L. J. Jordanova, pp. 51–85. London: Free Association Books.

Plummer, K. 1995. *Telling Sexual Stories: Power, Change and Social Worlds*. London: Routledge.

———, ed. 1981. *The Making of the Modern Homosexual*. London: Hutchinson.

Porter, R. 1985. The Patient's View. Doing Medical History from Below. *Theory and Society* 14:175–98.

———. 1987. "The Secrets of Generation Display'd:" Aristotle's Master-piece in Eighteenth-Century England. In *'Tis Nature's Fault: Unauthorized Sexuality During the Enlightenment*, edited by R. B. Maccubbin, pp. 1–21. Cambridge: Cambridge University Press.

———. 1990. Libertinism and Promiscuity. In *Don Giovanni: Myths of Seduction and Betrayal*, edited by J. Miller, pp. 1–19. New York: Schocken.

———, ed. 1997. *Rewriting the Self: Histories from the Middle Ages to the Present*. London: Routledge.

Porter, R., and L. Hall. 1995. *The Facts of Life: The Creation of Sexual Knowledge in Britain, 1650–1950*. New Haven: Yale University Press.

Porter, R., and M. Teich, eds. 1994. *Sexual Knowledge, Sexual Science: The History of Attitudes to Sexuality*. Cambridge: Cambridge University Press.

Portig, G. 1894. *Schiller in seinem Verhältnis zur Freundschaft und Liebe sowie in seinem inneren Verhältnis zu Goethe*. Hamburg: Rowohlt.

Prosser, J. 1998. Transsexuals and the Transsexologists: Inversion and the Emergence of Transsexual Subjectivity. In *Sexology in Culture: Labelling Bodies and Desires*, edited by L. Bland and L. Doan, pp. 116–31. Cambridge: Polity Press.

Pynsent, R. 1989. *Decadence and Innovation. Austro-Hungarian Life and Art at the Turn of the Century*. London: Weidenfeld and Nicholson.

Rabinbach, A. 1990. *The Human Motor: Energy, Fatigue, and the Origins of Modernity*. New York: Basic Books.

Radkau, J. 1998. *Das Zeitalter der Nervosität. Deutschland zwischen Bismarck und Hitler*. Munich: Carl Hanser.

Rey, M. 1987. Parisian Homosexuals Create a Lifestyle, 1700–1750: The Police Archives. In *'Tis Nature's Fault: Unauthorized Sexuality During the Enlightenment*, edited by R. B. Maccubbin, pp. 179–91. Cambridge: Cambridge University Press.

Risse, G. B., and J. H. Warner. 1992. Reconstructing Clinical Activities: Patient Records in Medical History. *Social History of Medicine* 5:183–205.

Robinson, P. 1976. *The Modernization of Sex: Havelock Ellis, Alfred Kinsey, William Masters and Virginia Johnson*. New York: Harper & Row.

Roemer, A. 1892. Das Sittengesetz vor dem Richterstuhl einer ärztlichen Autorität. In *Streitfragen. Wissenschaftliches Fachorgan der deutschen Sittlichkeitsvereine* 1: 5–15.

Roodenburg, H. 1988. "Venus Minsieke Gasthuis." Over seksuele attitudes in de achttiende-eeuwse Republiek. In *Van Sappho tot de Sade. Momenten in de geschiedenis van de seksualiteit*, edited by J. Bremmer, pp. 80–99. Amsterdam: Wereldbibliotheek.

Rosario, V. A. 1997. *The Erotic Imagination: French Histories of Perversity*. New York: Oxford University Press.

———, ed. 1997. *Science and Homosexualities*. New York: Routledge.

Rosenwald, G., and R. Ochberg, eds. 1992. *Storied Lives: The Cultural Politics of Self-Understanding*. New Haven: Yale University Press.

Rothman, D. J. 1971. *The Discovery of the Asylum: Social Order and Disorder in the New Republic*. Boston: Little, Brown.

Rousseau, G. 1987. The Pursuit of Homosexuality in the Eighteenth Century: "Utterly Confused Category" and/or Rich Repository? In *'Tis Nature's Fault: Unauthorized Sexuality During the Enlightenment*, edited by R. B. Maccubbin, pp. 132–68. Cambridge: Cambridge University Press.

Russelman, G. H. E. 1983. *Van James Watt tot Sigmund Freud. De opkomst van het stuwmodel van de zelfexpressie*. Deventer: Van Loghum Slaterus.

Russet, C. E. 1989. *Sexual Science: The Victorian Construction of Womanhood*. Cambridge: Harvard University Press.

Salvetti, M. E. 1984. *Gefässpsychopathologie bei Richard von Krafft-Ebing (1840–1902*. Bern: Huber.

Sass, H., and S. Herpertz. 1995. Personality Disorders. In *A History of Clinical Psychiatry: The Origin and History of Psychiatric Disorders*, edited by G. E. Berrios and R. Porter, pp. 633–44. London: Athlone.

Schiebinger, Londa. 1989. *The Mind Has No Sex?: Women in the Origins of Modern Science*. Cambridge: Harvard University Press.

Schmiedebach, H.-P. 1986. *Psychiatrie und Psychologie im Widerstreit. Die Auseinandersetzungen in der Berliner medicinisch-psychologischen Gesellschaft (1867–1899)*. Husum: Matthiessen.

Schmitt, W. 1983. Das Modell der Naturwissenschaft in der Psychiatrie im Übergang vom 19. zum 20. Jahrhundert. *Berichte zur Wissenschaftsgeschichte* 6:89–101.

Schorske, C. 1980. *Fin-de-Siècle Vienna: Politics and Culture*. New York: Knopf.

Schrenk, Martin. 1973. *Über den Umgang mit Geisteskranken. Die Entwicklung der psychiatrischen Therapie vom 'moralischen Regime' in England und Frankreich zu den 'psychischen Curmethoden' in Deutschland*. Berlin: Springer.

Schüle, H. 1902. Nekrolog Richard von Krafft-Ebing. *Zeitschrift für Psychiatrie* 60:305–29.

Scull, A. 1979. *Museums of Madness: The Social Organization of Insanity in Nineteenth Century England*. London: St. Martin's Press.

———. 1989. *Social Order/Mental Disorder: Anglo-American Psychiatry in Historical Perspective*. London: Routledge.

Sengoopta, C. 1992. Science, Sexuality, and Gender in the Fin de Siècle: Otto Weininger as Baedecker. *History of Science* 30:249–79.

———. 2000. *Otto Weininger: Sex, Science, and Self in Imperial Vienna*. Chicago: University of Chicago Press.

Sennett, R. 1974. *The Fall of Public Man*. New York: Knopf.

Shorter, E. 1975. *The Making of the Modern Family*. New York: Basic Books.

———. 1989. Women and Jews in a Private Nervous Clinic in Late-Nineteenth-Century Vienna. *Medical History* 33:149–83.

———. 1990. Private Clinics in Central Europe 1850–1933. *Social History of Medicine* 3:159–95.

———. 1992. *From Paralysis to Fatigue. The History of Psychosomatic Illness in the Modern Era.* New York: Free Press.

———. 1997. *A History of Psychiatry: From the Era of the Asylum to the Age of Prozac.* New York: John Wiley.

Shortland, M. 1987. Courting the Cerebellum: Early Organological and Phrenological Views of Sexuality. *British Journal of the History of Science* 20:173–99.

Showalter, E. 1987. *The Female Malady. Women, Madness, and English Culture, 1830–1980.* New York: Pantheon Books.

———. 1991. *Sexual Anarchy. Gender and Culture at the Fin de Siècle.* London: Bloomsbury.

Sievert, H. 1984. *Das Anomale Bestrafen. Homosexualität, Strafrecht und Schwulenbewegung im Kaiserreich und in der Weimarer Republik.* Hamburg: Ergebnisse-Verlag.

Silverstolpe, F. 1987. Benkert Was Not a Doctor. On the Nonmedical Origin of The Homosexual Category in the Nineteenth Century. In *Homosexuality, Which Homosexuality. History,* vol. I, pp. 206–20. Amsterdam: Vrije Universiteit.

Smith, R. 1981. *Trial by Medicine: Insanity and Responsibility in Victorian Trials.* Edinburgh: Edinburgh University Press.

Söldner, F. 1903. Nachruf Krafft-Ebing. *Psychiatrisch-neurologische Wochenschrift* 5:221–25.

Solomon, R. C. 1987. Sex, Contraception and Conceptions of Sex. In *The Contraceptive Ethos: Reproductive Rights and Responsibilities,* edited by W. B. Bondeson, H. T. Engelhardt, and S. F. Spicker, pp. 223–40. Dordrecht: Reidel.

Somerville, S. B. 1998. Scientific Racism and the Invention of the Homosexual Body. In *Sexology in Culture: Labelling Bodies and Desires,* edited by L. Bland and L. Doan, pp. 60–76. Cambridge: Polity Press.

Sommer, K. 1998. *Die Strafbarkeit der Homosexualität von der Kaiserzeit bis zum Nationalsozialismus. Eine Analyse der Straftatbestände im Strafgesetzbuch und in den Reformentwürfen (1871–1945).* Frankfurt am Main: Peter Lang.

Stanton, D.C. 1992. *Discourses of Sexuality: From Aristotle to AIDS.* Ann Arbor: University of Michigan Press.

Stark, G. D. 1981. Pornography, Society, and the Law in Imperial Germany. *Central European History* 14:200–29.

Stein, E., ed. 1990. *Forms of Desire: Sexual Orientation and the Social Constructionist Controversy.* New York: Garland.

Stekel, W. 1950. *The Autobiography of Wilhelm Stekel: The Life Story of a Pioneer Psychoanalyst.* Edited by E. A. Gutheil. New York: Liveright Publishing Corporation.

Sterz, H. 1903. Nekrolog R. von Krafft-Ebing. *Mitteilungen des Vereins der Ärzte in Steiermark,* 61–65.

Stockinger, J. 1979. Homosexuality and the French Enlightenment. In *Homosexualities and French Literature: Cultural Contexts/Critical Texts,* edited by G. Stambolian and E. Marks, pp. 161–85. Ithaca, N.Y.: Cornell University Press.

Stone, L. 1982. *The Family, Sex and Marriage in England 1500–1800*. Harmondsworth: Pelican.

Storr, M. 1998. Transformations: Subjects, Categories and Cures in Krafft-Ebing's Sexology. In *Sexology in Culture: Labelling Bodies and Desires*, edited by L. Bland and L. Doan, pp. 11–26. Cambridge: Polity Press.

Sulloway, F. J. 1979. *Freud. Biologist of the Mind. Beyond the Psychoanalytic Legend*. New York: Basic Books.

Swales, P. J. 1983. *Freud, Krafft-Ebing, and the Witches: The Role of Krafft-Ebing in Freud's Flight into Fantasy*. Privately published by the author.

Szasz, T. S. 1971. *The Manufacture of Madness: A Comparative Study of the Inquisition and the Mental Health Movement*. London: Routledge & Kegan Paul, Paladin.

———. 1972. *The Myth of Mental Illness: Foundations of a Theory of Personal Conduct*. London: Granada.

———. 1980. *Sex by Prescription*. Garden City, N.Y.: Doubleday.

Szeps-Zuckerkandl, B. 1939. *Ich erlebte fünfzig Jahre Weltgeschichte*. Stockholm: Bermann-Fischer Verlag.

Tagespost 332. 1902.

Taylor, C. 1994. *Sources of the Self: The Making of Modern Identity*. Cambridge: Cambridge University Press.

Theis, W., and A. Sternweiler. 1984. Alltag im Kaiserreich und in der Weimarer Republik. In *Eldorado. Homosexuelle Frauen und Männer in Berlin 1850–1950. Geschichte, Alltag und Kultur*, edited by M. Bollé, pp. 48–73. Berlin: Fröhlich & Kaufmann.

Timms, E. 1986. *Karl Kraus. Apocalyptic Satirist. Culture and Catastrophe in Habsburg Vienna*. New Haven: Yale University Press.

Trilling, L. 1972. *Sincerity and Authenticity*. Cambridge: Harvard University Press.

Trumbach, R. 1978. *The Rise of the Egalitarian Family: Aristocratic Kinship and Domestic Relations in Eighteenth-Century England*. New York: Academic Press.

———. 1986. Sodomitical Subcultures, Sodomitical Roles, and the Gender Revolution of the Eighteenth Century: The Recent Historiography. In *'Tis Nature's Fault: Unauthorized Sexuality During the Enlightenment*, edited by R. B. Maccubbin, pp. 109–21. Cambridge: Cambridge University Press.

———. 1989a. The Birth of the Queen: Sodomy and the Emergence of Gender Equality in Modern Culture 1660–1750. In *Hidden from History: Reclaiming the Gay and Lesbian Past*, edited by M. B. Duberman, M. Vicinus, and G. Chauncey, pp. 129–40. New York: New American Library.

———. 1989b. Gender and the Homosexual Role in Modern Western Culture: The 18th and 19th Centuries Compared. In *Homosexuality, Which Homosexuality?*, by D. Altman et al., pp. 149–69. Amsterdam: Dekker/Schorer, GMP Publishers.

———. 1994. The Origin and Development of the Modern Lesbian Role in the Western Gender System: Northwestern Europe and the United States 1750–1990. *Historical Reflections* 20:287–320.

———. 1998. *Sex and the Gender Revolution: Heterosexuality and the Third Gender in Enlightenment London*. Chicago: University of Chicago Press.

Turner, R. H. 1976. The Real Self: From Institution to Impulse. *American Journal of Sociology* 81:989–1016.

Ulrichs, C. H. 1898 (1864a). *'Vindicta'. Kampf für Freiheit und Verfolgung*. Leipzig: Max Spohr.

———.1898 (1864b). *'Formatrix'. Anthropologische Studien über urnische Liebe*. Leipzig: Max Spohr.

———.1898 (1869a). *'Incubes'. Urningsliebe und Blutgier* Leipzig: Max Spohr.

———.1898 (1869b). *'Argonauticus'. Zastrow und die Urninge des pietistischen, ultramontanen und freidenkenden Lagers*. Leipzig: Max Spohr.

———.1898 (1879). *'Kritische Pfeile'. Denkschrift über die Bestrafung der Urningsliebe*. Leipzig: Max Spohr.

Vance, C. 1989. Social Construction Theory: Problems in the History of Sexuality. In *Homosexuality, Which Homosexuality?*, by D. Altman et al., pp. 13–34. Amsterdam: Dekker/Schorer, GMP Publishers.

van der Meer, T. 1995. *Sodoms zaad in Nederland. Het ontstaan van homoseksualiteit in de vroegmoderne tijd*. Nijmegen: SUN.

van Ussel, J. 1968. *Geschiedenis van het seksuele probleem*. Meppel: Boom.

———. 1975. *Intimiteit*. Deventer: Van Loghum Slaterus.

Verplaetse, J. 1999. Vrouwenpijn en mannenplezier: de antifeministische wortels van sadomasochisme in de Belle Epoque. *Ethiek en maatschappij* 2–3:29–78.

Verwey, G. 1985. *Psychiatry in an Anthropological and Biomedical Context: Philosophical Presuppositions and Implications of German Psychiatry 1820–1870*. Dordrecht: Reidel.

———. 1995. Freud en de psychiatrie rond 1900. *Nederlands Tijdschrift voor Geneeskunde* 139:2187–190.

Vicinus, M. 1989. 'They Wonder to Which Sex I Belong': The Historical Roots of the Modern Lesbian Identity. In *Homosexuality, Which Homosexuality?*, by D. Altman et al., pp. 171–98. Amsterdam: Dekker/Schorer, GMP Publishers.

Wagner, N. 1987. *Geist und Geschlecht. Karl Kraus und die Erotik der Wiener Moderne*. Frankfurt am Main: Suhrkamp.

Wagner, P. 1987. The Discourse on Sex—Or Sex as Discourse: Eighteenth-Century Medical and Paramedical Erotica. In *Sexual Underworlds of the Enlightenment*, edited by G. S. Rousseau and R. Porter, pp. 46–68. Manchester: Manchester University Press.

Wagner-Jauregg, J. 1902. Festrede aus Anlass des 30jährigen Professoren-Jubiläums von Hofrat v. Krafft-Ebing. *Wiener klinische Wochenschrift* 15:318–19.

———. 1903. Richard Freiherr von Krafft-Ebing. In *Die Feierliche Inauguration des Rektors der Wiener Universität für das Studienjahr 1903/1904*, edited by J. Schipper, pp. 40–42. Vienna: Selbstverlag der Universität.

———. 1908. Richard v. Krafft-Ebing. *Wiener medizinische Wochenschrift* 58: 2305–11.

———. 1950. *Lebenserinnerungen*. Vienna: Springer.

Walkowitz, J. R. 1992. *City of Dreadful Delight: Narratives of Sexual Danger in Late-Victorian London*. Chicago: University of Chicago Press.

Walter, H. 1983. Richard von Krafft-Ebing. In *Vorläufer der Tiefenpsychologie*, edited by J. Rattner, pp. 255–81. Vienna: Europa Verlag.

Weeks, J. 1981. *Sex, Politics & Society: The Regulation of Sexuality Since 1800*. London: Longman.

———. 1983. *Coming Out: Homosexual Politics in Britain, from the Nineteenth Century to the Present*. London: Quartet Books.

————. 1985. *Sexuality and Its Discontents. Meaning, Myths and Modern Sexualities*. London: Routledge.

Weininger, O. 1912. *Geschlecht und Charakter. Eine principielle Untersuchung*. Vienna: Braumüller.

Wettley, A., and W. Leibbrand. 1959. *Von der "Psychopathia sexualis" zur Sexualwissenschaft*. Stuttgart: Ferdinand Enke.

Williams, R. 1982. *Dreamworlds*. Berkeley: University of California Press.

Wilson, E. 1991. *The Sphinx in the City: Urban Life, the Control of Disorder, and Women*. Berkeley: University of California Press.

Worbs, M. 1983. *Nervenkunst. Literatur und Psychoanalyse im Wien der Jahrhundertwende*. Frankfurt am Main: Europäische Verlagsanstalt.

Zweig, S. 1943. *The World of Yesterday: An Autobiography*. New York: Viking Press.

INDEX

Aarts, J., 267
abstinence, 21, 70, 284
Ackerknecht, E. H., 91n
adultery, 233
alcoholic dementia, 109n
alcoholism, 30, 54, 87, 108
algolagnia, 45, 61, 179
alienist, 79–80
Allerhand, J., 76n
anatomy, 25, 90, 114, 279
anatomy, brain, 101, 114, 116
androgyny, 48, 60, 67, 251–52
anesthesia, sexual, 44, 62–63, 70, 249n, 284
animism, 45n
Anna O. *See* Pappenheim, Bertha
anorexia nervosa, 45
anthropophagy, 44
anti-Semitism, 96, 97n
appetite, 67–68
Aristotle, 21–22
art (modernist), 259, 261, 263–64, 267–69
association theory, 183
asylum, 15, 17, 42, 76, 80–85, 90, 93–94,
    124–25, 129, 133, 135–37, 140, 145,
    159, 263; lunatic, 13, 139, 178
atavism, 183
Augustine, 21–22
autobiographical disclosure, 219, 221
autobiography, 2, 11–12, 14–17, 117, 122,
    129–30, 140n, 148–50, 165, 167, 170,
    176, 179, 190–91, 195–97, 199, 212,
    215–18, 220–23, 228–30, 232, 248, 279;
    modern, 216–17, 220, 223; sexual, 225
autoerotism, 71
avant-garde, Viennese, 267

Bachofen, Johann Jakob, 262
Bahr, Hermann, 263
Ball, Benjamin, 45
Barker-Benfield, G. J., 33, 57n
Bataille, Georges, 275
Baudelaire, Charles, 205
Baumeister, R. F., 218
Beard, George M., 92
Bech, H., 253
Belot, Adolphe, 149
Benedikt, Moritz, 94–96, 123, 186, 275
Benkert, Karl Maria, 67, 69. *See also* Kert-
    beny, Karl Maria
Bentham, Jeremy, 211
Berger, P., 91n
Berner, P., 88n
Bernheim, Hippolyte, 120
Berrios, G. E., 41, 87, 116
bestiality, 21–22, 35, 39–40, 45, 47, 50, 134
Bildung, 204, 221
Billroth, Theodor, 123, 262
Binet, Alfred, 45, 49, 58, 61–62, 64, 120,
    183, 279
Binswanger, Ludwig, 116
Birken, L., 239, 254
birth control. *See* contraception
bisexuality, 48, 66, 158, 278
Bleuler, Eugen, 116
Bleys, R. C., 46n
Bloch, Iwan, 46, 58, 71
bondage, sexual, 175n, 182–83, 205
bourgeois society, nineteenth-century, 217–
    18, 232, 237–38, 244–45, 248, 254, 259,
    261, 268, 282
Brecher, E. M., 7

318

INDEX

shoplifting, 206, 238
Shorter, Edward, 8, 12, 81, 91, 93n, 102, 109n, 116, 119–20, 124, 234n
Shortland, M., 39
Showalter, E., 9, 204, 267
Sievert, H., 35, 37n, 144n
Silverstolpe, F., 44, 212
sin, 21–23, 25, 28, 36, 42, 43, 52, 67, 106
Smith, R., 40n
social control, 10–13, 56
social utilitarianism, 26, 28–29
Socrates, 247
sodomy, 21–22, 27, 36, 37–39, 44, 231, 233, 241–42, 244–46, 248–49
Söldner, F., 76n, 94
Solomon, R. C., 235
Somerville, S. B., 46n
Sommer, K., 35, 37n, 144n
somnambulism, 86
Stadion, Count Emerich von, 149
Stanton, D. C., 2, 14n
Stark, G. D., 187
Stefanowski, Dimitri, 175n
Stein, E., 14n
Steinach, Eugen, 280
Stekel, W., 94
stercoracism, 45, 50, 152–53
Sternweiler, A., 254n
Sterz, H., 76n
Stichl, Anton, 93–94, 124
Stockinger, J., 26
Stone, L., 234n
Stopes, Marie, 284
Storr, M., 65
Stransky, E., 94
Sturm und Drang, 245–46
suffering, 226–29
suicide, 54, 134, 136, 149, 154, 181, 198, 200, 262
Sulloway, F. J., 67, 89n
Sulzenbacher, H., 37n, 141n, 144n, 249, 254n
Swales, P. J., 89n
Symonds, John Addington, 46
syphilis, 90–91, 109
Szasz, Thomas, 7–10
Szeps-Zuckerkandl, B., 94, 123

tabes, 87, 90, 109n
talking cure, 124
Tamassia, Arrigo, 45
Tardieu, Ambroise, 38
Tarnowsky, Benjamin, 45

Taylor, C., 218
Theis, W., 254n
therapy, 91, 101–2, 107, 120–22, 124; dietary, 91; light, 91
third sex. See gender, third
Thomas Aquinas, 22, 35
Thomson, J. Arthur, 32
Timms, E., 260n, 261
Tissot, Samuel August, 27
Toulmin, Stephen, 8, 260n, 264
transsexuality, 11, 48, 67, 251
transvestism, 48, 67, 189, 242, 244
travesty, 49, 194, 243, 251
tribady/tribadism, 39, 231
Trilling, L., 217, 219
Trumbach, Randolph, 234n, 241–43
Turner, R. H., 218
typology, 216

Ulrichs, Karl Heinrich, 44, 47, 66–67, 69, 139, 144, 148, 165, 172, 192, 246, 249, 252
unisexuality, 45
uranism, 44, 66, 139, 144, 159, 166, 168, 170, 206
urning, 138, 139, 142, 144–45, 147–50, 158–59, 161, 163–68, 170–72, 174, 179–80, 189–90, 192–94, 195–203, 207, 225–28, 237, 241, 244–45, 249–52, 254, 264–65
urolagnia, 47, 71

van der Meer, T., 241n
van Ussel, J., 40n, 235
Vance, C., 14n
van de Velde, Theodoor, 284
Verplaetse, J., 58, 182n, 267
Verwey, G., 100, 116, 119
Vicinus, M., 207, 244
Vico, Giambattista, 216
violence, 236–38; sexual, 134, 172, 178, 236
Virchow, Rudolf, 78
Voltaire, 25
von Gudden, Bernhard , 94n
von Suttner, Bertha, 96
voyeurism, 45, 235–36, 257

Wagner, N., 261
Wagner, P., 27, 231–32, 236
Wagner, Richard, 110, 246, 262, 267
Wagner-Jauregg, Julius, 76n, 89n, 96, 98, 186